Managing Chronic Conditions in Older Adults with Cardiovascular Disease

Editors

MICHAEL W. RICH
CYNTHIA BOYD
JAMES T. PACALA

CLINICS IN GERIATRIC MEDICINE

www.geriatric.theclinics.com

May 2016 • Volume 32 • Number 2

ELSEVIER

1600 John F. Kennedy Boulevard • Suite 1800 • Philadelphia, Pennsylvania, 19103-2899

http://www.theclinics.com

CLINICS IN GERIATRIC MEDICINE Volume 32, Number 2
May 2016 ISSN 0749–0690, ISBN-13: 978-0-323-44465-1

Editor: Jessica McCool
Developmental Editor: Colleen Viola

Clinics in Geriatric Medicine (ISSN 0749-0690) is published quarterly by Elsevier Inc., 360 Park Avenue South, New York, NY 10010-1710. Months of issue are February, May, August, and November. Business and Editorial Offices: 1600 John F. Kennedy Blvd., Suite 1800, Philadelphia, PA 191023-2899. Periodicals postage paid at New York, NY, and additional mailing offices. Subscription prices are $265.00 per year (US individuals), $557.00 per year (US institutions), $100.00 per year (US student/resident), $370.00 per year (Canadian individuals), $706.00 per year (Canadian institutions), $195.00 per year (Canadian student/resident), $390.00 per year (international individuals), $706.00 per year (international institutions), and $195.00 per year (international student/resident). Foreign air speed delivery is included in all *Clinics* subscription prices. All prices are subject to change without notice. POSTMASTER: Send address changes to *Clinics in Geriatric Medicine,* Elsevier Health Sciences Division, Subscription Customer Service, 3251 Riverport Lane, Maryland Heights, MO 63043. **Telephone: 1-800-654-2452 (U.S. and Canada); 314-447-8871 (outside U.S. and Canada). Fax: 314-447-8029. E-mail:** journalscustomerservice-usa@elsevier.com **(for print support) or** journalsonlinesupport-usa@elsevier.com **(for online support)**.

Reprints. For copies of 100 or more, of articles in this publication, please contact the Commercial Reprints Department, Elsevier Inc., 360 Park Avenue South, New York, New York 10010-1710. Tel.: 212-633-3874; Fax: 212-633-3820, E-mail: reprints@elsevier.com.

Clinics in Geriatric Medicine is covered in *MEDLINE/PubMed (Index Medicus), EMBASE/Excerpta Medica, Current Contents/Clinical Medicine (CC/CM), and the Cumulative Index to Nursing & Allied Health Literature*.

Contributors

EDITORS

MICHAEL W. RICH, MD, FACC, AGSF
Professor, Department of Medicine, Washington University School of Medicine, St Louis, Missouri

CYNTHIA BOYD, MD, MPH
Associate Professor, Department of Medicine, Johns Hopkins University School of Medicine, Baltimore, Maryland

JAMES T. PACALA, MD, MS, AGSF
Professor and Associate Head, Department of Family Medicine and Community Health, University of Minnesota Medical School, Minneapolis, Minnesota

AUTHORS

KAREN P. ALEXANDER, MD
Duke Clinical Research Institute, Duke University Medical Center, Durham, North Carolina

JOAKIM ALFREDSSON, MD, PhD
Departments of Cardiology and Medical and Health Sciences, Linköping University, Linköping, Sweden; Duke Clinical Research Institute, Duke University Medical Center, Durham, North Carolina

SUSAN P. BELL, MBBS, MSCI
Assistant Professor, Department of Medicine, Division of Cardiovascular Medicine; Division of Geriatric Medicine, Center for Quality Aging, Vanderbilt University Medicine Center, Nashville, Tennessee

NINA L. BLACHMAN, MD
Instructor, Division of Geriatric Medicine and Palliative Care, Department of Medicine, New York University School of Medicine, New York, New York

CAROLINE S. BLAUM, MD, MS
Diane and Arthur Belfer Professor of Geriatrics; Director, Division of Geriatric Medicine and Palliative Care, Department of Medicine; Professor, Department of Population Health, Langone Medical Center, New York University, New York, New York

MICHAEL A. CHEN, MD, PhD
Associate Professor of Medicine, Cardiology, Harborview Medical Center, University of Washington School of Medicine, Seattle, Washington

KUMAR DHARMARAJAN, MD, MBA
Section of Cardiovascular Medicine, Department of Internal Medicine, Yale University School of Medicine; Center for Outcomes Research and Evaluation, Yale-New Haven Hospital, New Haven, Connecticut

SHANNON M. DUNLAY, MD, MS
Division of Cardiovascular Diseases, Department of Internal Medicine, Mayo Clinic; Division of Health Care Policy and Research, Department of Health Sciences Research, Mayo Clinic, Rochester, Minnesota

JESSICA ESTERSON, MPH
Project Director, Section of Geriatrics, Department of Medicine, Yale School of Medicine, New Haven, Connecticut

MARGARET C. FANG, MD, MPH
Associate Professor of Medicine, Division of Hospital Medicine, University of California, San Francisco, San Francisco, California

ROSIE FERRIS, MPH
Research Coordinator, Division of Geriatric Medicine and Palliative Care, Department of Medicine; Department of Population Health, Langone Medical Center, New York University, New York, New York

DANIEL E. FORMAN, MD, FACC, FAHA
Section of Geriatric Cardiology, University of Pittsburgh Medical Center; Geriatric Research, Education, and Clinical Center, VA Pittsburgh Healthcare System, Pittsburgh, Pennsylvania

ROBERT GOLDBERG, PhD
Professor, Department of Quantitative Health Sciences; Professor of Medicine, Division of Cardiovascular Medicine, Department of Medicine, Meyers Primary Care Institute, University of Massachusetts Medical School, Worcester, Massachusetts

JERRY H. GURWITZ, MD
Professor, Division of Geriatric Medicine, Department of Medicine, Meyers Primary Care Institute; Department of Quantitative Health Sciences, University of Massachusetts Medical School, Worcester, Massachusetts

JAMES N. KIRKPATRICK, MD, FACC, FASE
Faculty, Cardiology, Bioethics and Humanities, Regional Heart Center, University of Washington Medical Center, Seattle, Washington

BRIAN R. LINDMAN, MD, MS, FACC
Assistant Professor of Medicine, Cardiovascular Division, Washington University School of Medicine, St Louis, Missouri

HILLARY D. LUM, MD, PhD
Assistant Professor of Medicine, VA Eastern Colorado Geriatric Research Education and Clinical Center (GRECC), Denver, Colorado; Division of Geriatric Medicine, Department of Medicine, University of Colorado School of Medicine, Aurora, Colorado

WILLIAM L. LYONS, MD
Professor, Internal Medicine, Division of Geriatrics and Gerontology, University of Nebraska Medical Center, Omaha, Nebraska

ARIELA R. ORKABY, MD
Geriatrician and Fellow in Preventive Cardiology, Division of Cardiology, VA Boston Healthcare System; Division of Aging, Brigham and Women's Hospital, Boston, Massachusetts

ESTHER PAK, MD
Fellow, Palliative Care, Hospital of the University of Pennsylvania, Philadelphia, Pennsylvania

ANNA L. PARKS, MD
Department of Medicine, University of California, San Francisco, San Francisco, California

JAY N. PATEL, MD
Department of Medicine, Washington University School of Medicine, St Louis, Missouri

PHILIP POSNER, PhD
Oak Ridge Institute of Science Education, Oak Ridge Associated Universities, Oak Ridge, Tennessee; National MS Society, National Capitol Chapter

MARCEL E. SALIVE, MD, MPH
Division of Geriatrics and Clinical Gerontology, National Institute on Aging, National Institutes of Health, Bethesda, Maryland

AVANTIKA A. SARAF, MPH
Division of Cardiovascular Medicine, Department of Medicine; Division of Geriatric Medicine, Center for Quality Aging, Vanderbilt University Medicine Center, Nashville, Tennessee

REBECCA L. SUDORE, MD
Associate Professor, Department of Medicine, Division of Geriatrics, San Francisco Veterans Affairs Medical Center, University of California, San Francisco, California

MARY E. TINETTI, MD
Gladys Philips Crofoot Professor of Medicine and Public Health; Chief, Section of Geriatrics, Department of Medicine, Yale School of Medicine, Yale School of Public Health, New Haven, Connecticut

MAYRA TISMINETZKY, MD, PhD
Assistant Professor, Division of Geriatric Medicine, Department of Medicine, Meyers Primary Care Institute; Assistant Professor of Quantitative Health Sciences, University of Massachusetts Medical School, Worcester, Massachusetts

JOYCE WALD, DO, FACC
Faculty, Cardiology, Perelman Center for Advanced Medicine, Hospital of the University of Pennsylvania, Philadelphia, Pennsylvania

Contents

Preface: Working Together in the Care of Patients with Cardiovascular Disease and Multimorbidity **xiii**

Michael W. Rich, Cynthia Boyd, and James T. Pacala

Epidemiology of Multimorbidity in Older Adults with Cardiovascular Disease **215**

Susan P. Bell and Avantika A. Saraf

Multimorbidity is the most significant condition affecting older adults, and it impacts every component of health care management and delivery. Multimorbidity significantly increases with age. For individuals with a diagnosis of cardiovascular disease, multimorbidity has a significant effect on the presentation of the disease and the diagnosis, management, and patient-centered preferences in care. Evidence-based therapeutics have focused on cardiovascular focused morbidity. Over the next 25 years, the proportion of adults aged 65 and older is estimated to increase threefold. The needs of these patients require a fundamental shift in care from single disease practices to a more patient-centered framework.

Magnitude and Impact of Multimorbidity on Clinical Outcomes in Older Adults with Cardiovascular Disease: A Literature Review **227**

Mayra Tisminetzky, Robert Goldberg, and Jerry H. Gurwitz

The authors aim to synthesize the current literature on the magnitude and impact of multimorbidity on clinical outcomes in older adults with cardiovascular disease (CVD). Most studies reported a significant association between the number of morbidities and the risk of dying. Multimorbidity was assessed either by counting the number of conditions or by use of the Charlson or Elixhauser indices. There are limited data available on the magnitude and impact of multimorbidity on clinical outcomes in patients with CVD and essentially no data on universal health outcomes (eg, health-related quality of life, symptom burden, and function).

Advance Care Planning and Goals of Care Communication in Older Adults with Cardiovascular Disease and Multi-Morbidity **247**

Hillary D. Lum and Rebecca L. Sudore

This article provides an approach to advance care planning (ACP) and goals of care communication in older adults with cardiovascular disease and multi-morbidity. The goal of ACP is to ensure that the medical care patients receive is aligned with their values and preferences. In this article, the authors outline common benefits and challenges to ACP for older adults with cardiovascular disease and multimorbidity. Recognizing that these patients experience diverse disease trajectories and receive care in multiple health care settings, the authors provide practical steps for multidisciplinary teams to integrate ACP into brief clinic encounters.

Patient Priority–Directed Decision Making and Care for Older Adults with Multiple Chronic Conditions **261**

Mary E. Tinetti, Jessica Esterson, Rosie Ferris, Philip Posner, and Caroline S. Blaum

Older adults with multiple conditions receive care that is often fragmented, burdensome, and of unclear benefit. An advisory group of patients, caregivers, clinicians, health system engineers, health care system leaders, payers, and others identified three modifiable contributors to this fragmented, burdensome care: decision making and care focused on diseases, not patients; inadequate delineation of roles and responsibilities and accountability among clinicians; and lack of attention to what matters to patients and caregivers (ie, their health outcome goals and care preferences). The advisory group identified patient priority–directed care as a feasible, sustainable approach to addressing these modifiable factors.

Multimorbidity in Older Adults with Heart Failure **277**

Kumar Dharmarajan and Shannon M. Dunlay

Multimorbidity is common among older adults with heart failure and creates diagnostic and management challenges. Diagnosis of heart failure may be difficult, as many conditions commonly found in older persons produce dyspnea, exercise intolerance, fatigue, and weakness; no singular pathognomonic finding or diagnostic test differentiates them from one another. Treatment may also be complicated, as multimorbidity creates high potential for drug-disease and drug-drug interactions in settings of polypharmacy. The authors suggest that management of multimorbid older persons with heart failure be patient, rather than disease-focused, to best meet patients' unique health goals and minimize risk from excessive or poorly-coordinated treatments.

Multiple Chronic Conditions in Older Adults with Acute Coronary Syndromes **291**

Joakim Alfredsson and Karen P. Alexander

Older adults presenting with acute coronary syndromes (ACSs) often have multiple chronic conditions (MCCs). In addition to traditional cardiovascular (CV) risk factors (ie, hypertension, hyperlipidemia, and diabetes), common CV comorbidities include heart failure, stroke, and atrial fibrillation, whereas prevalent non-CV comorbidities include chronic kidney disease, anemia, depression, and chronic obstructive pulmonary disease. The presence of MCCs affects the presentation (eg, increased frequency of type 2 myocardial infarctions [MIs]), clinical course, and prognosis of ACS in older adults. In general, higher comorbidity burden increases mortality following MI, reduces utilization of ACS treatments, and increases the importance of developing individualized treatment plans.

Multimorbidity in Older Adults with Aortic Stenosis **305**

Brian R. Lindman and Jay N. Patel

Aortic stenosis is a disease of older adults; many have associated comorbidities. With the aging of the population and the emergence of transcatheter aortic valve replacement as a treatment, clinicians will increasingly be confronted with aortic stenosis and multimorbidity, making the evaluation, management, and treatment of aortic stenosis more complex. To optimize patient-centered clinical outcomes, new treatment paradigms are needed that recognize the import and influence of multimorbidity on patients with aortic stenosis. The authors review the prevalence of medical and aging-related comorbidities in patients with aortic stenosis, their impact on outcomes, and discuss how they influence management and treatment decisions.

Multimorbidity in Older Adults with Atrial Fibrillation **315**

Michael A. Chen

Older adults with atrial fibrillation often have multiple comorbid conditions, including common geriatric syndromes. Pharmacologic therapy, whether for rate control or rhythm control, can result in complications related to polypharmacy in patients who are often on multiple medications for other conditions. Because of uncertainty about the relative risks and benefits of rate versus rhythm control (including antiarrhythmic or ablation therapy), anticoagulation, and procedural treatments (eg, ablation, left atrial appendage closure, pacemaker placement) in older patients with multimorbidity, shared decision-making is essential. However, this may be challenging in patients with cognitive dysfunction, high fall risk, or advanced comorbidity.

Anticoagulation in Older Adults with Multimorbidity **331**

Anna L. Parks and Margaret C. Fang

The number of patients with atrial fibrillation (AF) who are of advanced age or have multiple comorbidities is expected to increase substantially. Older patients with AF generally gain a net benefit from anticoagulation. Guidelines typically recommend anticoagulation. There are multiple challenges in the safe use of anticoagulation in frail patients, including bleeding risk, monitoring and adherence, and polypharmacy. Although there are options for chronic oral anticoagulation, clinicians must understand the unique advantages and disadvantages of these medications when developing a management plan. This article reviews issues surrounding the appropriate use and selection of anticoagulants in complex older patients with AF.

Approach to Evaluating the Multimorbid Patient with Cardiovascular Disease Undergoing Noncardiac Surgery **347**

William L. Lyons

Older patients undergo more inpatient and outpatient procedures than do younger individuals, and their risk of suffering undesired outcomes is greater. The performance of a productive preoperative assessment entails more than the application of the sundry clinical practice guidelines relating to a patient's various medical diagnoses. A better approach involves adoption of a physiologically integrated, whole-person assessment that takes into account the patient's cognitive function, mood, physical function and mobility (including the possibility of frailty), social support, nutritional status, and medication use. This article outlines such an approach and highlights the many gaps in the current evidence base.

Assessing Risks and Benefits of Invasive Cardiac Procedures in Patients with Advanced Multimorbidity **359**

Ariela R. Orkaby and Daniel E. Forman

Age-related cardiovascular disease in older adults is more likely to occur in combination with other age-related diseases, with mounting interactive complexity as multiple morbidities accumulate. Although invasive cardiac procedures are frequently recommended for cardiovascular disease, their value is less certain in the context of age-related intricacies of care. Tools for risk assessment before invasive procedures are insensitive to risks corresponding to the unique challenges of older adults. Recognizing multimorbidity and other age-related risks provide opportunities to intervene and moderate dangers. By refocusing risk assessment in terms of patient-centered goals, the fundamental utility of invasive cardiac procedures may be reconsidered and alternative therapies prioritized.

Integrating Care Across Disciplines **373**

Nina L. Blachman and Caroline S. Blaum

Interdisciplinary care teams are important in managing older patients. Geriatric patients with cardiovascular problems represent a unique paradigm for interdisciplinary teams, and patients benefit from the assistance of physicians, nurses, social workers, pharmacists, and therapists collaborating on treatment plans. Teams work on the inpatient and outpatient sides and at patients' homes to maximize function and prevent readmissions to the hospital.

Multimorbidity and End of Life Care in Patients with Cardiovascular Disease **385**

Esther Pak, Joyce Wald, and James N. Kirkpatrick

The care of patients with severe cardiovascular disease and multimorbidity entails complex medical decision-making especially at the end of life. Proven therapies must be incorporated into the context of patient preferences, values, and goals to achieve effective titration of medications and appropriate initiation and withdrawal of cardiac device therapies. As patients decline in the terminal stages, it is important to modify medical and device therapies in accordance with goals and values, and with hemodynamic changes, increasing multimorbidity, and accumulating symptom burden. The provision of effective end of life care for those with cardiovascular disease and multimorbidity requires cooperation between palliative care, specialty care, and primary care.

Future Research Directions for Multimorbidity Involving Cardiovascular Diseases **399**

Marcel E. Salive

Multimorbidity, defined as the co-occurrence of two or more chronic conditions, increases with age and may be found in approximately two-thirds of older adults in population studies, commonly including a variety of cardiovascular risk factors and chronic diseases. This article offers a research agenda for cardiovascular disease from a patient-centered multimorbidity perspective. Definitional issues remain for multimorbidity, along with high interest in understanding the inter-relationships between aging, diseases, treatments, and organ dysfunction in the development and progression of multimorbidity. Clinical trials, practice-based and population-based observational studies, and linkages of big data can play a role in improving health outcomes among persons with multimorbidity.

Index **409**

CLINICS IN GERIATRIC MEDICINE

FORTHCOMING ISSUES

August 2016
Infectious Diseases in Geriatric Medicine
Thomas T. Yoshikawa and
Dean C. Norman, *Editors*

November 2016
Geriatric Pain Management
M. Carrington Reid, *Editor*

February 2017
Rheumatic Diseases in Older Adults
James D. Katz and Brian Walitt, *Editors*

RECENT ISSUES

February 2016
Geriatric Oncology
Arati V. Rao and Harvey Jay Cohen, *Editors*

November 2015
Geriatric Urology
Tomas Lindor Griebling, *Editor*

August 2015
Nutrition in Older Adults
John E. Morley, *Editor*

ISSUE OF RELATED INTEREST

Medical Clinics of North America, July 2015 (Vol. 99, No. 4)
Management of Cardiovascular Disease
Deborah Wolbrette, *Editor*
http://www.medical.theclinics.com/

Preface

Working Together in the Care of Patients with Cardiovascular Disease and Multimorbidity

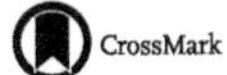

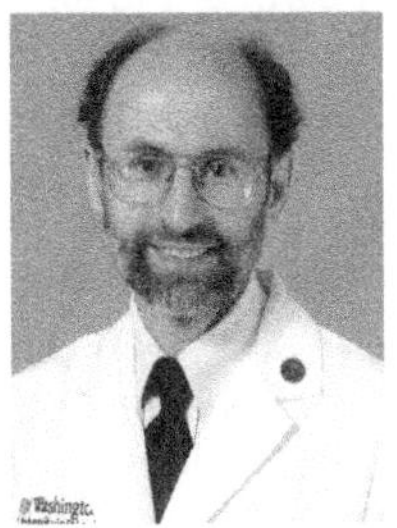

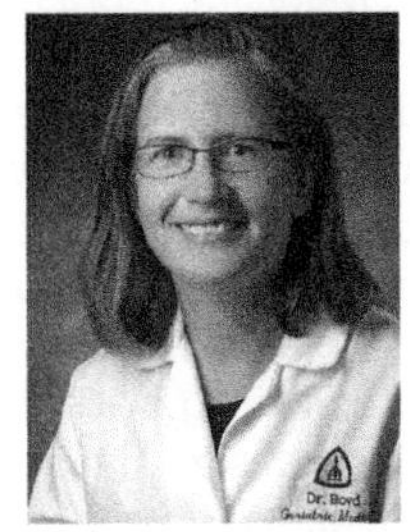

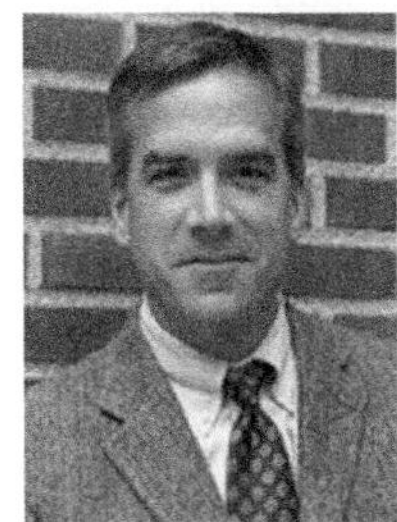

Michael W. Rich, MD, FACC, AGSF
Cynthia Boyd, MD, MPH
James T. Pacala, MD, MS, AGSF
Editors

More than 70% of older adults have cardiovascular disease (CVD), and the vast majority of these have multiple coexisting conditions; indeed, more than 50% of older adults have multimorbidity (MM), defined as three or more chronic conditions. Tremendous advances in the diagnosis and treatment of CVD over the past five decades have culminated in the publication of numerous evidence-based guidelines, which have contributed to improved cardiovascular care and clinical outcomes. However, positive results from the "guideline age" have been tempered by two factors that have been increasingly recognized by cardiologists and geriatricians: (1) most patients with CVD are elderly and also have MM, increasing the likelihood that treatment of their CVD will exacerbate other chronic conditions; and (2) most guideline recommendations, based on evidence from studies with restrictive inclusion criteria or nonrepresentative enrollment, do not account for complicating effects from coexisting conditions and treatments.

The overlap between CVD and MM mandates that cardiologists must practice geriatrics, and that geriatricians and other clinicians caring for older adults must practice cardiology. In doing so, each specialty must bridge the cultural gap between the two, starting with recognizing each other's basic philosophical orientation. Employing admittedly crude generalizations, cardiology can be characterized as a diagnosis-driven, largely interventional practice that ultimately seeks to fix a single problem. Geriatrics is a function-driven, noninterventional practice that focuses on minimizing the morbidity generated by multiple conditions. When it comes to pharmacotherapy, a cardiologist's first impulse is, "What medications can I start?," while a geriatrician's first thought is, "What medications can I stop?" If placed in the arena of sports, cardiologists would be on offense, while geriatricians would be on defense.

Fortunately, the two specialties have begun to recognize the value of each's approach and what can be learned by working together to improve the health of older adults. On

Clin Geriatr Med 32 (2016) xiii–xiv
http://dx.doi.org/10.1016/j.cger.2016.02.001

February 9–10, 2015, the American College of Cardiology, the American Geriatrics Society, and the National Institute on Aging cosponsored a workshop on Multimorbidity in Older Adults with CVD, bringing together experts in both fields to review current evidence, identify knowledge gaps, prioritize a research agenda, promote interdisciplinary strategies to address research needs, and foster the career development of junior investigators in CVD and MM. On May 14, 2015, a preconference session entitled, "How Do We Achieve Patient-Centered Care for the Complex Older Cardiology Patient?," was presented at the Annual Scientific Meeting of the American Geriatrics Society.

This issue of *Clinics in Geriatric Medicine* represents an outgrowth of the above efforts to expand our knowledge of caring for older adults with CVD and MM. Experts from the fields of cardiology and geriatrics have been recruited to author the articles of this issue to provide clinicians and researchers with state-of-the-art information on the care of and research needs for this prominent patient population. The first two articles, by Bell and Saraf and Tisminetzky and colleagues, focus on the epidemiology and impact of CVD and MM.The next two articles, by Lum and Sudore and Tinetti and colleagues, present approaches to achieving patient-centered, goal-oriented care for these patients. The next five articles focus on management of specific common cardiovascular conditions in persons with MM. Dr Lyons and Drs Orkaby and Forman address the evaluation of older adults with CVD and MM who are being considered for invasive procedures. The article written by Blachman and Blaum offers strategies for optimizing interprofessional team care, while the article written by Pak and colleagues deals with end-of-life care. Dr Salive presents a research agenda for continuing this important work in the final article. It is our hope that health care professionals will use the information and perspectives presented herein to advocate for older adults with CVD and MM through improved team care of patients, development of guidelines that account for complexities of coexisting conditions, and promotion of further research.

Michael W. Rich, MD, FACC, AGSF
Department of Medicine
Washington University School of Medicine
660 South Euclid Avenue
Campus Box 8086
St Louis, MO 63110, USA

Cynthia Boyd, MD, MPH
Department of Medicine
Johns Hopkins University School of Medicine
Mason F. Lord Building, Center Tower, 7th Floor
5200 Eastern Avenue
Baltimore, MD 21224, USA

James T. Pacala, MD, MS, AGSF
Department of Family Medicine
and Community Health
University of Minnesota Medical School
420 Delaware Street SE
MMC 381
Minneapolis, MN 55455, USA

E-mail addresses:
mrich@wustl.edu (M.W. Rich)
cyboyd@jhmi.edu (C. Boyd)
pacal001@umn.edu (J.T. Pacala)

Epidemiology of Multimorbidity in Older Adults with Cardiovascular Disease

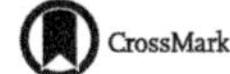

Susan P. Bell, MBBS, MSCI[a,b,*], Avantika A. Saraf, MPH[a,b]

KEYWORDS

• Older adults • Multimorbidity • Cardiovascular disease • Chronic conditions

KEY POINTS

- Multimorbidity, the presence of 2 or more chronic conditions, is the most common disease process impacting older adults.
- The prevalence of multimorbidity increases with age such that it is prevalent in more than 70% of adults aged 75 years and older.
- Assessment of multimorbidity should also include presence of geriatric syndromes.
- Multimorbidity is common in the presence of cardiovascular disease, especially heart failure, where 50% of Medicare beneficiaries have 5 or more coexisting chronic conditions.
- Multimorbidity has a substantial impact on disease management, quality of life, health care costs, and health care use.

INTRODUCTION

The proportion of adults aged 65 and over is increasing rapidly and older adults will comprise approximately 19% of the US population by 2030, including 19 million adults over the age of 85.[1] The result of this remarkable demographic shift imposes significant implications for overall future health care management where age is a driving factor in a multitude of disease processes, including cardiovascular disease (CVD), and contributes the most substantial risk. In 2013, CVD was responsible for more than 17 million deaths globally, an increase of 5 million (40%) annually since 1990, despite increasing advances in cardiovascular treatments and health care delivery.[2] The overwhelming driver of this increase can be attributed to population aging (55%) and to a

[a] Division of Cardiovascular Medicine, Department of Medicine, Vanderbilt University Medicine Center, Nashville, TN, USA; [b] Division of Geriatric Medicine, Center for Quality Aging, Vanderbilt University Medical Center, Nashville, TN, USA

* Corresponding author. Division of Cardiovascular Medicine, Center for Quality Aging, 2525 West End Avenue, Suite 350, Nashville, TN 37203.

E-mail address: susan.p.bell@vanderbilt.edu

Clin Geriatr Med 32 (2016) 215–226

http://dx.doi.org/10.1016/j.cger.2016.01.013 geriatric.theclinics.com

lesser extent population growth (25%). In the United States, CVD affects approximately 40 million individuals over the age of 65 and remains the leading cause of morbidity and mortality.[3,4]

The increasing prevalence of coexisting disease processes in this aging population further adds to the complexity and challenges facing patients with CVD and the providers that care for them. The diagnosis and management of CVD in older adults requires an in-depth understanding of the interplay between patient heterogeneity, the accumulation and activity of chronic and acute conditions, functional status, pharmacology, and social factors. However, the use of single disease practice guidelines remains as the standard of care across health care settings, irrespective of age and presence of multiple coexisting chronic conditions.[5,6] In fact, the most common chronic coexisting condition in older adults is the presence of multimorbidity, the coexistence of 2 or more chronic conditions.[7] The concept of multimorbidity differs from the familiar framework of comorbidity in that at any 1 time several conditions may be equally important and overlapping in management strategies and require comparable intensity and simultaneous management strategies to achieve optimal patient-centered outcomes and quality of life. This article examines the epidemiologic relationships and importance of multimorbidity in older adults with CVD.

PREVALENCE OF MULTIMORBIDITY

Multimorbidity rapidly increases with age such that it is prevalent in more than 70% of individuals 75 years or older.[8] The accumulation of chronic conditions as a result of genetics, lifestyle choices, environmental factors, treatment of prior conditions (eg, heart failure as an adverse consequence of chemotherapy regimens), and aging itself culminates in a vastly heterogenic older population of adults that require balancing the management of multiple medical problems. By the age of 65 years more than 60% of adults will have 2 or more chronic conditions, more than 25% will have 4 or more chronic conditions, and almost 10% will have 6 or more (**Fig. 1**).[8] These rates increase by each decade and result in more than 50% over individuals 85 years and older

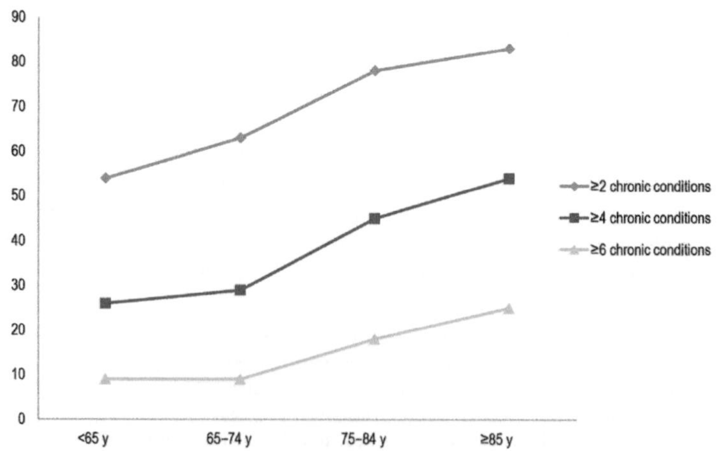

Fig. 1. Percentage of Medicare fee-for service beneficiaries by number of multiple chronic conditions and age (2010) showing increasing prevalence of multimorbidity with increasing age. (*Data from* Centers for Medicare & Medicaid Services. Chronic conditions overview. Available at: https://www.cms.gov/Research-Statistics-Data-and-Systems/Statistics-Trends-and-Reports/Chronic-Conditions/CC_Main.html. Accessed November 25, 2015.)

suffering from 4 or more chronic conditions and 25% with 6 or more chronic conditions.[8] The prevalence is high across all racial and ethnic groups; however, the pattern of multimorbidity by race changes over the age spectrum.[9] Through ages 50 to 59 years, multimorbidity is more common in blacks than in whites, and is higher in whites as compared with Asians. Furthermore, the presence of significant multimorbidity (≥5 conditions) through ages 50 to 59 is higher in blacks as compared with whites and Asians. In adults 60 and older, the relationship of 5 or more conditions seems to change, with multimorbidity being more common in whites as compared with blacks and Asians.[9]

Multimorbidity is extremely common and rapidly increases in a similar pattern with age in both men and women. **Fig. 2** demonstrates the patterns of increasing numbers of chronic conditions (≥2, ≥4, and ≥6 conditions) in men and women younger than 65 years of age and 65 years and older.[8] In 1 study among-community dwelling individuals, the prevalence of 5 or more conditions is more common in men over the age of 60 as compared with women,[9] but this finding is not consistent with other reported data that have demonstrated in Medicare beneficiaries (fee-for-service claims) the prevalence of multimorbidity is slightly higher in women compared with men.[8,9] In addition, the combinations of chronic diseases are different in men and women, with men more likely to have cancer, CVD, and cardiovascular risk factors (hypertension, diabetes mellitus, and hyperlipidemia) as compared with women, who had a higher prevalence of arthritis and depression.[10]

MULTIMORBIDITY AND GERIATRIC SYNDROMES

Evaluation of the impact of multimorbidity should not only include the contributing effects of chronic coexisting diagnoses, but also the prevalence of common and frequently underreported geriatric syndromes. Geriatric syndromes represent a group of clinical conditions involving multiple organ systems and that sometimes share common causative factors.[11,12] These include a number of conditions that, unlike traditional syndromes, do not fit a discrete metabolic, pathologic, or genetic disease

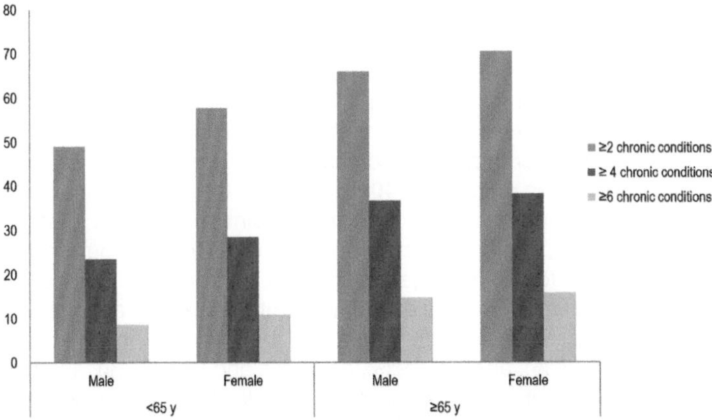

Fig. 2. Age-and sex-associated prevalence of multimorbidity by number of chronic conditions demonstrating the higher prevalence of number of chronic conditions above 65 as compared with below 65 and the higher prevalence of multimorbidity in women as compared with men. (*Data from* Centers for Medicare & Medicaid Services. Chronic conditions overview. Available at: www.cms.gov/Research-Statistics-Data-and-Systems/Statistics-Trends-and-Reports/Chronic-Conditions/CC_Main.html. Accessed November 25, 2015.)

category. Examples of geriatric syndromes include falls, cognitive impairment, delirium, weight loss, anorexia, pressure ulcers, functional decline, frailty, and depressive symptoms.[13] Their impact on quality of life, dependence, and disability is considerable. The presence and number of geriatric syndromes are independently associated with a risk for adverse outcomes such as functional decline, the acquisition of additional syndromes, hospital admissions, and mortality.[14,15] Despite the contributing role of geriatric syndromes in the presentation, management, and outcome of primary disease presentations, they are often underrecognized and seldom the focus of hospital and outpatient treatment.[11] In addition, geriatric syndromes may also impact compliance and tolerance of common therapies used in the management of CVD (ie, diuretics and antihypertensive therapy in the management of heart failure may precipitate worsening of falls and incontinence).

Frailty

Frailty encompasses a biological decline across multiple interrelated organ systems and a subsequent loss of reserve in response to stressors, such as acute illness, and can result in a poor tolerance to CVD and/or to CVD therapy. The estimated prevalence of frailty in community dwelling older adults 65 and older is approximately 7%, but increases to 20% in individuals over 80.[16] In older patients hospitalized with CVD, especially heart failure, it is estimated that the prevalence is greater than 50%.[17] Frailty is an independent predictor of a wide range of CVD, including subclinical CVD,[18] coronary artery disease, congestive heart failure,[19] and CVD mortality[20] and confers a 2- to 3-fold increased risk of adverse events and mortality.

MULTIMORBIDITY AND CARDIOVASCULAR DISEASE

CVD affects approximately 40 million individuals in the United States over the age of 65 and remains the leading cause of morbidity and mortality within that population both in the United States and globally.[2,4] Among Medicare beneficiaries with a diagnosis of CVD, the burden of multimorbidity is significant, with more than 50% of individuals that carry a diagnosis of heart failure or stroke also having 5 or more coexisting chronic medical conditions.[8] **Fig. 3** shows the prevalence of coexisting chronic conditions in 6 of the most frequently managed diagnoses in cardiovascular medicine. It demonstrates the high prevalence (>50%) of 3 or more additional chronic conditions with each diagnosis highlighting the complexity of managing CVD in older adults.[8,10] For example, in older adults with ischemic heart disease, heart failure, stroke, and atrial fibrillation, the most common concomitant conditions are arthritis, anemia, and diabetes mellitus and rates range from 40% to 50%.[10] Other common chronic conditions include chronic kidney disease, cognitive impairment, chronic obstructive lung disease, and depression, each of which much be considered when developing individual treatment strategies for the management of CVD. In the case of coronary heart disease, common management strategies such as beta-blockade, antiplatelet therapy, antihypertensives, and statin therapy[21] may not be tolerated in an individual with chronic lung disease (25%), anemia (39%), dizziness and falls (35%), and mobility difficulties (40%).[22] **Table 1** highlights a few of the complexities and considerations managing an individual with systolic heart failure and a number of cardiac (hypertension, ischemic heart disease, and atrial fibrillation), noncardiac (chronic obstructive pulmonary disease, chronic kidney disease) coexisting conditions and a number of common geriatric syndromes (incontinence, falls, and mobility impairment).

Fundamental knowledge gaps in management of CVD in older adults in the context of multimorbidity lies in our reliance on evidence-based guidelines derived from

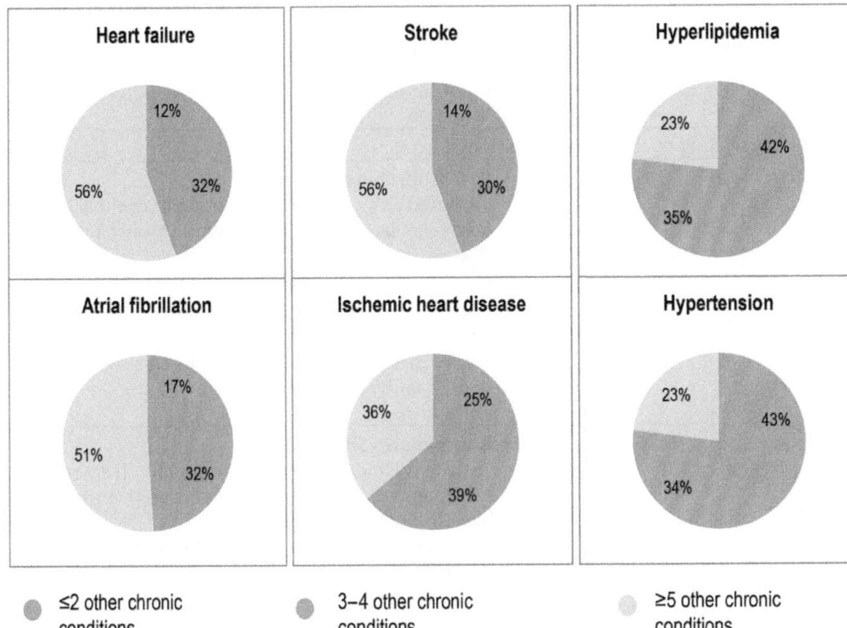

Fig. 3. Number of coexisting chronic conditions among Medicare fee for service beneficiaries with common cardiovascular diagnoses. (*Data from* Centers for Medicare & Medicaid Services. Chronic conditions overview. Available at: www.cms.gov/Research-Statistics-Data-and-Systems/Statistics-Trends-and-Reports/Chronic-Conditions/CC_Main.html. Accessed November 25, 2015; and Arnett DK, Goodman RA, Halperin JL, et al. AHA/ACC/HHS strategies to enhance application of clinical practice guidelines in patients with cardiovascular disease and comorbid conditions: from the American Heart Association, American College of Cardiology, and US Department of Health and Human Services. J Am Coll Cardiol 2014;64(17):1851–56.)

clinical trials that have largely recruited participants that are not proportionately representative of the majority of older patients managed by medical providers. More than one-half of clinical trials focused on the management of coronary artery disease failed to include any participant over the age of 75 years.[23] Furthermore, individuals over the age of 75 make up less than 10%[23] of those included in any of the trials despite representing 25% to 32% of the population included in registries.[24] **Table 2** shows baseline patient characteristics of individuals from the Global Registry of Acute Coronary Events (GRACE) registry, a multinational, prospective registry that describes the epidemiology, management practices, and in-hospital outcomes and changes over time therein, of patients with the entire spectrum of acute coronary syndromes (ACSs). In comparison, the corresponding baseline characteristic prevalence is shown for 3 ACS focused clinical trials (Comparison of Primary Angioplasty and Pre-hospital Fibrinolysis in Acute Myocardial Infarction [CAPTIM],[25] Clopidogrel in Unstable angina to prevent Recurrent Events [CURE][26] and Global Use of Strategies To Open Occluded Coronary Arteries IV—Acute Coronary Syndrome [GUSTO IV ACS][27]). The comparison demonstrates that on average individuals in clinical trials are younger with a much smaller proportions older than 65, and older than 75, as compared with the ACS registry. They also have much lower prevalence of significant risk factors for adverse events, such as the presence of heart failure, diabetes mellitus, and prior

Table 1
Factors affecting management of heart failure with significant multimorbidity

	Estimated Prevalence (%)	Drug–Disease, Drug–Drug, and Disease–Disease Interactions
Cardiovascular disease coexisting conditions		
Hypertension	85.6[10]	• Orthostatic hypotension • Increased risk of falls with treatment: optimal tolerated medical therapy limited with chronic kidney disease
Ischemic heart disease	72.1[10]	• Intolerance of beta-blocker therapy owing to fatigue • Decreased exertional symptoms owing to mobility impairment • Intolerance of statins owing to muscle aches • Heart healthy diet may increase unintentional weight loss
Atrial fibrillation	28.8[10]	• Anticoagulation monitoring • Toxicity with impaired renal or hepatic clearance • Anticoagulation and antiplatelet therapy increases bleeding risk • Increased dizziness from medications (propafonone, flecanide) • Nausea and reduced appetite (amiodarone) • Adherence to diet for Coumadin therapy may reduce compliance with heart healthy diet
Chronic noncardiac coexisting conditions		
Chronic kidney disease	44.8[10]	• Diuretic resistance • Increase risk of contrast induced nephrotoxicity with angiography • Increased bleeding risk with antiplatelet therapies • Increased stroke risk • Advanced kidney disease will limit heart failure therapies and increase volume retention • General fatigue, vomiting, and loss of appetite will increase weight loss and sarcopenia
Chronic obstructive pulmonary disease	30.9[10]	• Intolerance of beta-blockers • Beta agonist therapy may increase heart rate • Steroid treatment may promote fluid retention • Exacerbation of chronic obstructive pulmonary disease and heart failure common and difficult to discriminate primary trigger
Geriatric syndromes		
Incontinence	50[34]	• Anticholinergic effects of incontinence treatment may increase confusion and impair cognition • Medications may increase dry mouth leading to increased oral intake • Assessment of fluid balance using input:output ratio impaired • Reduced compliance with diuretic therapy through fear of incontinence • Reduced social activities and physical activity • Increased risk of falls owing to urgency

(*continued on next page*)

Table 1
(continued)

	Estimated Prevalence (%)	Drug–Disease, Drug–Drug, and Disease–Disease Interactions
Mobility impairment	>57[35]	• Reduced physical activity increases cardiovascular risk, increased frailty, and increased risk of falls • Reduced mobility impairs compliance with daily weights and access to heart healthy diet
Falls	35[36]	• Reduced mobility owing to fear of falls • Increased risk of injury with antiplatelet and anticoagulation therapy
Weight loss	7–9[37]	• Side effects of medications may reduce calorie intake (metallic taste, nausea, vomiting, gastrointestinal upset) • Impaired pharmacodynamics leading to overdosing of standard medications and increased side effects

Data from Refs.[10,34–37]

stroke. In addition, there is no report and a low anticipated prevalence of significant risk factors such as falls, cognitive impairment, disability, and functional decline.

IMPACT OF MULTIMORBIDITY AND CARDIOVASCULAR DISEASE

Although the incidence of multimorbidity in older adults increases, there remain few data to inform clinicians on how to best care for older adults with multimorbidity and CVD. Advances in medical research and technology have evolved around the single disease—focused model resulting in a significant reduction in morbidity and mortality from those specific disease processes (ie, reduction in mortality after an acute myocardial infarction). However, in comparison very little attention has been devoted to coexisting and equally important multiple chronic conditions in a single patient. **Fig. 4** compares the traditional single disease focused conceptual framework with a more patient-centered multimorbidity model.[28] In the comorbid model approach, a single CVD diagnosis is the primary and index disease and all other conditions are viewed as secondary and less significant processes to be considered in the management. As a consequence, clinical practice guidelines focus mainly on treating the primary CVD and when comorbid conditions are considered, recommendations highlight pairs of disease processes such as atrial fibrillation and diabetes mellitus or heart failure and chronic kidney disease. Moreover, standard practice guidelines do not provide specific guidance to a provider managing an acute exacerbation of heart failure with acute on chronic kidney disease, poorly controlled diabetes mellitus, atrial fibrillation with recurrent falls, and inadequate social support. The multimorbid conceptual framework demonstrates a more patient-centric approach to managing CVD in the context of multiple chronic conditions, geriatric syndromes, functional status, and social determinants of health. In this framework, the presenting CVD represents the smallest component of managing the patient with increasing complexity with each layer of impacting factors.

Older adults with multimorbidity are frequently seen by numerous general and specialist providers and use many services to manage individual diseases that may be inefficient, burdensome, and duplicative. Increasing multimorbidity is associated with higher 30-day readmission rates. Despite contributing to only 14% of the Medicare population, individuals with 6 or more chronic conditions have 30-day hospital readmission rates of more than 25% and make up 70% of the population that is

Table 2
Comparison of baseline characteristics in GRACE ACS registry and ACS focused clinical interventional trials

	GRACE Registry[24]			Clinical Trials		
Patient Characteristics	**STEMI**	**NSTEMI**	**Unstable Angina**	**CAPTIM Study[25]**	**CURE Trial[26]**	**GUSTO IV ACS Trial[27]**
Age (y), median (mean)	64	68	66	58	(64)	(65)
>65 (%)	51	60	57	—	49	—
>75 (%)	25	32	27	10	—	22.7
Male (%)	72	67	62	82.5	62	62
Prior myocardial infarction (%)	19	33	41	8.2	32	30
Heart failure (%)	7	14	14	Not reported	7.4	8
Diabetes mellitus (%)	21	27	25	11.1	22.8	22
Hypertension (%)	50	59	65	33.9	59	51
Hypercholesterolemia (%)	35	42	51	51	Not reported	30
Body mass index (kg/m^2)	27	27	27	Not reported	Not reported	Mean weight 77 kg
Prior stroke (%)	6	10	9	Not reported	4.4	3

Abbreviations: ACS, acute coronary syndrome; CAPTIM, Comparison of Primary Angioplasty and Pre-hospital Fibrinolysis in Acute Myocardial Infarction; CURE, Clopidogrel in Unstable angina to prevent Recurrent Events; GRACE, Global Registry of Acute Coronary Events; GUSTO V ACS, Global Use of Strategies To Open Occluded Coronary Arteries IV—Acute Coronary Syndrome; NSTEMI, non–ST-elevation myocardial infarction; STEMI, ST-elevation myocardial infarction.

Data from Refs.[24–27]

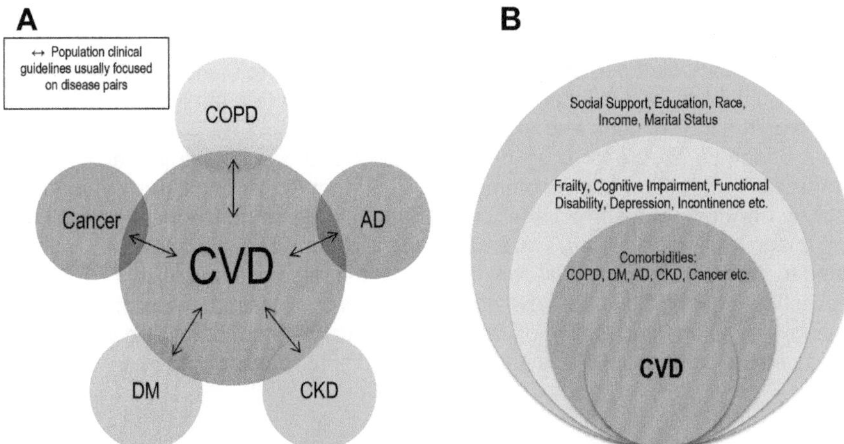

Fig. 4. Conceptual model of comorbidity versus multimorbidity in the context of cardiovascular disease (CVD). (*A*) Comorbid conceptual framework demonstrating the traditional disease-centered approach to understanding disease processes. Clinical practice guidelines are based on this framework where at most when comorbid conditions are considered they focus on disease pairs, such as CVD and diabetes mellitus or CVD and chronic kidney disease. (*B*) Multimorbid conceptual framework demonstrating a more patient-centric approach to managing CVD in the context of multiple chronic conditions, geriatric syndromes, functional status and social determinants of health. AD, Alzheimer disease; CKD, chronic kidney disease; COPD, chronic obstructive pulmonary disease; DM, diabetes mellitus.

readmitted. **Fig. 5** shows the impact of multimorbidity on rates of readmissions in Medicare beneficiaries by increasing number of chronic conditions.[8] Further, multimorbidity is also associated with much higher levels of per capita Medicare spending (**Fig. 5**B), where individuals with 6 or more chronic conditions cost more than 3 times the average per capita spending.[8]

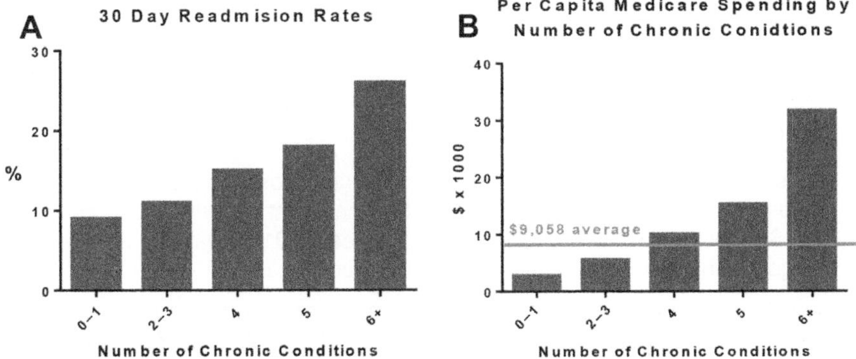

Fig. 5. (*A*) Readmission rates for fee-for-service Medicare beneficiaries by number of chronic conditions showing that readmission rates increase with increasing number of chronic conditions. (*B*) Per capita spending for Medicare beneficiaries by number of chronic conditions showing that individuals with 6 or more chronic conditions cost more than 3 times the average spending rate. (*Data from* Centers for Medicare & Medicaid Services. Chronic conditions overview. Available at: www.cms.gov/Research-Statistics-Data-and-Systems/Statistics-Trends-and-Reports/Chronic-Conditions/CC_Main.html. Accessed November 25, 2015.)

Poor care coordination and integration of care can also result in unsafe and competing management strategies by providers that may lead to multiple prescriptions for medications. Each provider will frequently adhere to standard of care clinical practice guidelines for individual chronic diseases, which frequently leads to burdensome monitoring regimens and significant polypharmacy.[29] As a consequence, the patient becomes at risk for drug–drug interactions, drug–disease interactions, and therapeutic competition (the recommended treatment for 1 condition may adversely affect and/or compete with another coexisting).[30] Adverse consequences, including poor adherence, adverse drug events, hospitalization, and mortality, are not only related to the number of medications, but also to the regimen complexity.[31,32] Studies have estimated that 50% of older adults are taking at least 1 medication with no ongoing indication, and many of these drugs are initiated during hospitalization, such as stress ulcer prophylaxis and antipsychotics for delirium.[33]

SUMMARY

Multimorbidity is the most significant and common condition affecting older adults and impacts every component of health care management and delivery. The prevalence of multimorbidity significantly increases with age and is prevalent in more than 70% of individuals 75 years or older. It represents the most common coexisiting disease process in older adults and impacts the complexity of all aspects of disease management. For individuals with a diagnosis of CVD, multimorbidty has a significant effect on the presentation of the disease, the diagnosis, management and the patient-centered preferences in care. Conventional assessment of cardiovascular and therapeutic risk is based on extrapolation of guidelines developed from evidence demonstrated in younger individuals and fails to weight the increased burden of complications and multimorbidity. In addition, evidence-based therapeutics have focused almost solely on cardiovascular focused morbidity (ie, changes in ejection fraction, number of reperfusion events) and while excluding outcomes such as functional status, maintenance of independence, and quality of life that may be of equal or more importance to an older adult. Over the next 25 years, the proportion of adults aged 65 and older is estimated to increase 3-fold, and with that remarkable change will come the complexities of managing this population. The resulting needs of these patients will require a fundamental shift in traditional care from single disease practices to a more patient-centered framework.

REFERENCES

1. Vincent GK, Velkoff VA. The next four decades: the older population in the United States: 2010 to 2050. Washington, DC: US Department of Commerce, Economics and Statistics Administration; US Census Bureau; 2010. Available at: www.aoa.acl.gov/Aging_Statistics/future_growth/future_growth.aspx.
2. Roth GA, Forouzanfar MH, Moran AE, et al. Demographic and epidemiologic drivers of global cardiovascular mortality. N Engl J Med 2015;372(14):1333–41.
3. Go AS, Mozaffarian D, Roger VL, et al. Heart disease and stroke statistics–2013 update: a report from the American Heart Association. Circulation 2013;127(1):e6.
4. Mozaffarian D, Benjamin EJ, Go AS, et al. Heart disease and stroke statistics-2015 update: a report from the American Heart Association. Circulation 2015;131(4):e29.

5. Boyd CM, Vollenweider D, Puhan MA. Informing evidence-based decision-making for patients with comorbidity: availability of necessary information in clinical trials for chronic diseases. PLoS One 2012;7(8):e41601.
6. Fihn SD, Gardin JM, Abrams J, et al. 2012 ACCF/AHA/ACP/AATS/PCNA/SCAI/STS guideline for the diagnosis and management of patients with stable ischemic heart disease: a report of the American College of Cardiology Foundation/American Heart Association task force on practice guidelines, and the American College of Physicians, American Association for Thoracic Surgery, Preventive Cardiovascular Nurses Association, Society for Cardiovascular Angiography and Interventions, and Society of Thoracic Surgeons. J Am Coll Cardiol 2012;60(24):e44–164.
7. Tinetti ME, Fried TR, Boyd CM. Designing health care for the most common chronic condition—multimorbidity. JAMA 2012;307(23):2493–4.
8. Centers for Medicare & Medicaid Services. Chronic conditions overview. Available at: www.cms.gov/Research-Statistics-Data-and-Systems/Statistics-Trends-and-Reports/Chronic-Conditions/CC_Main.html. Accessed November 25, 2015.
9. Rocca WA, Boyd CM, Grossardt BR, et al. Prevalence of multimorbidity in a geographically defined American population: patterns by age, sex, and race/ethnicity. Mayo Clin Proc 2014;89(10):1336–49.
10. Arnett DK, Goodman RA, Halperin JL, et al. AHA/ACC/HHS strategies to enhance application of clinical practice guidelines in patients with cardiovascular disease and comorbid conditions: from the American Heart Association, American College of Cardiology, and US Department of Health and Human Services. J Am Coll Cardiol 2014;64(17):1851–6.
11. Inouye SK, Studenski S, Tinetti ME, et al. Geriatric syndromes: clinical, research, and policy implications of a core geriatric concept. J Am Geriatr Soc 2007;55(5):780–91.
12. Tinetti ME, Inouye SK, Gill TM, et al. Shared risk factors for falls, incontinence, and functional dependence: unifying the approach to geriatric syndromes. JAMA 1995;273(17):1348–53.
13. Lee PG, Cigolle C, Blaum C. The co-occurrence of chronic diseases and geriatric syndromes: the health and retirement study. J Am Geriatr Soc 2009;57(3):511–6.
14. Buurman BM, Hoogerduijn JG, de Haan RJ, et al. Geriatric conditions in acutely hospitalized older patients: prevalence and one-year survival and functional decline. PLoS One 2011;6(11):e26951.
15. Anpalahan M, Gibson S. Geriatric syndromes as predictors of adverse outcomes of hospitalization. Intern Med J 2008;38(1):16–23.
16. Fried LP, Tangen CM, Walston J, et al. Frailty in older adults: evidence for a phenotype. J Gerontol A Biol Sci Med Sci 2001;56(3):M146–56.
17. Afilalo J, Karunananthan S, Eisenberg MJ, et al. Role of frailty in patients with cardiovascular disease. Am J Cardiol 2009;103(11):1616–21.
18. Newman AB, Gottdiener JS, McBurnie MA, et al. Associations of subclinical cardiovascular disease with frailty. J Gerontol A Biol Sci Med Sci 2001;56(3):M158–66.
19. Cacciatore F, Abete P, Mazzella F, et al. Frailty predicts long-term mortality in elderly subjects with chronic heart failure. Eur J Clin Invest 2005;35(12):723–30.
20. Ekerstad N, Swahn E, Janzon M, et al. Frailty is independently associated with short-term outcomes for elderly patients with non-ST-segment elevation myocardial infarction. Circulation 2011;124(22):2397–404.
21. Williams MA, Fleg JL, Ades PA, et al. Secondary prevention of coronary heart disease in the elderly (with emphasis on patients > or =75 years of age): an

American Heart Association scientific statement from the Council on Clinical Cardiology Subcommittee on Exercise, Cardiac Rehabilitation, and Prevention. Circulation 2002;105:1735–43.

22. Boyd CM, Leff B, Wolff JL, et al. Informing clinical practice guideline development and implementation: prevalence of coexisting conditions among adults with coronary heart disease. J Am Geriatr Soc 2011;59(5):797–805.
23. Lee PY, Alexander KP, Hammill BG, et al. Representation of elderly persons and women in published randomized trials of acute coronary syndromes. JAMA 2001; 286(6):708–13.
24. Steg PG, Goldberg RJ, Gore JM, et al. Baseline characteristics, management practices, and in-hospital outcomes of patients hospitalized with acute coronary syndromes in the Global Registry of Acute Coronary Events (GRACE). Am J Cardiol 2002;90(4):358–63.
25. Bonnefoy E, Lapostolle F, Leizorovicz A, et al. Primary angioplasty versus prehospital fibrinolysis in acute myocardial infarction: a randomised study. Lancet 2002;360(9336):825–9.
26. Yusuf S, Zhao F, Mehta SR, et al. Effects of clopidogrel in addition to aspirin in patients with acute coronary syndromes without ST-segment elevation. N Engl J Med 2001;345(7):494–502.
27. Simoons ML, GUSTO IV-ACS Investigators. Effect of glycoprotein IIb/IIIa receptor blocker abciximab on outcome in patients with acute coronary syndromes without early coronary revascularisation: the GUSTO IV-ACS randomised trial. Lancet 2001;357(9272):1915–24.
28. Boyd CM, Fortin M. Future of multimorbidity research: how should understanding of multimorbidity inform health system design. Public Health Rev 2010;32(2): 451–74.
29. Boyd CM, Darer J, Boult C, et al. Clinical practice guidelines and quality of care for older patients with multiple comorbid diseases: implications for pay for performance. JAMA 2005;294(6):716–24.
30. Lorgunpai SJ, Grammas M, Lee D, et al. Potential therapeutic competition in community-living older adults in the US: use of medications that may adversely affect a coexisting condition. PLoS One 2014;9(2):e89447.
31. Lau DT, Kasper JD, Potter D, et al. Hospitalization and death associated with potentially inappropriate medication prescriptions among elderly nursing home residents. Arch Intern Med 2005;165(1):68–74.
32. Claxton AJ, Cramer J, Pierce C. A systematic review of the associations between dose regimens and medication compliance. Clin Ther 2001;23(8):1296–310.
33. Morandi A, Vasilevskis E, Pandharipande PP, et al. Inappropriate medication prescriptions in elderly adults surviving an intensive care unit hospitalization. J Am Geriatr Soc 2013;61(7):1128–34.
34. Palmer MH, Hardin SR, Behrend C, et al. Urinary incontinence and overactive bladder in patients with heart failure. J Urol 2009;182(1):196–202.
35. Wong CY, Chaudhry SI, Desai MM, et al. Trends in comorbidity, disability, and polypharmacy in heart failure. Am J Med 2011;124(2):136–43.
36. Stenhagen M, Ekström H, Nordell E, et al. Falls in the general elderly population: a 3-and 6-year prospective study of risk factors using data from the longitudinal population study 'Good ageing in Skane'. BMC Geriatr 2013;13(1):81.
37. Pocock SJ, McMurray JJ, Dobson J, et al. Weight loss and mortality risk in patients with chronic heart failure in the candesartan in heart failure: assessment of reduction in mortality and morbidity (CHARM) programme. Eur Heart J 2008; 29(21):2641–50.

Magnitude and Impact of Multimorbidity on Clinical Outcomes in Older Adults with Cardiovascular Disease

A Literature Review

Mayra Tisminetzky, MD, PhD[a,b], Robert Goldberg, PhD[b,c],
Jerry H. Gurwitz, MD[a,b,*]

KEYWORDS

• Multimorbidity • Elderly • Clinical outcomes • Cardiovascular disease

KEY POINTS

- Multimorbidity is highly prevalent in older adults with cardiovascular disease and is related to higher levels of health care use and mortality.
- There are inconsistencies in the manner in which multimorbidity has been characterized in older adults presenting with cardiovascular disease.
- Limited data exist on the impact of multimorbidity on universal health outcomes (eg, health-related quality of life, symptom burden, and function) in older adults with cardiovascular disease.

INTRODUCTION

Approximately two-thirds of American men and women 65 years of age and older have been diagnosed with cardiovascular disease (CVD).[1] CVD in older men and women adversely impacts quality of life, and it is the leading cause of death in older

Meyers Primary Care Institute is a joint endeavor of University of Massachusetts Medical School, Reliant Medical Group, and Fallon Health, all of Worcester, MA.
The authors have no conflicts of interest to disclose. Drs J.H. Gurwitz and M. Tisminetzky are supported by award number 1R24AG045050 from the National Institute on Aging, Advancing Geriatrics Infrastructure & Network Growth (AGING-1R24AG045050). Partial salary support was provided to Dr R. Goldberg by National Institutes of Health Grant 1U01HL105268–01 and R01 HL35434.
[a] Division of Geriatric Medicine, Department of Medicine, Meyers Primary Care Institute, University of Massachusetts Medical School, 425 North Lake Avenue, Worcester, MA 01605, USA; [b] Department of Quantitative Health Sciences, University of Massachusetts Medical School, 425 North Lake Avenue, Worcester, MA 01605, USA; [c] Division of Cardiovascular Medicine, Department of Medicine, Meyers Primary Care Institute, University of Massachusetts Medical School, 425 North Lake Avenue, Worcester, MA 01605, USA
* Corresponding author. Meyers Primary Care Institute, 630 Plantation Street, Worcester, MA 01605.
E-mail address: jerry.gurwitz@umassmed.edu

Clin Geriatr Med 32 (2016) 227–246
http://dx.doi.org/10.1016/j.cger.2016.01.014 geriatric.theclinics.com

Americans. As the US population has aged, the prevalence of CVD has increased dramatically, together with other chronic conditions.[2–4] There is increasing awareness that older individuals with CVD and multiple chronic conditions experience higher levels of health care use and poorer outcomes.[4–10] Moreover, the clinical management of persons with CVD with multiple chronic conditions can be especially challenging due to complex therapeutic regimens, the involvement of multiple health care providers, and competing priorities impacting decision-making in the care of these patients.[11]

Despite the high prevalence of CVD and multimorbidity in the elderly, there remains a lack of consensus regarding how best to assess and measure multimorbidity and to determine how the presence of multiple chronic conditions impacts clinical outcomes.[11] The aim of this article is to review the current literature on the magnitude and impact of multimorbidity on clinical outcomes in older adults with CVD.

METHODS

Search Strategy and Information Sources

The available published literature was reviewed by searching the electronic databases Medline, PubMed, Medline Plus, and Embase, for the time period January 2005 through August 2015. The authors used the following search terms: *cardiovascular disease*, *myocardial infarction*, *heart failure*; *comorbidities*, *multimorbidity*, *multiple chronic conditions*; *clinical outcomes*, *mortality*, *hospital readmission*, *rehospitalization.* Search limits were used in each database to restrict the search to clinical studies, articles in the English language, and studies in the last 10 years (excluding animal studies) (Appendix 1).

In addition to the electronic search of these databases, the authors hand-searched the references of original articles. All references identified by the above searches were merged into a single bibliographic database.

After compiling the search results of the databases, the yield obtained by hand-searching, and removing duplicate articles, the studies were reviewed by the coauthors. One of the reviewers independently examined the titles and abstracts to determine eligibility for inclusion. If the title and abstract appeared to be potentially relevant by one of the raters, the article was marked for a full text review. Any article that was marked as unsure by the rater was also marked for full text review.

The studies reviewed in the report included patients 18 years or older with confirmed CVD cared for in the hospital and clinic setting. Excluded were case reports, letters to the editors, or situations where only an abstract was provided. (See PRISMA [Preferred Reporting Items for Systematic Reviews and Meta-Analyses] checklist for details.)

PRISMA 2009 checklist

Section/Topic	#	Checklist Item	Reported on Page #
Title			
Title	1	Identify the report as a systematic review, meta-analysis, or both.	1
Abstract			
Structured summary	2	Provide a structured summary including, as applicable: background; objectives; data sources; study eligibility criteria, participants, and interventions; study appraisal and synthesis methods; results; limitations; conclusions and implications of key findings; systematic review registration number.	4

(*continued on next page*)

(*continued*)

Section/Topic	#	Checklist Item	Reported on Page #
Introduction			
Rationale	3	Describe the rationale for the review in the context of what is already known.	5
Objectives	4	Provide an explicit statement of questions being addressed with reference to participants, interventions, comparisons, outcomes, and study design (PICOS).	6
Methods			
Protocol and registration	5	Indicate if a review protocol exists, if and where it can be accessed (e.g., Web address), and, if available, provide registration information including registration number.	NA
Eligibility criteria	6	Specify study characteristics (e.g., PICOS, length of follow-up) and report characteristics (e.g., years considered, language, publication status) used as criteria for eligibility, giving rationale.	7
Information sources	7	Describe all information sources (e.g., databases with dates of coverage, contact with study authors to identify additional studies) in the search and date last searched.	6
Search	8	Present full electronic search strategy for at least one database, including any limits used, such that it could be repeated.	6
Study selection	9	State the process for selecting studies (i.e., screening, eligibility, included in systematic review, and, if applicable, included in the meta-analysis).	7 and figure 1
Data collection process	10	Describe method of data extraction from reports (e.g., piloted forms, independently, in duplicate) and any processes for obtaining and confirming data from investigators.	7
Data items	11	List and define all variables for which data were sought (e.g., PICOS, funding sources) and any assumptions and simplifications made.	NA
Risk of bias in individual studies	12	Describe methods used for assessing risk of bias of individual studies (including specification of whether this was done at the study or outcome level), and how this information is to be used in any data synthesis.	NA
Summary measures	13	State the principal summary measures (e.g., risk ratio, difference in means).	RR/OR/HR/ Pearson correlation coefficient
Synthesis of results	14	Describe the methods of handling data and combining results of studies, if done, including measures of consistency (e.g., I^2) for each meta-analysis.	NA
Risk of bias across studies	15	Specify any assessment of risk of bias that may affect the cumulative evidence (e.g., publication bias, selective reporting within studies).	NA
Additional analyses	16	Describe methods of additional analyses (e.g., sensitivity or subgroup analyses, meta-regression), if done, indicating which were pre-specified.	NA

(*continued on next page*)

(continued)

Section/Topic	#	Checklist Item	Reported on Page #
Results			
Study selection	17	Give numbers of studies screened, assessed for eligibility, and included in the review, with reasons for exclusions at each stage, ideally with a flow diagram.	8 and figure 1
Study characteristics	18	For each study, present characteristics for which data were extracted (e.g., study size, PICOS, follow-up period) and provide the citations.	Table 1
Risk of bias within studies	19	Present data on risk of bias of each study and, if available, any outcome level assessment (see item 12).	Table 3
Results of individual studies	20	For all outcomes considered (benefits or harms), present, for each study: (a) simple summary data for each intervention group (b) effect estimates and confidence intervals, ideally with a forest plot.	Table 4A, B and C
Synthesis of results	21	Present results of each meta-analysis done, including confidence intervals and measures of consistency.	NA
Risk of bias across studies	22	Present results of any assessment of risk of bias across studies (see Item 15).	NA
Additional analysis	23	Give results of additional analyses, if done (e.g., sensitivity or subgroup analyses, meta-regression [see Item 16]).	NA
Discussion			
Summary of evidence	24	Summarize the main findings including the strength of evidence for each main outcome; consider their relevance to key groups (e.g., healthcare providers, users, and policy makers).	9-11
Limitations	25	Discuss limitations at study and outcome level (e.g., risk of bias), and at review-level (e.g., incomplete retrieval of identified research, reporting bias).	12
Conclusions	26	Provide a general interpretation of the results in the context of other evidence, and implications for future research.	12
Funding			
Funding	27	Describe sources of funding for the systematic review and other support (e.g., supply of data); role of funders for the systematic review.	NA

From Moher D, Liberati A, Tetzlaff J, Altman DG, The PRISMA Group. Preferred Reporting Items for Systematic Reviews and Meta-Analyses: The PRISMA Statement. PLoS Med 2009;6(6): e1000097.

RESULTS

Search Results

A total of 261 articles were identified from the initial literature search; after 204 duplicates were removed, and 57 articles were excluded on the basis of title and abstract review, 36 articles were retrieved for more detailed assessment. Of these, 15 studies met the inclusion criteria (**Fig. 1**). No additional articles were identified from the references of the included articles.

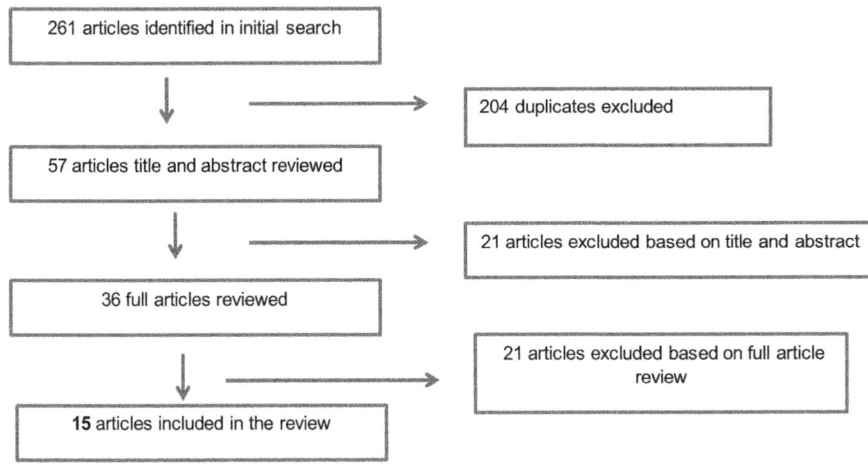

Fig. 1. Search strategy.

Study Characteristics

The characteristics of included articles are detailed in **Table 1**. Five studies included patients with acute myocardial infarction, and 10 included patients with heart failure as the cardiovascular condition of interest. Six of the included studies were retrospective cohort studies,[3,9,10,13,17] 4 were cross-sectional,[5,12,19,20] 3 were prospective cohort studies,[15,21,22] and 2 were randomized controlled trials.[16,18] Seven were US-based studies[3,5,9,10,17,19,21]; non-US-based studies (n = 8) were performed in Canada[14,18] and several European countries, including Italy,[20] Spain,[12] Portugal,[13] Denmark,[16] France,[15] and the Netherlands.[22] Eleven studies used medical records for data collection,[3,5,9,10,12–16,21,22] 3 used claims-based data,[17,19,20] and one group of investigators analyzed data on multimorbidity collected in the context enrolling subjects in a large randomized controlled trial (SOLVD [Studies of Left Ventricular Dysfunction]).[18]

Study sample sizes ranged from 93[22] to more than 182,000[19] participants; 8 of the 15 studies[3,5,9,10,16–19] included less than 1000 subjects. All 15 studies provided information about the average age of the study sample, which ranged from 59[18] to 83[13] years; the percentage of women ranged from 5%[3] to 80%.[15] Six of the 7 US-based studies[3,5,9,10,19,21] provided data on race/ethnicity, and most subjects in those studies was Caucasian.

Assessment and Magnitude of Multimorbidity

The number of chronic conditions was assessed by simple counts of chronic conditions[3,5,9,10,13,15–19,21] (n = 11), by combination of the Elixhauser and Charlson indices[12] (n = 1), and by the Charlson index alone[14,20,22] (n = 3) (**Table 2**). The prevalence of chronic conditions ranged from at least one additional morbidity in 10%[5] to 77%[9] of persons; the frequency of 4 or more additional chronic conditions ranged from 5%[9] to 60%.[21] The most common morbidities considered were diabetes,[3,15,21] chronic kidney disease,[3,16,17,19,21] anemia,[3,15,16] chronic obstructive pulmonary disease,[3,16,21] and dementia/cognitive impairment.[3,19,21]

Multimorbidity and Clinical Outcomes

All the studies reviewed found a positive association between the cumulative effect of multimorbidity and the risk of dying (**Tables 3–6**). Three studies reported a significant

Table 1
Study population characteristics

Authors, Country	Setting	Condition	Population Characteristics	Study Design, Time Period
Lichtman et al,[5] 2007, USA	19 Medical centers (academic, inner city, and nonuniversity hospitals)	AMI	N: 3907. Mean age: 64 y, 40% women, 60% white	Cross-sectional data collected from January 2003 to June 2004
Gili et al,[12] 2011, Spain	2 Major hospitals (ICU; department of cardiology and internal medicine)	AMI	N: 5275. Mean age: 72 y	Cross-sectional data collected from 2003 to 2009
Picarra et al,[13] 2011, Portugal	1 Hospital (cardiology department)	AMI	N:132 Mean age: 83 y, 55% men	Retrospective data collected from January 2005 to December 2007
McManus et al,[9] 2012, USA	11 Medical centers in central MA	AMI	N: 9581. Mean age: 70 y, 57% men, 93% Caucasian	Retrospective data collected from 1990 to 2007
Chen et al,[10] 2013, USA	11 Medical centers in central MA	AMI	N: 2972. Mean age: 71 y, 55% men, 93% Caucasian	Retrospective data collected from 2003 to 2007
Clarke et al,[14] 2011, Canada	1 Tertiary care HF ambulatory clinic in	HF	N: 824. Mean age 64 y, 69% men, Mean EF: 33%	Retrospective data collected from December 1998 to December 2004
Maréchaux et al,[15] 2011, France	1 Hospital	HF	N: 98. Mean age: 76 y, 80% women. 64% had low EF	Prospective data collected from October 2005 to September 2007
Mogensen et al,[16] 2011, Denmark	70 Different hospitals in Denmark, Norway, and Sweden	HF	N: 8507. Mean age 72 y, 40% women	Two RCTs data collected for one study (Denmark) from 1993 to 1996 and the other (multisite in Europe) from 2001 to 2002
Ather et al,[3] 2012, USA	Ambulatory clinics of the US Department of Veterans Affairs	HF	N: 2843 preserved and 6599 with reduced HF. Mean age 70 y, 95% men. 77% white	Retrospective data collected from October 2000 to September 2002

Oudejans et al,[22] 2012, The Netherlands	2 Regional hospitals (geriatric outpatient clinics)	HF	N: 93. Mean age: 83 y, 40% men	Prospective data collected from July 2003 to July 2010
Smith et al,[17] 2013, USA	4 Health plans in CA, CO, OR, MA, and WA	HF	N: 24,331; 14,579 with preserved and 9752 with reduced HF. Mean age: 74 y, 48% women	Retrospective data collected from January 2005 to December 2008
Bohm et al,[18] 2014, Canada	23 Medical centers in the US, Canada, and Belgium	HF	SOLVD prevent N: 4228. Mean age: 59 y, 89% men 87% white; SOLVD treatment N: 2569 Mean age: 61 y, 80% men 80% white	RCTs data collected from June 1986 to March 1989
Lee et al,[19] 2014, USA	Agency of Healthcare Research and Quality Inpatient Sample (4390 hospitals; 44 states)	HF	N: 192,327 hospitalizations for HF. Mean age: 73 y, 51% women, 68% white	Cross-sectional data collected during 2009
Buck et al,[20] 2015, Italy	Cardiovascular centers (28 provinces in northern Italy)	HF	N: 628 Mean age 73 y, men 58%	Cross-sectional data collected from 2011 to 2012
Murad et al,[21] 2015, USA	4 Centers, NC, CA, MA, and PA	HF	N: 558 Mean age: 79 y, 52% men, 87% white	Prospective data collected from 1989 to 1990 to 2nd wave 1992 to 1993 to 2002

Abbreviations: AMI, acute myocardial infarction; EF, ejection fraction; HF, heart failure; ICU, intensive care unit; RCT, randomized controlled trial.
Data from Refs.[3,5,9,10,12–22]

Table 2
Assessment of multimorbidity

Method	Assessment of MCCs	Data Source	Prevalence of MCCS
Count of MCCs	Simple count of acute non-cardiac-related conditions[5]	Medical records	Non-CVD-related conditions prevalence: 7%. Most prevalent chronic conditions were: pneumonia (18%); gastrointestinal bleeding (16%), and stroke (10%)[5]
	Simple counts of non-CVD conditions[13]	Medical records	57% of patients had at least one non-CVD-related condition. Hypertension (80%); diabetes (34%); AMI (30%); AF (22%) were the most prevalent MCCs[13]
	Simple counts of CVD-related conditions[9]	Medical records; physician's progress notes	17% of patients had 3 or more CVD-chronic conditions. Most common dyad of CVD-related conditions was: hypertension and diabetes (12%)[9]
	Simple counts of CVD and non-CVD-related conditions[10]	Medical records	25% of patients had 4 or more cardiac and 16% had 2 or more non-cardiac-related conditions. Hypertension (75%) and renal disease (22%) were the most prevalent morbidities[10]
	Simple counts of CVD-related conditions[15]	Medical records; patient reports	Most prevalent MCCs were: hypertension (90%); HF (49%); AF (45%); diabetes (48%)[15]
	Simple counts of CVD and non-CVD-related conditions[16]	Medical records	Most prevalent CVD-related conditions were previous AMI (34%); hypertension (25%); COPD (23%); AF (22%); diabetes (16%)[16]
	Simple count of non-CVD-related conditions[3]	Electronic medical records; clinicians reports	Most prevalent conditions were: hypertension (70%); renal disease (49%); diabetes (45%); AF (35%); COPD (34%); psychiatric disorders (28%)[3]
	Simple counts of MCCs[17]	Cardiovascular Research Network PRESERVE study	Most prevalent chronic conditions were: hypertension (80%); hyperlipidemia (68%); COPD (42%); AF (38%)[17]
	Simple counts of MCCs[18]	Investigators' case report forms	In SOLVD prevention 46% had 2 or more MCCs. In SOLVD treatment 60% patients had 2 or more MCCs. Most prevalent MCCs: diabetes (26% vs 15%) and chronic kidney disease (41% vs 26%) in the SOLVD prevention and treatment, respectively[18]
	Counts and clusters of MCCs[19]	Discharge records using AHRQ software	Average number of MCCs: 7.5. Most prevalent morbidities were: hypertension (68%); renal disease (39%); COPD (36%); diabetes (34%); anemia (28%); AMI (16%)[19]
	Counts of CVD and non-CVD-related conditions[21]	Medical records	60% of study sample had >3 MCCs. Hypertension (82%); diabetes (29%); COPD (20%) were the most prevalent chronic conditions[21]

Indexes	Charlson and Elixhauser scores[12]	Medical records	Hypertension (49%); arrhythmias (35%); HF (25%) were the most prevalent chronic conditions[12]
	Charlson index[14]	Electronic database; medical records	Charlson score of >6 presented in 13% of the study population. Most prevalent chronic conditions: AMI (60%); hypertension (54%); diabetes (48%); AF (31%); COPD (22%)[14]
	Charlson index[22]	Practitioner's reports; hospital information system	Most prevalent MCCs were: hypertension (42%); AF (39%); COPD (27%); cognitive impairment (27%); diabetes (27%)[22]
	Charlson index[20]	Electronic database; medical records	76% of study sample had 1 morbidity. Most prevalent morbidities were: AF (46%); ACS (40%); COPD (38%); diabetes (36%); anemia (24%); renal disease (19%)[20]

Abbreviations: ACS, acute coronary syndrome; AF, atrial fibrillation; AHRQ, Agency for Healthcare Research and Quality; AMI, acute myocardial infarction; COPD, chronic obstructive pulmonary disease; HF, heart failure; MCCs, multiple chronic conditions.

Data from Refs.[3,5,9,10,12–22]

Table 3
Assessment of outcomes and limitations (see Tables 4–6 for detailed findings)

	Data Source	Outcome Findings	Study Limitations
Long-term mortality	Medical records, death certificates at state and local divisions of Vital Statistics[9]	30-d and 1-y mortality HR increased proportionally with number of MCCs (see **Table 5**)	Limited generalizability due to mostly white population. Potential misclassification; data on MCCs were abstracted from medical records without validation[9]
	Electronic database; death certificates from Department of Health[14]	Number of MCCs was highly associated with the risk of non-sudden but not with sudden death (see **Table 5**)	Limited generalizability: one ambulatory clinic included in study. Charlson index was calculated from data from medical records without validation[14]
	Medical records[15]	Risk of dying and hospitalizations was associated with the presence of diabetes and anemia, but not with hypotension (see **Table 6**)	Small sample size. Only 3 chronic conditions were included in the study. Composite endpoint makes it difficult to compare the impact of chronic conditions. No validation of outcomes[15]
	Danish Central Personal Registry[16]	Risk of dying was associated with the presence of diabetes, AF, COPD, anemia, and chronic kidney disease (see **Table 5**)	Limited generalizability due to the restricted criteria of the 2 RCTs. Study data outdated. Misclassification, no validation on MCCs data[16]
	5 National VA databases[3]	Risk of dying was associated with the presence of diabetes, AF, COPD, anemia, liver disease, dementia, and chronic kidney disease (see **Tables 4–6**)	Limited generalizability, 90% of the study sample were men from a VA. Potential misclassification due to data on non-CVD conditions and mortality were abstracted from electronic medical records without validation[3]
	Hospital medical records and practitioner's reports[22]	Risk of dying was associated with a Charlson score of ≥4 (see **Table 5**)	Small sample size. No information on the distribution of MCCs in the study sample. Potential misclassification due to data on MCCs and mortality without validation[22]
	Death certificates, Social Security files, and hospital databases[17]	Risk of dying and hospitalization was significant for those with severe kidney disease (see **Tables 5** and **6**)	Potential misclassification due to data collected without validation. Limited generalizability, only insured individuals were included in the study[17]
	Investigators' data forms[18]	4-y mortality HR increased proportionally with number of MCCs in both study participants (see **Tables 5** and **6**)	Outdated data (data were collected in early 1990s); limited generalizability due to RCT with very restricted criteria[18]
	Medical records (unclear)[21]	Risk of dying was associated with the presence of diabetes, cerebrovascular disease, depression, COPD, functional and cognitive impairment, and chronic kidney disease (see **Table 5**)	Potential misclassification due to the characteristics of the study design and no validation of MCCs or mortality. Data might be outdated (patients enrolled early 1990s follow-up ended in 2002)[21]

In-hospital mortality	Medical records, Social Security Death Master file[5]	Risk of dying was associated with the presence of MCCs (see **Table 4**)	Potential missing data and misclassification due to abstraction of medical records without validation. Differential (longer) follow-up for those with CVD-related conditions[5]
	Medical records[12]	"Higher" scores on the Charlson and Elixhauser were associated with a higher risk of dying (see **Table 4**)	Charlson and Elixhauser scores were calculated based on discharge data without validation. No data on study sample demographic characteristics, limited generalizability[12]
	Medical records[13]	Mortalites were higher in those with as compared with those without MCCs (see **Table 4**)	Small sample size. Unclear how data on mortality were collected/validated. Data on comorbidities were abstracted from medical records without validation, potential misclassification[13]
	Medical records, death certificates at state and local divisions of Vital Statistics[10]	Mortality ORs increased proportionally with number of MCCs (see **Table 4**)	Limited generalizability, mostly white patients from one geographic area. Potential misclassification due to data on MCCs without validation[10]
	Medical records[19]	Risk of dying was associated with the presence of several MCCs/Charlson score, or patient profile (see **Table 4**)	Limited generalizability, due to the use of hospitalizations instead of patient as unit of analysis. Potential misclassification due to using administrative data without validation[19]
Hospitalization	Medical records[20]	Risk of hospitalization higher and lower quality of life (physical and emotional) in those with MCCs (see **Table 6**)	Limited generalizability, only symptomatic patients were included in this study. No validation of the different "exposures"[20]

Abbreviations: AF, atrial fibrillation; COPD, chronic obstructive pulmonary disease; MCCs, multiple chronic conditions; RCT, randomized controlled trial; VA, Veterans Administration.

Data from Refs.[3,5,9,10,12–22]

Table 4
In-hospital case fatality rates (detailed)

Crude CFRs			Adjusted CFRs			
MCCs Counts	**CVD-related Conditions**	**Non-CVD-related Conditions**	**MCCs Counts**	**CVD-related Conditions**	**Non-CVD-related Conditions**	**Charlson/Elixhauser**
MCCs+: 17% MCCs−: 4%[13]	—	Patients with: 21% Patients w/o: 3%[5]	—	—	ORs (95% CI) for those with multimorbidity: 5.0 (3.3; 7.7)[5]	—
0: 3.7% 1: 6.1% 2: 10.6% 3: 11.2% 4 or +: 14.2%[10]	—	—	—	ORs (95% CI) for those with: 1: 1.31 (0.67; 2.57); 2: 2.00 (1.05; 3.82); 3: 2.14 (1.10; 4.20); 4 or +: 2.80 (1.43; 5.49)[10]	ORs (95% CI) for those with: 1: 1.24 (1.03; 1.50); 2: 1.63 (1.12; 2.37); 3 or +: 1.76 (1.11; 2.78)[10]	—
	—	—	RR (95% CI): for those with 7 or + MCCs: 1.03 (1.02; 1.04)[19]	—	—	RR (95% CI) Charlson score of 5 or +: 1.16 (1.08; 1.25)[19]
	—	—	—	ORs (95% CI) for those with: HF: 2.97 (2.47; 3.56) Arrhythmias: 1.61 (1.36; 1.93)[12]	—	High Elixhauser score $\geq$2.4: ORs: 1.14 (1.07; 1.22)[12]
	For those with: HF preserved: 20% HF reduced: 25%[3]	—	—	—	—	—

Abbreviations: HF, heart failure; MCCs, multiple chronic conditions; RR, relative risk.
Data from Refs.[3,5,10,12,13,19]

association between unspecified multimorbidity and long-term mortality.[9,14,18] One study found a significant association between a score of 4 or more on the Charlson index and long-term mortality.[22] Three studies found a significant association between number of morbidities and the hospital case fatality rate (CFR),[5,10,13] and one study reported a significant association between a higher Charlson score and hospital CFR.[12] As an example, of the positive association between number of morbidities and long-term mortality, one study found that in a cohort of 9500 patients hospitalized due to an acute myocardial infarction, 1-year mortality odds ratio (ORs) ranged from 1.16 (1.01; 1.34) to 2.31 (1.92; 2.78) for those presenting with 1 or 4 or more chronic conditions, respectively, as compared with those without any chronic conditions.[9] Another study found that patients with heart failure and hypertension had a hazard ratio (HR) for death of 1.32 (1.12; 1.54), and those presenting with heart failure and diabetes had an HR of 1.55 (1.28; 1.88), as compared with those without these chronic conditions.[18]

Another study demonstrated a positive association between the number of morbidities and hospital CFRs; the ORs ranged from 2.00 (95% confidence interval [CI]: 1.05, 3.82) to 2.80 (1.43, 5.49) in those patients with acute myocardial infarction and presenting with 2 or 4 or more chronic conditions, respectively, as compared with those without any morbidities.[10] As an example of studies that examined the impact of specific chronic conditions on mortality, in a cohort of 5275 patients that had experienced a previous hospitalization for an acute myocardial infarction, researchers reported ORs of 2.97 (2.47, 3.56) for those with heart failure and ORs of 1.61 (1.36; 1.93) for those with arrhythmias as compared with patients without these conditions.[12]

Of note, the authors identified only one study that reported on outcomes falling into the category of "universal outcomes."[20] In a cohort of 628 patients with heart failure, the investigators found a statistically significant association between the overall burden of comorbidity, as assessed by the Charlson comorbidity index, and worse physical and emotional quality of life (Pearson's correlation coefficients were reported for this analysis; for example, for emotional quality of life, the coefficient decreased from 0.16 in those with one to 0.04 in those with 4 chronic conditions based on the Charlson index.)[20]

DISCUSSION

In this review, it was found that there is a significant association between number and types of chronic conditions and the risk of dying; the most frequent morbidities examined were diabetes, chronic kidney disease, anemia, chronic pulmonary disease, and dementia/cognitive impairment. Whereas the findings highlight the very high prevalence of multimorbidity in patients with CVD, and the association of the cumulative effect of number of chronic conditions with outcomes such as mortality or the risk of rehospitalization, only very limited data are available on the magnitude and impact of multimorbidity on universal health outcomes, such as symptom burden, functional capacity, and self-rated health among older adults with CVD.

Despite the high prevalence of CVD, and additional chronic conditions in these individuals, the findings suggest that there is a lack of consistency in the manner in which the burden of multimorbidity is assessed and characterized.[3,5,10,12–22] Although several different approaches exist for measuring multimorbidity, none of these is considered to be a "gold standard." Simply counting morbidities is seemingly straightforward; however, this approach does not take into account the clinical severity of a condition or the varying impact across conditions. Comorbidity indices are relatively easy to apply, but may also lack sufficient specificity to adequately characterize the complexity of patients presenting with multimorbidity and CVD. Summary scores

Table 5
Long-term case fatality rates (detailed)

MCCs Counts	CVD-related Conditions	Non-CVD-related Conditions	Charlson/Elixhauser
30-d ORs for those with: 1: 1.19 (0.93; 1.35); 2: 1.49 (1.23; 1.80); 3: 1.64 (1.32; 2.03); 4 or + :1.68 (1.28; 2.21);	HR (95% CI) for those with: Hypertension + diabetes 30-d: 1.09 (0.85; 1.39) Hypertension + diabetes 1-y: 1.27 (1.06; 1.50)[9]	—	—
1-y ORs for those with: 1: 1.16 (1.01; 1.34); 2: 1.62 (1.41; 1.87); 3: 1.94 (1.66; 2.26); 4 or + : 2.31 (1.91; 2.78)[9]	HR (95% CI) for those with: AF: 1.30 (1.06; 1.60); Diabetes: 1.31 (1.01; 1.61)[16]	HR (95% CI) for those with: COPD: 1.46 (1.37; 1.55); Anemia: 1.29 (1.13; 1.48); Chronic kidney disease: 1.36 (1.13; 1.63)[16]	—
	—	HR (95% CI) for those with severe kidney disease: HF preserved EF: 1.67 (1.41; 1.76); HF reduced EF: 2.15 (1.87; 2.48)[17]	—
(4-y) mortality ORs for those with: 1: 1.48 (1.10; 2.00); 2: 2.02 (1.43; 2.85); 3: 2.80 (1.85; 4.22); 4 or +: 4.95 (3.02; 8.11)[18]	HR (95% CI) for those with: Hypertension: 1.32 (1.12; 1.54) Diabetes: 1.55 (1.28; 1.88)[18]	HR (95% CI) for those with: COPD:1.73 (1.30; 2.31)[18]	—
	—	—	3-y HR (95% CI) for those with: Charlson score of 3–4: 1.5 (0.7; 2.9); Charlson score of 4 or + 4.0 (1.9; 8.8) (1–2 score-referent group)[22]
	—	—	HR (95% CI) for those with: Charlson score ≥4: Non-sudden death: 2.78 (2.09; 3.70); Sudden death: 0.49 (0.19; 1.28)[14]

	—	HR (95% CI) for those with: Chronic kidney disease: HF preserved: 1.28 (1.07; 1.53) HF restricted EF 1.25 (1.12; 1.38); Anemia: HF preserved: 1.35 (1.13; 1.61) HF restricted EF: 1.42 (1.28; 1.57), COPD: HF preserved: 1.61 (1.36; 1.91) HF restricted EF: 1.23 (1.11; 1.37), Liver disease: HF preserved: 2.31 (1.48; 3.62) HF restricted EF: 1.41 (1.05; 1.89); Dementia: HF preserved: 1.75 (1.21; 2.51) HF restricted EF: 1.48 (1.16; 1.90)[3]	—
	HR (95% CI) for those with: Diabetes: 1.64 (1.33; 2.03) Cerebrovascular disease: 1.53 (1.22; 1.92)[21]	HR (95% CI) for those with: Chronic kidney disease: 1.32 (1.07; 1.62) Depression: 1.44 (1.09; 1.90), Functional impairment: 1.30 (1.04; 1.63), Cognitive impairment: 1.33 (1.02; 1.73).[21]	—

Abbreviations: AF, atrial fibrillation; COPD, chronic obstructive pulmonary disease; HF, heart failure; MCCs, multiple chronic conditions.
Data from Refs.[3,9,14,16–18,21,22]

Table 6
Hospitalization rates and adjusted analysis findings (detailed)

Hospitalization Rates Unadjusted	MCCs Counts	CVD-related Conditions	Non-CVD-related Conditions	Charlson/Elixhauser
40% at least 1 admission[20]	—	—	HR (95% CI) for those with: Severe kidney disease HF preserved EF: 1.32 (1.24; 1.41) HF reduced EF: 1.47 (1.35; 1.60)[17]	—
	HR (95% CI) for those with: 1: 1.14 (0.95; 1.75); 2: 1.47 (1.20; 1.80); 3: 1.66 (1.31; 2.10); 4 or +: 2.09 (1.59; 2.75)[18]	HR (95% CI) for those with: Hypertension: 1.15 (1.06; 1.25) Diabetes: 1.31 (1.18; 1.46)[18]	HR (95% CI) for those with: COPD: 1.53 (1.30; 1.80)[18]	—
	—	—	—	Pearson correlation Charlson score 1: 0.21 score 2: 0.16; score 3: 0.18; score 4 or +: 0.18[20]
For those with: HF preserved: 50% HF reduced: 49%[3]	—	—	—	—
Hospitalization + CFRs				
24% with 1 admission[15]	—	HR (95% CI) for those with: Diabetes: 1.76 (1.03; 3.00)[15]	HR (95% CI) for those with: Hypotension: 0.98 (0.97; 0.99); Anemia: 2.52 (1.32; 5.05)[15]	—

Abbreviations: COPD, chronic obstructive pulmonary disease; HF, heart failure; MCCs, multiple chronic conditions.
Data from Refs.[3,15,17,18,20]

derived from various indices of multimorbidity can also be challenging to apply and integrate into clinical decision-making relevant to the care of individual patients.

Although the use of claims data to characterize multimorbidity in large populations in a "real-world" setting may be highly efficient, these data are often inadequate to fully and accurately characterize the severity of disease and time of initial diagnosis of chronic conditions and pose substantial challenges in addressing outcomes such as health-related quality of life, symptom burden, and function.

A relatively recent systematic review aimed to compare multimorbidity measures using administrative data.[23] The most common instrument used was the Charlson index, followed by the Elixhauser index. The investigators concluded that "the performance of a given comorbidity measure depends on the patient group and outcome" being assessed.[23] Future studies, combining data from claims databases and supplemented by other sources of data, such as electronic health records, may serve to improve the current understanding of the impact of multimorbidity on clinical outcomes in older adults with CVD.

The overarching aim of this review was to summarize findings from studies examining the association between the presence of multiple chronic conditions and clinical outcomes in patients with CVD. All the studies included in this review found a positive significant association between the burden of multimorbidity and short- and long-term mortality. Although prior literature has suggested that multimorbidity plays an important role in quality of life and other universal health outcomes, in this review, only one study examined quality of life associated with the presence of multimorbidity.[20]

In, 2011, the National Institute on Aging, in collaboration with the Agency for Healthcare Research and Quality, convened an expert panel on health outcome measures for older persons with multimorbidity. The goal of this effort was to develop recommendations for the content of a core set of well-validated universal patient-centered outcome measures that could be routinely assessed in health care settings.[24] Among the recommended health outcomes to be measured were symptom burden, physical function and mobility, mental health outcomes, cognitive function, and social health outcomes. This expert panel concluded that universal outcome measures have emerged as a strong complement to disease-specific measures for comparative effectiveness research among older adults with multimorbidity.[24] The panel also suggested that the routine assessment of these measures would facilitate meaningful and interpretable results that could be used by patients and providers to better communicate the balance between benefit and risk of various interventions. Furthermore, another recent study evaluated function-related indicators in administrative claims data from the US Medicare beneficiaries with a hospitalization for acute myocardial infarction during 2007.[25] The investigators suggested that an "expanded concept of general illness severity that incorporates indicators of potentially diminished functional status can better capture the heterogeneity of patients with multimorbidity."[25]

Several limitations of this review must be acknowledged. This review was limited to studies published in English. The extent to which the inability to review studies published in languages other than English affected the findings is unknown. Because this review included only peer-reviewed publications, there is a potential for introducing possible publication bias. Because the authors allowed for heterogeneity of the multimorbidity assessment measures included in this review, a quantitative meta-analysis was not feasible. Finally, because most participants in the included studies were white, the generalizability of the findings to other race/ethnic groups may be limited. Future studies should examine potential racial and ethnic differences in the magnitude and impact of multimorbidity on clinical outcomes in patients presenting with CVD.

SUMMARY

Although multimorbidity is highly associated with the risk of dying in patients with CVD, there are only very limited data on the impact of multimorbidity on universal health outcomes (ie, health-related quality of life, symptom burden, and function). In addition, the review of the literature suggests a profound lack of consistency in the manner in which the burden of multimorbidity has been assessed and characterized across studies. Capturing the true complexity of older patients with CVD remains an ongoing challenge. Until that challenge is addressed, the value of available research on multimorbid patients with CVD for informing clinical decision-making is questionable.

REFERENCES

1. FASTSTATS - Heart Disease. Available at: http://www.cdc.gov/nchs/fastats/heart-disease.htm. Accessed February 21, 2016.
2. Saczynski JS, Go AS, Magid DJ, et al. Patterns of comorbidity in older patients with heart failure: the cardiovascular research network preserve study. J Am Geriatr Soc 2013;61(1):26–33.
3. Ather S, Chan W, Bozkurt B, et al. Impact of noncardiac comorbidities on morbidity and mortality in a predominantly male population with heart failure and preserved versus reduced ejection fraction. J Am Coll Cardiol 2012; 59(11):998–1005.
4. Vogeli C, Shields AE, Lee TA, et al. Multiple chronic conditions: prevalence, health consequences, and implications for quality, care management, and costs. J Gen Intern Med 2007;22(Suppl 3):391–5.
5. Lichtman JH, Spertus JA, Reid KJ, et al. Acute noncardiac conditions and in-hospital mortality in patients with acute myocardial infarction. Circulation 2007; 116(17):1925–30.
6. Ani C, Pan D, Martins D, et al. Age- and sex-specific in-hospital mortality after myocardial infarction in routine clinical practice. Cardiol Res Pract 2010;2010: 752–65.
7. Braunstein JB, Anderson GF, Gerstenblith G, et al. Noncardiac comorbidity increases preventable hospitalizations and mortality among Medicare beneficiaries with chronic heart failure. J Am Coll Cardiol 2003;42(7):1226–33.
8. Sachdev M, Sun JL, Tsiatis AA, et al. The prognostic importance of comorbidity for mortality in patients with stable coronary artery disease. J Am Coll Cardiol 2004;43(4):576–82.
9. McManus DD, Nguyen HL, Tisminetzky M, et al. Multiple cardiovascular comorbidities and acute myocardial infarction: temporal trends (1990–2007) and impact on death rates at 30 days and 1 year. Clin Epidemiol 2012;4:115–23.
10. Chen H-Y, Saczynski JS, McManus DD, et al. The impact of cardiac and noncardiac comorbidities on the short-term outcomes of patients hospitalized with acute myocardial infarction: a population-based perspective. Clin Epidemiol 2013;5: 439–48.
11. Boyd CM, Leff B, Wolff JL, et al. Informing clinical practice guideline development and implementation: prevalence of coexisting conditions among adults with coronary heart disease. J Am Geriatr Soc 2011;59(5):797–805.
12. Gili M, Sala J, López J, et al. Impact of comorbidities on in-hospital mortality from acute myocardial infarction, 2003-2009. Rev Esp Cardiol 2011;64(12):1130–7.
13. Piçarra BC, Santos AR, Celeiro M, et al. Non-cardiac comorbidities in the very elderly with acute myocardial infarction: prevalence and influence on management and in-hospital mortality. Rev Port Cardiol 2011;30(4):379–92.

14. Clarke B, Howlett J, Sapp J, et al. The effect of comorbidity on the competing risk of sudden and nonsudden death in an ambulatory heart failure population. Can J Cardiol 2011;27(2):254–61.
15. Maréchaux S, Six-Carpentier MM, Bouabdallaoui N, et al. Prognostic importance of comorbidities in heart failure with preserved left ventricular ejection fraction. Heart Vessels 2011;26(3):313–20.
16. Mogensen UM, Ersbøll M, Andersen M, et al. Clinical characteristics and major comorbidities in heart failure patients more than 85 years of age compared with younger age groups. Eur J Heart Fail 2011;13(11):1216–23.
17. Smith DH, Thorp ML, Gurwitz JH, et al. Chronic kidney disease and outcomes in heart failure with preserved versus reduced ejection fraction: the Cardiovascular Research Network PRESERVE Study. Circ Cardiovasc Qual Outcomes 2013;6(3): 333–42.
18. Böhm M, Pogue J, Kindermann I, et al. Effect of comorbidities on outcomes and angiotensin converting enzyme inhibitor effects in patients with predominantly left ventricular dysfunction and heart failure. Eur J Heart Fail 2014;16(3):325–33.
19. Lee CS, Chien CV, Bidwell JT, et al. Comorbidity profiles and inpatient outcomes during hospitalization for heart failure: an analysis of the U.S. nationwide inpatient sample. BMC Cardiovasc Disord 2014;14:73–82.
20. Buck HG, Dickson VV, Fida R, et al. Predictors of hospitalization and quality of life in heart failure: a model of comorbidity, self-efficacy and self-care. Int J Nurs Stud 2015;52:1714–22.
21. Murad K, Goff DC Jr, Morgan TM, et al. Burden of comorbidities and functional and cognitive impairments in elderly patients at the initial diagnosis of heart failure and their impact on total mortality: the Cardiovascular Health Study. JACC Heart Fail 2015;3(7):542–50.
22. Oudejans I, Mosterd A, Zuithoff NP, et al. Comorbidity drives mortality in newly diagnosed heart failure: a study among geriatric outpatients. J Card Fail 2012; 18(1):47–52.
23. Sharabiani MT, Aylin P, Bottle A. Systematic review of comorbidity indices for administrative data. Med Care 2012;50(12):1109–18.
24. Working Group on Health Outcomes for Older Persons with Multiple Chronic Conditions. Universal health outcome measures for older persons with multiple chronic conditions. J Am Geriatr Soc 2012;60(12):2333–41.
25. Chrischilles E, Schneider K, Wilwert J, et al. Beyond comorbidity: expanding the definition and measurement of complexity among older adults using administrative claims data. Med Care 2014;52(Suppl 3):S75–84.

APPENDIX 1: MEDLINE SEARCH STRATEGY

Search	String
#1	Cardiovascular disease [title/abstract]
#2	Myocardial infarction [title/abstract]
#3	Heart failure [title/abstract]
#4	#1 OR #2 OR #3
#5	Comorbidities [title/abstract]
#6	Multimorbidity [title/abstract]
#7	Multiple chronic conditions [title/abstract]
#8	#5 OR #6 OR #7
#9	Clinical outcomes [title/abstract]
#10	Mortality [title/abstract]
#11	Hospital readmission [title/abstract]
#12	Rehospitalization [title/abstract]
#13	#9 OR #10 OR #11 OR #12
#14	#4 AND #8 AND #13
#15	#14 AND full text[sb] AND last 10 years [PDat] AND Humans

Advance Care Planning and Goals of Care Communication in Older Adults with Cardiovascular Disease and Multi-Morbidity

Hillary D. Lum, MD, PhD[a,b,*], Rebecca L. Sudore, MD[c]

KEYWORDS

- Advance care planning • Goals of care • Patient-doctor relationship
- Communication • Older adults • Cardiovascular disease • Multi-morbidity

KEY POINTS

- Advance care planning (ACP) involves a process of eliciting patients' values and life goals over time and then translating those values into appropriate medical care plans.
- ACP can help individuals receive medical care that is aligned with their values and improve patient-reported outcomes.
- ACP should be initiated early in the disease trajectory for patients with cardiovascular disease, even at the time of diagnosis, and account for how other chronic conditions impact their prognosis, personal values, and medical preferences.
- Multidisciplinary teams can promote ACP by
  - Assessing patients' readiness to engage
  - Asking about surrogate decision-makers
  - Engaging patients in discussions about values and preferences

Disclosure: The authors do not have commercial or financial conflicts of interest to disclose. This work was supported in by part by a Junior Faculty Career Development Award from the National Palliative Care Research Center (NPCRC).

[a] VA Eastern Colorado Geriatric Research Education and Clinical Center (GRECC), 1055 Clermont Streeet, Denver, CO, 80220, USA; [b] Division of Geriatric Medicine, Department of Medicine, University of Colorado School of Medicine, 12631 East 17th Avenue, B-179, Aurora, CO 80045, USA; [c] Division of Geriatrics, Department of Medicine, San Francisco Veterans Affairs Medical Center, University of California, SFVAMC 4150 Clement Street, #151R, San Francisco, CA 94121, USA

* Corresponding author. 12631 East 17th Avenue, B-179, Aurora, CO 80045.
E-mail address: Hillary.Lum@ucdenver.edu

Clin Geriatr Med 32 (2016) 247–260
http://dx.doi.org/10.1016/j.cger.2016.01.011 geriatric.theclinics.com
0749-0690/16/$ – see front matter Published by Elsevier Inc.

INTRODUCTION

Advance care planning (ACP) is relevant for the estimated 85.6 million American adults (>1 in 3) who have cardiovascular disease, including 85% of men and 86% of women older than 80 years.[1] Many of these individuals have more than one chronic condition (ie, multi-morbidity). For example, 86% of patients with heart failure have multi-morbidity, with hypertension, hyperlipidemia, and arrhythmias being common.[2,3] The American Geriatrics Society published guiding principles for the care of older adults with multi-morbidity, emphasizing a person-centered approach that includes patient preferences and current medical conditions.[4] Although the American Heart Association (AHA) emphasized the importance of ACP in heart failure, ACP and goals of care communication should be integrated into the care of all older adults with cardiovascular disease and multi-morbidity.[2]

This article defines ACP, discusses the benefits and challenges to ACP in older adults with cardiovascular disease and multi-morbidity, and provides practical steps for clinicians about assessing patients' readiness to engage in ACP, identifying surrogate decision-makers, and asking about values related to quality of life. The authors also provide practical guidance to documenting patients' preferences, translating these preferences into medical orders, and communicating these preferences with other providers.

What Is Advance Care Planning?

ACP is a process whereby people identify their values and preferences for medical care and designate a surrogate decision-maker in advance of a medical crisis or the loss of decision-making capacity.[5] The goal is to help patients receive medical care that is aligned with their preferences. **Table 1** provides common ACP terms and definitions. It is important to note that ACP includes several behaviors, such as considering treatment goals in light of personal values, completing advance directives, and communicating with families and clinicians[6] (**Fig. 1**). The ACP process may be started at any age and any stage of illness.[7] It may focus on designating a surrogate and discussing preferences for surrogate decision-making (eg, degree of leeway or flexibility when making decisions).[8] It may also focus on discussions about values related to quality of life and preferences for overall health states that patients may or may not find acceptable (eg, being bed bound or in a coma). Ideally, early, anticipatory ACP conversations between patients, surrogate decision-makers, and health care providers will prepare patients and families for in-the-moment goals of care conversations, such as decisions about the use or nonuse of life-sustaining treatments and unanticipated events.[2,8] Therefore, over time, ACP discussions and documentation may focus on specific goals of care for medical treatments, such as cardiopulmonary resuscitation (CPR) or the implantation of a left ventricular assist device (LVAD).[5,9]

The importance of focusing ACP on values identification and ongoing discussions, and not just a one-time documented advance directive, cannot be overstated.[10] Completing advance directive documents is only one part of ACP (see **Fig. 1**). Living wills often focus on preferences for life-sustaining procedures, such as CPR and mechanical ventilation in specific medical situations. As patients' clinical condition changes over time, their preferences and values may also change. Furthermore, in addition to CPR, patients and their loved ones may need to make many decisions that are not addressed in advance directives, such as whether to have pacemaker and/or implantable cardioverter defibrillator (ICD) placement; cardiac catheterization; advanced cardiac therapies, such as inotropes or LVADs; or nursing home placement. Values-focused discussions can help patients, surrogates, and clinicians with all the

Table 1
ACP terms and definitions

ACP Terms	Description of Terms
ACP	Process of considering and communicating personal values and goals related to medical care over time
Advance directive	Legal documents describing preferences for future care *and* appointing a surrogate to make health care decisions in the event of lack of decision-making capacity
Medical durable power of attorney	Legal document that appoints an agent to make future medical decisions; becomes effective only when patients become incapacitated
Surrogate decision-maker or health care proxy	A decision-maker that makes medical decisions when patients become incapacitated *and* the patients did not previously identify a medical durable power of attorney (Most states use a hierarchy system to designate a health care proxy, whereas a few states appoint a proxy that is agreed on by all interested parties.)
Living will	Documents an individual's wishes prospectively regarding initiating, withholding, and withdrawing certain life-sustaining medical interventions; effective when patients become incapacitated and have certain medical conditions
Cardiopulmonary resuscitation directive or do-not-resuscitate order	Documents preferences to refuse unwanted resuscitation attempts
Orders for life-sustaining treatment (ie, Physicians Orders for Life Sustaining Treatment)	Medical order set that translates patient preferences for life-sustaining therapies into orders (This form is intended for seriously ill people with life-limiting illnesses and is portable and transferable between health care settings.)

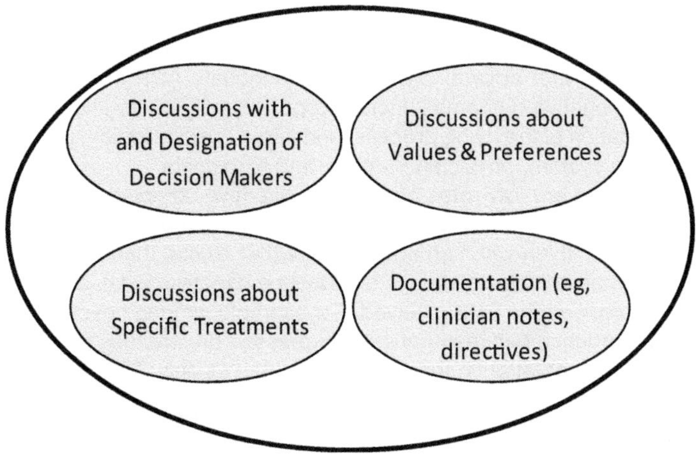

Fig. 1. Multiple aspects of ACP.

complex medical decisions that patients may face, not only decisions about particular medical procedures, such as CPR.

For older adults with cardiovascular diseases, the presence of other chronic conditions, such as diabetes mellitus, chronic obstructive pulmonary disease, osteoarthritis, cancer, or dementia, affect the individual's prognosis, quality of life, symptom burden, risks related to polypharmacy, and caregiver needs. Thus, ACP for older adults with cardiovascular diseases and multi-morbidity must use a tailored, person-centered approach that takes into account the full picture of patients' health and medical care, rather than being focused on a single disease in isolation.

Benefits of and Challenges to Advance Care Planning in Older Patients with Cardiovascular Disease and Multi-Morbidity

Benefits of ACP include

- Ability to identify, respect, and implement an individual's wishes for medical care, especially if the individual loses decision-making capacity[11]
- Sense of control over managing one's personal affairs, peace of mind, and decreased burden and conflict among loved ones[6]
- Improved patients' quality of life[12] and satisfaction with their clinicians who initiated ACP conversations[13]
- Decreased use of unwanted intensive medical interventions, hospitalizations, and CPR at the end of life[12,14]
- Fewer in-hospital deaths, more hospice use, and potentially lower Medicare costs among older adults with advance directives specifying comfort-oriented end-of-life care[15,16]
- Reduced stress, anxiety, and depression in surviving family members[17]
- New ability for clinician reimbursement for ACP conversations through the Centers for Medicare and Medicaid as of January 2026[18]

Challenges of advance care planning in older adults with cardiovascular disease

Despite the benefits of ACP and recommendations by the AHA to engage patients in ACP discussions, many older adults with cardiovascular disease and multi-morbidity die after extended periods of disability without discussing their preferences with family or clinicians. For example, only 12% of outpatient clinicians, including physicians, nurse practitioners, and physician assistants, caring for patients with heart failure reported having annual ACP discussions[19]; only 25% of patients hospitalized with heart failure reported discussing resuscitation preferences with their inpatient physician.[20] A recent review found that absent, delayed, or inadequate ACP communication was associated with negative outcomes, including poor quality of life and anxiety, family distress, prolongation of the dying process, undesired hospitalization, patient mistrust of the health care system, physician burnout, and high costs.[9]

Furthermore, there are low rates of advance directive completion in patients with heart failure (41%), severe aortic stenosis (47%), or individuals admitted to a cardiac care unit (26%).[21–23] Even when an advance directive exists, there is still poor correlation between what individuals state in an advance directive, what is documented in the medical record, and the care received. For example, among hospitalized patients in Canada, concordance between patients' expressed preferences for life-sustaining treatment and documentation in the medical record was only 30%.[24]

Patient and clinician barriers to advance care planning and goals of care communication

Patients face multiple barriers to engaging in an ACP process, such as[6,25]

- Fear of dying or finding it too difficult to think about end-of-life issues
- Fear of upsetting the doctor by desiring to discuss ACP
- Inability to plan for the future due to challenging life/social issues, including lack of an available surrogate decision-maker
- Limited knowledge of ACP or difficulty understanding advance directives

Clinicians caring for patients with cardiovascular disease and multi-morbidity also face significant barriers to ACP discussions. In a study of recently hospitalized patients with heart failure, outpatient clinicians, including cardiologists (22%), often missed opportunities to engage patients in ACP despite patients' comments or questions that could have prompted such discussions.[26] Clinician-reported barriers include lack of patient and family readiness, difficulty understanding the limitations and complications of life-sustaining treatments, lack of agreement among family members about goals of care, and patients' lack of capacity to make decisions about goals of care.[27] Other clinician barriers include lack of time, difficulty discussing prognosis, and discomfort and lack of confidence with ACP discussions.[10,19] Because patients with cardiovascular diseases may have highly variable disease trajectories, prognostic uncertainty is inevitable and should not, but often, limits attempts to engage patients in ACP.[2] However, because multi-morbidity in patients with cardiovascular disease is associated with higher mortality,[28] prognostic tools designed for older adults with multi-morbidity could help clinicians tailor ACP discussions.[29]

Practical Steps to Advance Care Planning in Older Adults with Cardiovascular Diseases

Clinicians can use practical and systematic steps to engage older adults with cardiovascular disease and multi-morbidity in the ACP process. **Box 1** provides clinical triggers for multidisciplinary health care team members to initiate ACP conversations. *These triggers reflect the complex needs that patients with multi-morbidity commonly face.*

Key steps to ACP include (1) assessing and addressing patients' readiness and barriers, (2) identifying surrogate decisions-makers, (3) asking about individuals' values related to quality of life and serious illness, (4) documenting ACP preferences, and (5) translating individuals' preferences into medical care plans. These steps, especially

Box 1
Triggers for ACP conversations in older adults with cardiovascular diseases

- New cardiovascular diagnosis and at (annual) routine visits
- Diagnosis of new medical comorbidities, especially depression or dementia
- Disease exacerbation prompting ED visits, hospitalizations, and other care transitions
- Increased symptoms and/or decreased quality of life
- New or worsening functional impairment or change in health status
- New cardiovascular instability (hypotension, azotemia, ICD shock)
- Consideration of advance cardiac therapy (ie, inotrope, LVAD)
- Changes in caregiver, family, or social situation

Abbreviations: ED, emergency department; ICD, internal cardioverter defibrillator.

Data from Allen LA, Stevenson LW, Grady KL, et al. Decision making in advanced heart failure: a scientific statement from the American Heart Association. Circulation 2012;125(15):1928–52; and Dunlay SM, Strand JJ. How to discuss goals of care with patients. Trends Cardiovasc Med 2015;26(1):36–43.

in the outpatient and inpatient setting, can be done individually and sequentially over time based on clinician time constraints and patients' clinical needs. Many of these steps can also be completed by multidisciplinary team members (eg, nurses, social workers, nurse practitioners, chaplains, psychologists, physicians, and other trained staff). **Table 2** provides an overview of key ACP steps and opportunities for health care team members to initiate ACP discussions across various stages of illness and health care settings. These steps emphasize a person-centered approach that focuses on the individual's personal values and life goals, rather than a single disease, symptom, or treatment decision.

Assessing and addressing patients' readiness and barriers to advance care planning

Engaging individuals in ACP begins with assessing patients' readiness. Studies show that patients are in varying stages of readiness to engage in ACP.[6,30] **Table 2** suggests brief opening questions that explore patients' readiness through understanding their past experiences with ACP and openness to ongoing discussions. Questions should be tailored to the individual's clinical context, such as what a new cardiovascular or other diagnosis may mean to them.

Barriers often need to be addressed before patients are ready to participate in ACP.[8,31] **Table 2** also provides examples of open-ended questions to help identify patient barriers to ACP. Understanding personal barriers (eg, fear of dying, fear of upsetting their doctor, lack of a suitable surrogate decision-maker) that patients experience can help tailor responses and communication to help overcome these barriers. When patients are not ready to engage in ACP, clinicians can ask about any increased medical, functional, or social support changes, such as the death of a spouse, that warrant involvement of multidisciplinary team members (ie, social worker, home health nurses, palliative care team). Most people, even if they are not ready to discuss a particular aspect of ACP, such as identifying a surrogate decision-maker, may be willing to explore nonthreatening topics, such as prior experiences of family and friends or their experiences with prior hospitalizations.

Identifying surrogate decision-makers

Designating and preparing a trusted surrogate decision-maker is the cornerstone of effective substitute decision-making in the event of patients' incapacity. This step is important, because 50% to 76% of people will require substitute decision-making at the end of life.[11] Surrogates, if prepared, are able to provide illustrations of patients' life stories to inform medical decision-making that represents the patients' values.[32]

Even if the clinician has limited time, **Table 2** provides language to help emphasize the importance of choosing a surrogate and discussing the concept of flexibility or leeway in surrogate decision-making.[13] Surrogates need to be asked to assume the responsibility; they need to agree to their role; there needs to be communication and documentation of surrogates as a medical power of attorney in the medical record.[8] One challenge of surrogate decision-making is that surrogates may not understand patients' values and preferences, especially as these preferences may change with changing health.[33] Clinicians can encourage patients and surrogates to have ongoing discussions with changes in health and as ACP is revisited over time.

Asking about values related to quality of life

Clinicians should initiate conversations that help patients articulate their personal values, life goals, and preferences regarding future medical care. **Table 2** provides questions for clinicians to help patients describe what quality of life means to them, reflect on trade-offs between quality of life and quantity of life, and consider their preferences for specific life-sustaining treatments.[10] For example, clinicians can ask

Table 2
Opportunities for ACP discussions across stages of illness and health care settings

Recommended ACP Steps	Setting and Timing	Description	Who can Initiate[a]	Example Questions
Assessing patients' readiness	At any stage in the illness trajectory and in any setting	Exploring patients' readiness to discuss ACP	PCP and/or cardiologist with assistance from multidisciplinary team (eg, social workers, nurses, facilitators)	• At this clinic/hospital, we ask all patients to plan for their future medical care in case they lose the ability to make their own medical decisions. Can we talk about this today? Is there anyone you would want with you when we talk about this? • Have you ever completed an advance directive, such as a living will? Can we review this? If you were to fill one out, have you thought about what you might say?
Addressing patient barriers	At any stage in the illness trajectory and in any setting	Identifying and addressing patients' concerns related to ACP	PCP and/or cardiologist (with multidisciplinary team)	• Are there things that you worry about when you think about planning for future medical care? • What makes it difficult to talk about such things with me or your loved ones?
Identifying surrogate decision-makers	At the time of diagnosis or referral to cardiologist	Identifying a trusted person as a surrogate decision-maker to help clinicians apply the patients' values to specific clinical situations	PCP and/or cardiologist (with multidisciplinary team)	• Is there someone you trust to help make medical decisions on your behalf, if you are not able to do so? • What have you talked about? or What would you tell this person is important about your medical care?

(*continued on next page*)

Table 2
(*continued*)

Recommended ACP Steps	Setting and Timing	Description	Who can Initiate[a]	Example Questions
Documenting ACP preferences	After ACP discussions, at any stage in the illness trajectory and in any setting	Documenting preferences in the medical record and/or advance directive (ie, medical power of attorney)	Clinician or trained team member involved in the ACP discussions	Because you have chosen (loved one) to help make decisions on your behalf if you are very sick and unable to talk with me, I recommend that you complete the medical power of attorney form to make it official.
Assess understanding of illness and discuss prognosis	During routine care, including cardiac device placement, procedures, or during hospitalization	Understanding the patients' understanding and providing disease trajectory education and prognosis	PCP and/or cardiologist[a]	• What have your doctors told you about your illness and what to expect? • Many people want to know their life expectancy or how long they may have to live. For each person we never know for sure, but based on your heart disease we do know general estimates. Knowing this information helps some people make medical decisions. Is this something you would want to know?
Asking about values related to quality of life	During routine care, including cardiac device placement or procedures or during hospitalization	Exploring the individual's values and priorities in life and discussing what constitutes an acceptable quality of life	PCP and/or cardiologist,[a] hospitalist, palliative care (with multidisciplinary team)	• What are you looking most forward to over the next few years. What gives your life meaning? • Do you know other people with heart disease? How have their experiences been? Are there parts of their experiences that help you decide what type of treatment you would or would not want for yourself? • I know you were just hospitalized with heart failure. What was that like for you and your family? • If you were in this situation again, what would you hope for? What would you be most worried about? Did this situation change the way you may be thinking about your care or ways of living that would or would not be acceptable to you?

Documenting ACP preferences	After ACP discussions, at any stage in the illness trajectory and in any setting	Documenting preferences in the medical record and/or advance directive (ie, living will)	Clinician or trained team member involved in the ACP discussions	Because you have told me what would be important to you about certain life-sustaining medical interventions if you have certain serious medical conditions, I recommend that you complete a living will to help your loved ones and health care providers known your preferences.
Translating patients' values into specific treatment plans	During hospital, ICU, or nursing home admission	Translating values into current medical care documents (ie, POLST form, CPR directive)	PCP, cardiologist,[a] intensivist, palliative care team, nursing home attending	Based on what you have told me about what is important to you in life, how you want to live, and the health states that are/are not acceptable to you, and based on the risks and benefits of this treatment, I would recommend (option).
Communicating with health care providers from other settings	During routine care and care transitions, including use of postacute care (ie, skilled nursing facility or home health)	Facilitating verbal and written communication of patients' preferences, including transfer across settings	PCP, cardiologist, nursing home provider, outpatient palliative care, (with multidisciplinary team)	Based on our conversation today, and the (advance directive we completed/the POLST form I completed), I am going to make a note and place these forms in your medical record. I would like to send a copy to your other providers and your hospital so they know your wishes.

Abbreviations: ICU, intensive care unit; PCP, primary care provider; POLST, Physician Orders for Life-Sustaining Treatment.

[a] The primary or cardiology providers may include physicians, advance practice nurses, physician assistants, and can be assisted by multidisciplinary team members, including trained facilitators who may be nurses, social workers, chaplains, health coaches, or patient navigators.

Data from Refs.[8,10,31]

patients about their values over time to help guide medical decisions, including whether certain health states would make life not worth living. Clinicians can also teach older adults to ask questions to help them participate in shared decision-making (eg, What are the risks? What are the benefits? What are the burdens?).[2] These discussions should incorporate asking about patients' understanding of their cardiovascular disease, as well as other conditions, and be tailored to their desire for information about disease trajectory and estimated prognosis.

Translating patient values into specific medical treatment plans

As patients experience worsening health and face decisions related to specific medical treatments, clinicians will continue ACP discussions and move to the next step of goals of care conversations. Best practices for conversations about goals of care for specific treatment preferences with patients with cardiovascular disease and multi-morbidity include[9,10]

- Eliciting decision-making preferences, including understanding wishes for family involvement in ACP discussions and decisions
- Reviewing previous discussions and advance directives
- Discussing prognostic information and anticipated outcomes for treatment options
- Understanding values, fears, and goals for the future
- Discussing and deciding on a treatment plan based on patients' values

Translating patients' values into specific treatment plans is especially important in the care of older adults with cardiovascular diseases and multi-morbidity. As patients and clinicians discuss patients' personal values related to quality of life, clinicians and the multidisciplinary team can provide recommendations for specific medical treatment plans that weigh benefits and harms in the context of the patients' preferences, all of their medical conditions, and their physical functioning. The treatment plan should align with the patients' values and preferences, help them reach their life goals, and avoid or minimize interactions within and among treatment conditions.[4]

Table 2 provides an example of translating patients' values into specific medical treatment plans. For instance, a clinician may recommend that patients consider ICD placement if they describe that living as long as possible, or to see their children graduate college, is very important to them. Alternatively, a clinician may not recommend an ICD for patients who state that being comfortable is their main priority, including avoiding medical interventions.

Common treatment plans for patients with cardiovascular diseases and multi-morbidity include

- General scope of care options: life-prolonging (ie, CPR and life-sustaining treatments), limited interventions (ie, hospitalization with limitations in the extent of medical intervention), or comfort care (ie, symptom relief)[34,35]
- Role of hospitalization and/or outpatient services like hospice[16]
- Role of CPR, including recommending for or against this procedure[36]
- Role of cardiac treatments and devices, such as pacemakers, ICDs, inotropic medications, and LVADs[37]

Clinicians can use Physician Orders for Life-Sustaining Treatment to translate ACP preferences into medical orders, such as CPR, scope of treatment, and artificial nutrition based on conversations with patients or surrogates.[35] These orders were designed to be most appropriate for patients with limited life expectancies and for those patients who want to limit specific medical interventions. These medical orders are legal documents that can followed in all settings (ie, home, clinic, hospital, nursing home).

Documenting patient preferences
Clinicians have 2 major roles in supporting documentation of ACP preferences. First, clinicians should use state-specific advance directives to enable patients to formally identify a surrogate decision-maker (ie, medical power of attorney) or document their preferences for future medical care (ie, living will). Clinicians should emphasize the importance of discussing the forms and sharing copies with the designated surrogate, other family and friends, and other clinicians. Secondly, clinicians and teams should help facilitate communication of patients' documented preferences with other health care providers, especially because older adults with cardiovascular disease and multi-morbidity may see a primary care provider and multiple specialists. Clinicians should document the content of ACP discussions in the medical record and alert other involved health care team members. Advance directives and out-of-hospital orders should be officially added to the medical record. Other clinic, hospital, or nursing home–based team members can help share documentation with other providers and across health care settings as well as help scanning documents into the medical record.

Team-Based Approaches to Advance Care Planning

Care teams can work together to systematically identifying patient, clinician, and health care system barriers to ACP and work to incorporate ACP over multiple visits. Existing clinic programs can be modified to support ACP. For example, ACP interventions (ie, patient-centered ACP tools, see later discussion) could be added to existing self-management, caregiver support, or transitions of care programs (ie, after heart failure–related hospitalizations). Because older adults with cardiovascular disease, especially those with heart failure, frequently experience care transitions, it is critical that ACP and goals of care conversations are relayed to all relevant health care team members. As patients engage in ACP and conversations about their goals of care with clinicians from multiple settings (inpatient, outpatient, home health, nursing home), these teams can work together to support ongoing discussions; education and counseling about risks, benefits, and burdens of medical treatment; and communication with patients, surrogates, and other clinicians as the patients' health status, needs, and preferences change over time.

Patient-Centered Advance Care Planning Tools and Approaches to Goals of Care Conversations

Recent advances in ACP include the development of accessible, evidence-based tools to assist patients and clinicians with knowledge and decision-making related to ACP.[38,39] An advantage of many of these patient-centered ACP tools is that they can help engage patients and families in ACP beyond clinical settings, even before seeing a clinician.

For patients

- PREPARE (https://www.prepareforyourcare.org/)[40] is an evidenced-based, video-based, and easy-to-use ACP Web site in English and Spanish that focuses on preparing patients for communication and decision-making. The Web site creates a tailored summary of the patients' values and preferences that can be used to jump-start the conversation with the clinician.
- ACP Decisions (http://www.acpdecisions.org/) includes ACP videos describing overall goals of care, CPR, and mechanical ventilation that can influence patients' and surrogates' preferences for end-of-life care.[34]

- The Conversation Project (http://theconversationproject.org/)[41] provides a written toolkit with values-based questions to help individuals start ACP conversations.
- Making Your Wishes Known (https://www.makingyourwishesknown.com/)[42] is an evidenced-based interactive computer program that assists individuals with ACP, including advance directive documentation.

For clinicians

- Serious Illness Conversation Guide (https://www.ariadnelabs.org/programs/serious-illness-care/) is a checklist to assist clinicians with key steps in ACP conversations.[9]
- ePrognosis (www.eprognosis.org) is a Web site with evidence-based geriatric prognostic indices that incorporate multi-morbidity.[29]

SUMMARY

Clinicians who care for older adults with cardiovascular disease and multi-morbidity can engage older adults in ACP through multiple brief discussions over time. ACP emphasizes choosing a surrogate decision-maker, identifying personal values, communicating values with surrogates and clinicians, translating preferences into specific medical treatment plans, and documenting preferences for future medical care. Although patients and clinicians face specific challenges related to ACP, multidisciplinary teams can incorporate practical steps into brief clinical encounters. Additionally, several patient-centered ACP tools are available to support patients and clinicians in engaging in ACP.

REFERENCES

1. Mozaffarian D, Benjamin EJ, Go AS, et al. Heart disease and stroke statistics–2015 update: a report from the American Heart Association. Circulation 2015;131(4):e29–322.
2. Allen LA, Stevenson LW, Grady KL, et al. Decision making in advanced heart failure: a scientific statement from the American Heart Association. Circulation 2012;125(15):1928–52.
3. Chamberlain AM, St Sauver JL, Gerber Y, et al. Multimorbidity in heart failure: a community perspective. Am J Med 2015;128(1):38–45.
4. Guiding principles for the care of older adults with multimorbidity: an approach for clinicians. Guiding principles for the care of older adults with multimorbidity: an approach for clinicians: American Geriatrics Society Expert Panel on the care of older adults with multimorbidity. J Am Geriatr Soc 2012;60(10):E1–25.
5. Sinuff T, Dodek P, You JJ, et al. Improving end-of-life communication and decision making: the development of a conceptual framework and quality indicators. J Pain Symptom Manage 2015;49(6):1070–80.
6. Fried TR, Bullock K, Iannone L, et al. Understanding advance care planning as a process of health behavior change. J Am Geriatr Soc 2009;57(9):1547–55.
7. IOM (Institute of Medicine). Dying in America: improving quality and honoring individual preferences near the end of life. Washington, DC: The National Academies Press; 2014.
8. Sudore RL, Fried TR. Redefining the "planning" in advance care planning: preparing for end-of-life decision making. Ann Intern Med 2010;153(4):256–61.

9. Bernacki RE, Block SD, American College of Physicians High Value Care Task Force. Communication about serious illness care goals: a review and synthesis of best practices. JAMA Intern Med 2014;174(12):1994–2003.
10. Dunlay SM, Strand JJ. How to discuss goals of care with patients. Trends Cardiovasc Med 2015;26(1):36–43.
11. Silveira MJ, Kim SY, Langa KM. Advance directives and outcomes of surrogate decision making before death. N Engl J Med 2010;362(13):1211–8.
12. Wright AA, Zhang B, Ray A, et al. Associations between end-of-life discussions, patient mental health, medical care near death, and caregiver bereavement adjustment. JAMA 2008;300(14):1665–73.
13. McMahan RD, Knight SJ, Fried TR, et al. Advance care planning beyond advance directives: perspectives from patients and surrogates. J Pain Symptom Manage 2013;46(3):355–65.
14. Fromme EK, Zive D, Schmidt TA, et al. Association between physician orders for life-sustaining treatment for scope of treatment and in-hospital death in Oregon. J Am Geriatr Soc 2014;62(7):1246–51.
15. Bischoff KE, Sudore R, Miao Y, et al. Advance care planning and the quality of end-of-life care in older adults. J Am Geriatr Soc 2013;61(2):209–14.
16. Ache K, Harrold J, Harris P, et al. Are advance directives associated with better hospice care? J Am Geriatr Soc 2014;62(6):1091–6.
17. Detering KM, Hancock AD, Reade MC, et al. The impact of advance care planning on end of life care in elderly patients: randomised controlled trial. BMJ 2010; 340:c1345.
18. Centers for Medicare and Medicaid Services. CMS finalizes 2016 Medicare payment rules for physicians, hospitals & other providers. 2015. Available at: https://www.cms.gov/Newsroom/MediaReleaseDatabase/Press-releases/2015-Press-releases-items/2015-10-30.html. Accessed October 31, 2015.
19. Dunlay SM, Foxen JL, Cole T, et al. A survey of clinician attitudes and self-reported practices regarding end-of-life care in heart failure. Palliat Med 2015; 29(3):260–7.
20. Krumholz HM, Phillips RS, Hamel MB, et al. Resuscitation preferences among patients with severe congestive heart failure: results from the SUPPORT project. Study to understand prognoses and preferences for outcomes and risks of treatments. Circulation 1998;98(7):648–55.
21. Butler J, Binney Z, Kalogeropoulos A, et al. Advance directives among hospitalized patients with heart failure. JACC Heart Fail 2015;3(2):112–21.
22. Nkomo VT, Suri RM, Pislaru SV, et al. Advance directives of patients with high-risk or inoperable aortic stenosis. JAMA Intern Med 2014;174(9):1516–8.
23. Kirkpatrick JN, Guger CJ, Arnsdorf MF, et al. Advance directives in the cardiac care unit. Am Heart J 2007;154(3):477–81.
24. Heyland DK, Barwich D, Pichora D, et al. Failure to engage hospitalized elderly patients and their families in advance care planning. JAMA Intern Med 2013; 173(9):778–87.
25. Schickedanz AD, Schillinger D, Landefeld CS, et al. A clinical framework for improving the advance care planning process: start with patients' self-identified barriers. J Am Geriatr Soc 2009;57(1):31–9.
26. Ahluwalia SC, Levin JR, Lorenz KA, et al. Missed opportunities for advance care planning communication during outpatient clinic visits. J Gen Intern Med 2012; 27(4):445–51.

27. You JJ, Downar J, Fowler RA, et al. Barriers to goals of care discussions with seriously ill hospitalized patients and their families: a multicenter survey of clinicians. JAMA Intern Med 2015;175(4):549–56.
28. Di Angelantonio E, Kaptoge S, Wormser D, et al. Association of cardiometabolic multimorbidity with mortality. JAMA 2015;314(1):52–60.
29. ePrognosis - estimating prognosis for elders. Available at: http://eprognosis.ucsf.edu/. Accessed September 1, 2015.
30. Fried TR, Redding CA, Robbins ML, et al. Stages of change for the component behaviors of advance care planning. J Am Geriatr Soc 2010;58(12):2329–36.
31. Sudore RL, Schickedanz AD, Landefeld CS, et al. Engagement in multiple steps of the advance care planning process: a descriptive study of diverse older adults. J Am Geriatr Soc 2008;56(6):1006–13.
32. Sulmasy DP, Snyder L. Substituted interests and best judgments: an integrated model of surrogate decision making. JAMA 2010;304(17):1946–7.
33. Shalowitz DI, Garrett-Mayer E, Wendler D. The accuracy of surrogate decision makers: a systematic review. Arch Intern Med 2006;166(5):493–7.
34. Volandes AE, Brandeis GH, Davis AD, et al. A randomized controlled trial of a goals-of-care video for elderly patients admitted to skilled nursing facilities. J Palliat Med 2012;15(7):805–11.
35. Physicians Orders for Life-Sustaining Treatment (POLST) Paradigm. Available at: http://www.polst.org/. Accessed July 26, 2014.
36. Blinderman CD, Krakauer EL, Solomon MZ. Time to revise the approach to determining cardiopulmonary resuscitation status. JAMA 2012;307(9):917–8.
37. Swetz KM, Kamal AH, Matlock DD, et al. Preparedness planning before mechanical circulatory support: a "how-to" guide for palliative medicine clinicians. J Pain Symptom Manage 2014;47(5):926–35.e6.
38. Butler M, Ratner E, McCreedy E, et al. Decision aids for advance care planning: an overview of the state of the science. Ann Intern Med 2014;161(6):408–18.
39. Austin CA, Mohottige D, Sudore RL, et al. Tools to promote shared decision making in serious illness: a systematic review. JAMA Intern Med 2015;175(7):1213–21.
40. Sudore RL, Knight SJ, McMahan RD, et al. A novel website to prepare diverse older adults for decision making and advance care planning: a pilot study. J Pain Symptom Manage 2013;47(4):674–86.
41. The Conversation Project. Available at: http://theconversationproject.org/starter-kit/intro/. Accessed October 13, 2012.
42. Green MJ, Levi BH. Development of an interactive computer program for advance care planning. Health Expect 2009;12(1):60–9.

Patient Priority–Directed Decision Making and Care for Older Adults with Multiple Chronic Conditions

Mary E. Tinetti, MD[a,b,*], Jessica Esterson, MPH[a],
Rosie Ferris, MPH[c,d], Philip Posner, PhD[e,f], Caroline S. Blaum, MD[c,d]

KEYWORDS

- Multiple chronic conditions • Fragmented and burdensome care • Patient priorities
- Patient's health outcome goals and care preferences • Patient priority–directed care
- Current care planning

KEY POINTS

- A majority of older adults have multiple chronic conditions. They receive care that is fragmented, of unclear benefit, burdensome, potentially harmful, and not always focused on what matters most to them.
- One cause of this poor-quality care is that each clinician caring for patients with multiple chronic conditions concentrates on managing different conditions and monitoring different disease-specific outcomes.
- One approach to improving care for patients with multiple chronic conditions is for clinicians to refocus care from treating individual diseases in isolation to achieving patients' specific health priorities, that is, a move from disease-based to patient priority–directed care.
- With patient priority–directed care, all clinicians integrate their care to help meet patients' specific, actionable, and achievable health outcome goals within the context of their care preferences.

Disclosure Statement: The authors have nothing to disclose.
Funding: Supported by grants from the John A. Hartford Foundation and the Patient-Centered Outcomes Research Institute.
[a] Section of Geriatrics, Department of Medicine, Yale School of Medicine, 333 Cedar Street, PO Box 208025, New Haven, CT 06520, USA; [b] Yale School of Public Health, 60 College Street, New Haven, CT 06520, USA; [c] Division of Geriatric Medicine and Palliative Care, Department of Medicine, Langone Medical Center, New York University, 462 First Avenue, C&D Building, Room CD612-613, New York, NY 10016, USA; [d] Department of Population Health, Langone Medical Center, New York University, 550 First Avenue, BCD612, New York, NY 10016, USA; [e] Oak Ridge Institute of Science Education, Oak Ridge Associated Universities, Oak Ridge, TN, USA; [f] National MS Society, National Capitol Chapter
* Corresponding author. Yale University School of Medicine, New Haven, CT.
E-mail address: mary.tinetti@yale.edu

Clin Geriatr Med 32 (2016) 261–275
http://dx.doi.org/10.1016/j.cger.2016.01.012 geriatric.theclinics.com
0749-0690/16/$ – see front matter

THE PROBLEM

A majority of older adults with cardiovascular diseases have multiple other chronic conditions.[1,2] Individuals with multiple chronic conditions are the major users of health care and are cared for by multiple clinicians.[3–5] The problems inherent in a siloed disease-based approach to decision making for persons with multiple chronic conditions is exemplified by Mrs Smith's experience.

> *Mrs. Smith is an 83-year-old woman with hypertension, prior myocardial infarction, atrial fibrillation, heart failure, diabetes, depression, peptic ulcer disease, and end-stage kidney disease. She currently takes 15 doses of 11 medications each day.*
>
> *Over 10 days, Mrs. Smith has her scheduled appointments with her primary care provider, cardiologist, endocrinologist, nephrologist, and psychiatrist. She complains to each of them of tiredness, decreased appetite, and weakness. She also reports feeling burdened by the multiple medications (which she thinks cause some of her symptoms), restricted diet, multiple health care visits, and frequent blood tests. Each of her clinicians, following state-of-the-art, evidence-based guideline recommendations, offers conflicting advice to increase, decrease, or stop the same medications. Her endocrinologist suggests that she start insulin, which would require more blood sugar monitoring and daily shots. Her nephrologist tells her she will have to start hemodialysis soon and needs to undergo placement of an arteriovenous fistula. After these health care visits, Mrs. Smith is still tired and weak but also frustrated that none of her clinicians addressed her concerns and confused by the many additional and conflicting recommendations. Her clinicians are frustrated because Mrs. Smith has not been adherent to her medication or diet regimens and is reluctant to follow the recommendations to start insulin or initiate hemodialysis. The clinicians are also frustrated that other clinicians have changed medications they prescribed. They are not sure how best to communicate with each other and no one seems to take overall responsibility for Mrs. Smith's care.*

Care Is Fragmented and Lacking in Accountability

Medicare patients, on average, see 2 primary care providers and 5 specialists a year.[6] A primary care provider whose practice consists of 30% Medicare patients with 4 or more chronic conditions must coordinate with 86 other providers in 36 practices.[7] These clinicians focus on subsets of a patient's diseases, tracking different disease-specific outcomes.[8] Accountability is unclear when there are multiple providers.[8] Primary care providers, specialists, and patients often do not understand each other's roles and responsibilities, which are not usually made explicit.[8,9]

Care Is of Unclear Benefit and Potential Harm

Older adults, in general, and those with multiple and complex conditions, in particular, are excluded from most randomized clinical trials (RCTs), including cardiovascular trials.[10,11] Older adults with multiple conditions may not accrue the same benefit from many treatments and interventions as healthier participants in RCTs.[12,13] As a result, existing disease guidelines may not apply to this large population of patients.[14,15] The dearth of valid evidence means individuals receive many treatments that are of unclear benefit.[16] Furthermore, these treatments may be harmful. Up to 20% of older adults receive at least 1 guideline-recommended medication, including several cardiovascular medications, that may adversely affect coexisting conditions.[17]

Care Is Burdensome

Patients and caregivers report that the increasing number and complexity of patient-related workload, such as medication, diet, and exercise regimens; health visits; and self-monitoring tasks, are burdensome, often as burdensome as the conditions themselves.[18–22] There are increasing calls for reducing the intensity of activities required of all patients with chronic conditions, in particular those with several coexisting conditions.[21–23]

Care May Not Focus on What Matters Most to Patients

Older adults with multiple chronic conditions, when faced with tradeoffs that require difficult choices, vary in their health outcome goals[24–29] and what they are willing and able to do to achieve those outcomes.[23,28] Care that focuses on treating individual diseases ignores these tradeoffs and may not be consistent with patients' own goals or care preferences. What clinicians consider nonadherence often occurs when patients' care preferences or health outcome goals are not considered.[24]

THE SOLUTION

Development of Patient Priority–Directed Care

Over 18 months, advisory groups of patients; caregivers; primary and specialty clinicians; health system leaders; payers; representatives of national patient, caregiver, and clinician organizations; and experts in practice change, health information technology (HIT), health system engineering and redesign, patient and caregiver engagement, patient goals ascertainment, and health policy were convened face-to-face and by webinars and conference calls to

- Identify modifiable contributors to fragmented, burdensome care for older adults with multiple chronic conditions
- Explore approaches that might address these contributors
- Provide their perspectives on challenges to, and opportunities for, addressing these contributors
- Identify the core elements for building a feasible, sustainable approach to improving the care and outcomes of older adults with multiple conditions by addressing the identified modifiable factors

To help drive the development and implementation of the approach, a subset of the advisory groups built a logic model (**Fig. 1**). The model describes the current problems to be addressed, the inputs needed to move toward patient priority–directed care, the activities that define the care, and the outcomes desired.

Identified Contributors

Three potentially modifiable factors contributing to fragmentation, care burden, and poor outcomes for older adults with multiple chronic conditions that the group elected to address were

- Decision making and care focused on diseases not patients
- Inadequate delineation of roles and responsibilities and accountability among clinicians
- Lack of attention to what matters to patients and caregivers (ie, their health outcome goals and care preferences)

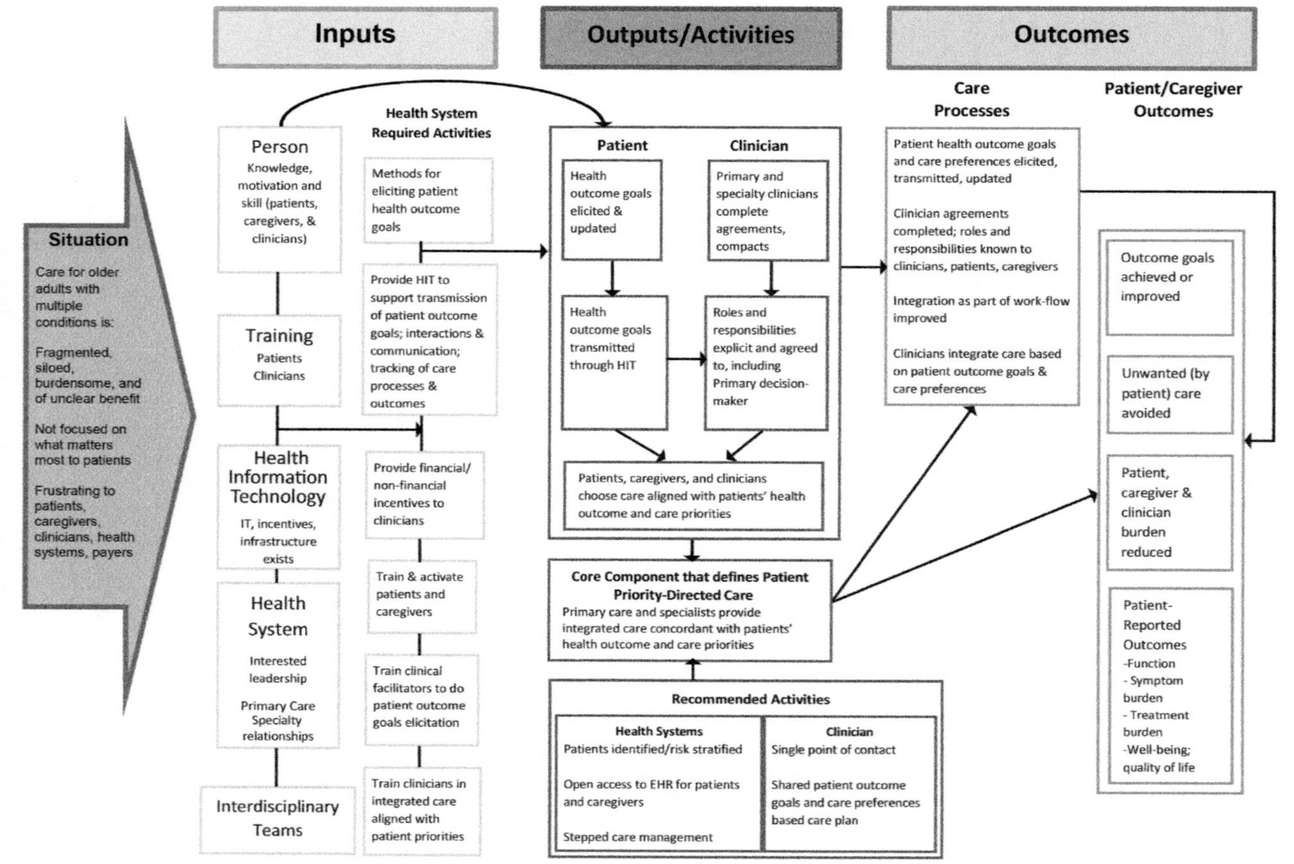

Fig. 1. Patient priority–directed care logic model.

Patient Priority–Directed Care As An Approach to Improve Care and Outcomes of Older Adults with Multiple Chronic Conditions

One strategy for addressing these 3 contributors is for all clinicians to align their care toward the same outcomes, patients' own specific health outcome goals being the obvious choice: move from disease-based to patient priority–directed care in which management of individual diseases becomes a means toward achieving each patient's health outcome goals rather than an end in of itself. The core elements that define patient priority–directed care are that patients identify their health outcome goals and care preferences. Primary and specialty care then is aligned around achieving these individualized goals and preferences.

- Health outcome goals are the personal health and life outcomes (eg, function, social activities, and symptom relief) that people hope to achieve through their health care.
- Care preferences refer to what individuals are able and willing to do to achieve their health outcomes and include activities, such as medication management, diet and exercise regimens, and health visits; diagnostic testing; and self-monitoring as well as the time, inconvenience, discomfort, money, and so forth inherent in completing these tasks.

Examples of specific health outcomes and patient workload activities and care preferences are listed in **Table 1**.

For Whom Is Patient Priority–Directed Care Beneficial?

The 60% to 70% of the population over age 65 years with multiple chronic conditions faces tradeoffs across conditions and many are burdened by their complex treatments. Individuals who are experiencing increased health care utilization, including office visits, emergency department visits, and hospitalizations, or who regret decisions, such as undergoing a procedure, may be particularly ready to consider their priorities and tradeoffs.[26,27] Although this older, complex population is most in need of an evolution from a siloed, disease-centric approach to patient priority–directed care, this approach would ensure patient-centered care for everyone. Benefits of priority-directed care include

- Improved health care value: Value is outcome (output) per cost (ie, input). From patients' perspective, care that focuses on achieving their own specific health outcome goals (output) within the context of what they are able and willing to do (inputs) is, by definition, the highest value care.[30]
- Decreased fragmentation and burden: When clinicians, patients, and caregivers all agree that a patient's own health outcome goals, rather than an assortment of separate disease-specific outcomes, guide and align care, conflicting recommendations across clinicians and conditions are minimized. Unnecessary burden and unwanted care are avoided if clinicians honor patients' care preferences. Determining which clinician should direct care becomes easier, further reducing fragmentation.
- Simplified decision making: The number of diagnostic and treatment options is confined to those most likely to address a patient's specific outcome goals and ability to adhere.
- Improved adherence: Patients are more likely to adhere to treatments aligned with their care preferences that are focused on achieving the outcomes they most desire.

Table 1
Patient health outcome goals and workload (care preferences)

Domains and Examples of Specific, Measurable, Actionable, Reliable and Timebound Health Outcomes	Domains and Examples of Patient Workload[a]
• Life prolongation (eg, see my grandson graduate from high school in 5 y) • Function (eg, walk 2 blocks without shortness of breath; live in my own home until I need help from someone at night). • Symptoms (eg, reduce back pain enough to perform morning activities without medications that cause drowsiness; get my appetite back and be able to eat the foods I like) • Well-being (eg, be as free from anxiety or uncertainty about cancer recurrence as possible) • Occupational/social roles (eg, work 3 more years; pick up my granddaughter from school)	• Interactions with clinicians (eg, number of clinicians, visits, recommendations; conflicting recommendations) • Health care utilization (eg, hospitalizations; ICU stays; emergency department visits) • Medication management (eg, complexity, number, dosing, and schedule; route—oral, inhalants, or injections; associated tasks [eg, laboratory testing and physiologic monitoring]; and adverse medication effects [eg, fatigue, dizziness, appetite, and diarrhea]) • Self-management tasks (eg, diet; exercise; monitor weights, blood pressure, and glucose) • Diagnostic and laboratory testing • Procedures (eg, scheduling, preparation, anxiety and discomfort, complications, and time to recovery) • Financial costs (eg, out-of-pocket expenses and uncompensated time off work)

Health outcome goals are the individual health outcomes that persons hope to achieve through their health care. To inform care, these health outcome goals must be SMART (that is, specific, measurable, actionable, reliable, and time bound). Health outcome goals are distinct from behavioral goals, such as stopping smoking, or disease goals, such as improved blood pressure.

[a] When understood as what patients are willing and able to do, these activities define care preferences. They are also referred to as treatment or care burden or workload.

Guiding principles and core elements of patient priority–directed care

The principles and core elements that guided the development and implementation of patient priority–directed care are

- Patient outcome goals and care preferences drive care and communication. The focus of decision making and care should change from disease based to patient priority based. This change will happen only if there is the expectation on everyone's part that patients and caregivers are active partners in decision making and care. Clinicians should align their care to achieve patients' outcome goals within their care preferences. Patients' goals and preferences should be shared in all communication, including consults and encounter notes.
- Roles and responsibilities are agreed to and accountability is established. Specific responsibilities for a patient's care should be assigned to the clinician (primary care or specialist) most qualified and available to deliver those aspects of care. All members of the team, including patients and caregivers, must be willing and able to carry out their agreed-on roles and responsibilities, which are determined by the patient's conditions, outcome goals, and care preferences. Accountability is assigned and agreed on for all processes and outcomes of care. One clinician must agree to be the quarterback, or primary decision

maker, who assures that all the care for a patient is aligned and is focused on achieving the patient's goals.

- Anticipatory guidance is provided; tradeoffs and uncertainty are acknowledged. Clinicians should prepare patients for anticipated events, trajectories, or situational crises. Knowledge and understanding of what might happen help patients and caregivers understand the need for establishing goals and preferences and better prepare them for informed decision making for acute or chronic care decisions that arise. The effect of many care options are unknown or uncertain for older adults with multiple chronic conditions. This uncertainty, which should be communicated, supports the need for shared decision making and for focusing on patient outcome goals.
- Information and care are integrated and shared. All clinicians work from an integrated plan based on patients' actionable and achievable health outcome goals and what they are willing to do to achieve them. Health technology is used effectively to provide patients' health priority–directed care.

Challenges and opportunities

Several challenges to, and complementary opportunities for, moving from a disease-based to patient priority–directed approach to care were identified through the planning process. These are summarized in **Table 2**.

Patient Priority–Directed Care and Advanced Care Planning

Patient priority–directed care complements advanced care planning (See Lum HD, Sudore RL: Advance care planning and goals of care communication in older adults with cardiovascular disease and multimorbidity, in this issue). Both depend on patients and their caregivers understanding what matters most to them and what they want from their health care. Both are ongoing processes, not discrete events. Both require clinicians to translate patients' goals into care options. Patient priority–directed care focuses on current care rather than future care; it is an approach for all clinicians to use in deciding which care within their area of expertise is most likely to help patients achieve their goals. While noting the importance of translating goals into care options, advanced care planning focuses on the patient goals component and on life-sustaining interventions and advanced illness. Patient priority–directed care expands on this by detailing the principles and approaches for how all clinicians can bridge and integrate disease-based and priority-based decision making across all conditions at all stages of illness.

Steps in Implementing Patient Priority–Directed Care

The authors currently are building and testing the workflow steps involved in articulating patient health outcome goals and translating them into care options, shared decision making, and care. Although detailed descriptions of all the steps are beyond the scope of this article, an overview of the decision-making process and care is provided in **Fig. 2**.

Key steps include

- Patients' health outcome goals and care preferences are elicited, documented, and transmitted. Patient priority–directed care begins with patients and caregivers identifying and communicating their health outcome goals and treatment and care preferences with the help of a trained and skilled member of the health care team. These outcome goals and care preferences then guide interactions among patients, caregivers, and clinicians and serve as the basis for selecting care options. Verbalizing their care preferences and outcome goals activates

Table 2
Challenges and opportunities for patient goals–directed care

Challenges and Barriers	Opportunities and Facilitators
Innovation fatigue; many simultaneous payment and delivery changes	Fit health system mission; address identified need; redesign of, not add-on to, workflow; local champion; strong business case
Care coordination, patient-centered medical homes, and other innovative models are already doing this	Complements these innovations; provides decision-making content for the structural innovations
Clinicians not trained; may be unable or unwilling to move from disease guideline–driven to goal and preference driven care; risk adverse	Start with clinicians who are able and willing to change; early successes will encourage other clinicians; local champions encourage the practice change until becomes routinized; clinicians must be prepared to provide patient priority–directed care for it to be successful
Some patients may interpret this approach as withholding care or providing less care	Ensure that clinicians and goal facilitators are well trained in goals and care preferences elicitation, not withholding care but rather tailoring care to patient's own stated goals and preferences
Patients may prioritize unrealistic goals; goals and preferences are unstable with patients' changing day to day	Trained clinicians prepare patients and work through values to specific, measurable, actionable, reliable, and timebound goals; aspirational goals may be motivating for some patients. Goals and preferences are reassessed periodically as are any clinical measures. Priority domains tend to be stable although specific level within domain changes with health status changes
EHRs inadequate to transmit goals and support goals-based integrated care among clinicians	Local modification of EHRs, until quality measures and financing incentives are in place
Clinical workflows may not allow time to tailor clinical care to individual goals; inadequate payment for communication time	Patient priority–directed care defines the workflow. Once trained, the workflow will be simplified because everyone is focused on same few outcomes. Once integrated into workflow, goal and preference elicitation is a constant, iterative process

Challenges and opportunities for health systems are discussed in the text.

and engages patients and caregivers and helps them understand their care, including their own priorities when faced with inherent tradeoffs.[24] To inform health decisions between all providers and across all settings, patient priority–directed care requires articulation of outcomes that are specific, measurable, actionable, reliable, and time bound (SMART). Patients are at different stages (See Lum HD, Sudore RL: Advance care planning and goals of care communication in older adults with cardiovascular disease and multimorbidity, in this issue) of readiness and require time and support to work through what matters most to them. A member of the clinical team, such as an advanced practice registered nurse (APRN) or physician assistant, with strong communication skills and training in goals elicitation, begins by helping patients and caregivers appreciate how understanding their health conditions and trajectories and knowing their goals and preferences can help them interact with their clinicians to get the

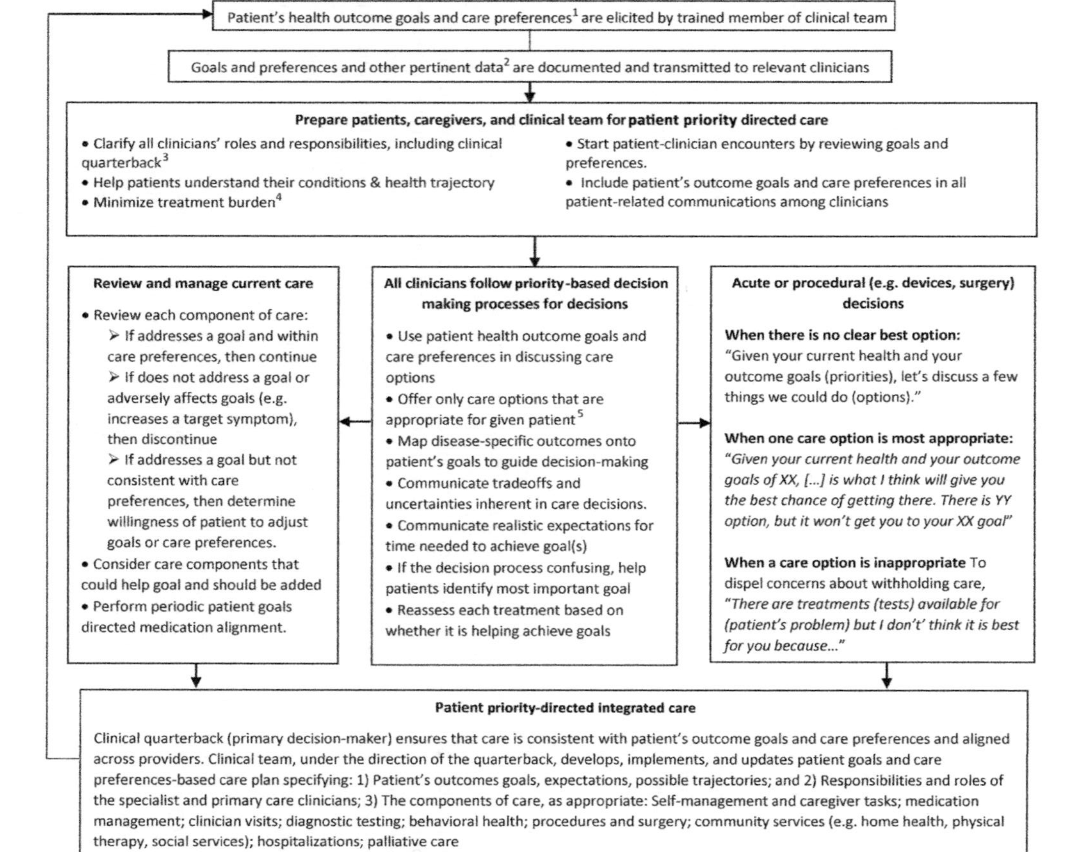
Patient's health outcome goals and care preferences[1] are elicited by trained member of clinical team
Goals and preferences and other pertinent data[2] are documented and transmitted to relevant clinicians
Prepare patients, caregivers, and clinical team for patient priority directed care
• Clarify all clinicians' roles and responsibilities, including clinical quarterback[3]
• Help patients understand their conditions & health trajectory
• Minimize treatment burden[4]
• Start patient-clinician encounters by reviewing goals and preferences.
• Include patient's outcome goals and care preferences in all patient-related communications among clinicians
Review and manage current care
• Review each component of care:
➢ If addresses a goal and within care preferences, then continue
➢ If does not address a goal or adversely affects goals (e.g. increases a target symptom), then discontinue
➢ If addresses a goal but not consistent with care preferences, then determine willingness of patient to adjust goals or care preferences.
• Consider care components that could help goal and should be added
• Perform periodic patient goals directed medication alignment.
All clinicians follow priority-based decision making processes for decisions
• Use patient health outcome goals and care preferences in discussing care options
• Offer only care options that are appropriate for given patient[5]
• Map disease-specific outcomes onto patient's goals to guide decision-making
• Communicate tradeoffs and uncertainties inherent in care decisions.
• Communicate realistic expectations for time needed to achieve goal(s)
• If the decision process confusing, help patients identify most important goal
• Reassess each treatment based on whether it is helping achieve goals
Acute or procedural (e.g. devices, surgery) decisions
When there is no clear best option:
"Given your current health and your outcome goals (priorities), let's discuss a few things we could do (options)."
When one care option is most appropriate:
"Given your current health and your outcome goals of XX, [...] is what I think will give you the best chance of getting there. There is YY option, but it won't get you to your XX goal"
When a care option is inappropriate To dispel concerns about withholding care, "There are treatments (tests) available for (patient's problem) but I don't' think it is best for you because..."
Patient priority-directed integrated care
Clinical quarterback (primary decision-maker) ensures that care is consistent with patient's outcome goals and care preferences and aligned across providers. Clinical team, under the direction of the quarterback, develops, implements, and updates patient goals and care preferences-based care plan specifying: 1) Patient's outcomes goals, expectations, possible trajectories; and 2) Responsibilities and roles of the specialist and primary care clinicians; 3) The components of care, as appropriate: Self-management and caregiver tasks; medication management; clinician visits; diagnostic testing; behavioral health; procedures and surgery; community services (e.g. home health, physical therapy, social services); hospitalizations; palliative care

care they want: "When your clinicians understand what you want out of your health care, they can offer you health care options that give you the best chance of reaching these goals." The goals facilitator then helps patients work through their values toward the specific goals they would like their health care to help them achieve, such as, "Walk upstairs to my bedroom without feeling short of breath." Patients are also prepared to discuss their current care with their clinicians within the context of their own specific goals and care preferences. As a result of the goals elicitation, patients are able to

- Identify 1 to 5 SMART goals to inform clinical decision making
- Understand aspects of their current care that they are willing and unwilling (or unable) to perform to achieve these goals
- Understand their health conditions, expected health trajectories, and key tradeoffs
- Become ready and able to engage with clinicians in translating goals and preferences into care decisions

The goals and preferences are documented in a readily accessible place in electronic health records (EHRs) and are updated as health status changes or major decisions are required.

- Clinicians provide care aligned with patients' goals and preferences (see **Fig. 2**). Patient priority–based care provides a decisional flow for all clinicians to use in reviewing and adjusting current chronic care and considering future acute procedural and chronic decisions. Patients' goals and care preferences form the basis

Fig. 2. Patient goals–directed decisional and care pathway. [1] Health outcome goals are patient's personalized health outcomes priorities, the feasible life goals that persons hope to achieve through their health care (eg, pain controlled to allow five hours of sleep most nights; able to walk >1 block without stopping; cognitively and physically able to care for grandchild). Care preferences refer to what people are able and willing to do and to tolerate when selecting or undergoing specific treatments, diagnostic evaluations, or procedures, they are the activities ("workload") involved in being a patient or caregiver (eg, adhering to medications, dietary recommendations, exercise regimens, visits and appointment; adverse effects, burden, discomfort of treatments; self-monitoring and self-management tasks). [2] Pertinent data includes the medical, functional, cognitive, social and other health and life contextual data needed to provide patient priority directed care. Goals and preference elicitation requires training and sufficient time to ensure that the goals elicited are specific, measureable, actionable, reliable, and time bound so as to form the basis for decision making and care. [3] Clinical quarterback: Predominant clinician who takes responsibility for ensuring care is integrated across clinicians and conditions and is consistent with patient's outcome goals and care preferences. [4] Minimize treatment and overall care burden: 1. Focus care on achieving goals for clinically dominant condition (eg, end stage or severely symptomatic). When a clinically dominant condition is present, reduce or eliminate treatments for other conditions unless this would compromise achievement of the patient's goals; 2. Determine least burdensome combination of treatments that is likely to achieve the goals and care preferences for concordant conditions; 3. If possible, begin with simple and quick interventions that address one or more patient goals; 4. If possible, stagger treatments or procedures rather than provide them all at once. [5] Appropriate care options: 1. Existing evidence is applicable to the individual patient; 2. Benefit likely within patient's expected life expectancy; 3. likely to help achieve the patient's own goals; 4. Not adversely affect coexisting conditions; and 5. Overall greater benefit than harm given the patients overall health. Options that do not meet these criteria should be discontinued or not offered (although should be mentioned if the patient prefers to hear all options).

of all communications between clinicians and between clinicians and patients. Care options are considered within the context not only of whether they are likely to improve survival or disease-specific outcomes but also whether they are likely to improve each patient's specific health goals and are consistent with what the patient is willing and able to do. Uncertainty and tradeoffs are acknowledged. A few key features include the following:

- Roles and responsibilities of each clinician, other members of the team, and clinical quarterback are identified.
- The patient's health outcome goals and care preferences are included in all communications among clinicians and used to drive all clinical decisions.
- Assessment and plan are framed by goals and care preferences; management of individual conditions is done within the context of meeting patent's outcome goals, not merely disease-specific outcomes.

Clinicians follow the priority-based decision-making processes outlined in **Fig. 2** for chronic and acute decisions. Implementing the steps outlined in the text and in **Fig. 2** requires training, tools, practice change, and workflow adaptation, all of which are under way.

What Is Needed to Support Implementation of Patient Priority–Directed Care

- Infrastructure: Population management, including risk stratification, interdisciplinary teams, care coordination, complex care management, and relationships with community services and facilities, such as long-term care, home care, and transportation providers, are essential. Agreements and compacts among clinicians must spell out roles and responsibilities and accountability. Because these characteristics match criteria for patient-centered medical homes, specialty neighborhoods, and accountable care organizations, many health systems have built the needed infrastructure.[31–33]
- HIT must support goal elicitation and primary and specialty care integration. Information tools, such as patient priority–based consult templates and problem lists, facilitate patient priority–based communication and interactions.
- Guidance and preparation for clinicians: Clinical education and training remain focused on managing discrete diseases. Clinical training needs to evolve to address multiple chronic conditions, the predominant condition in twenty-first century patients.[34] In the meantime, practicing clinicians need training and preparation. As for most practice changes, multiple strategies are needed. Early adopters will acquire the skills and adopt the new approach. Their successes will encourage other clinicians. Learning collaboratives, local champions, and point-of-care decision tools will help interested clinicians acquire the skills. Once the skills are acquired, clinicians will find that aligning around patients' outcome goals and care preferences provides a platform for interacting with patients and other clinicians, simplifying decision making and care for complex patients.
- Guidance and preparation for patients and caregivers: Some patients know their health goals and have experience in shared decision making. Others need support and guidance from the member of the team doing the goals elicitation and from their other clinicians to move from passive recipient of care to active partner. Effective goals elicitation is geared to each patient's state of readiness.
- Acquire patient outcome–based evidence to inform goals-based guidelines: Translating patients' goals into care options is a challenging component of patient priority–directed care. Current guidelines are based on disease-specific outcomes or survival. Observational studies and RCTs need to measure the

effect of interventions on the universal, patient-centered outcome categories (function, symptoms, and so forth) that define most people's health outcome priorities.[34,35] The fact that chronic conditions exert their effects on these patient-centered outcomes will facilitate this evidence development.[35] Guidelines must then incorporate decision algorithms based on these universal, patient-centered health outcomes as well as other considerations, such as competing conditions and life expectancy, relevant to the care of individuals with multiple conditions.[14,15] In the meantime, decision pathways that link common patient outcome goals and care preferences to specific care options for common chronic conditions (eg, anticoagulation with atrial fibrillation and β-blockers for heart failure) and for acute procedural decisions (eg, implantable cardioverter defibrillator and dialysis) will guide clinicians' movement from disease-based to priority-based decision making.

- Financial incentives: Although challenging under a fee-for-service payment model, integrated health systems and health systems operating under shared savings or risk models have financial incentives to align primary and specialty care with patients' goals and care preferences. As more patients are cared for by providers and facilities operating under values-based models, the interest in this type of care is likely to increase. Health systems will want to know that upfront costs in patient and clinician training, the clinical time to complete the goals elicitation, and the HIT costs result in a good return on the investment.
- Quality metrics that reflect patients' goals and preferences: The quality metrics that measure clinicians' performances and drive value-based payments remain largely disease based. The plethora of disease-based metrics discourages patient-centered decision making and has the unintended consequence of compounding treatment burden for older adults who must adhere to multiple disease guideline recommendations. Increasingly, organizations recognize that the burgeoning number of disease-based and event-based metrics are counterproductive and not patient centered.[36,37] The next generation of metrics should reflect what matters to patients, such as Were outcome goals ascertained and addressed? and Was the burden of care minimized and unwanted and unnecessary care avoided? The need to ascertain patient-reported outcomes, such as function, symptoms, and well-being, is also recognized.

Patient Priority–Directed Care for Mrs Smith

With the help of an APRN trained in goals elicitation, Mrs Smith identifies her primary outcome goals as sufficient improvement in her fatigue and weakness that she can walk 2 blocks and in her appetite so she can enjoy her favorite foods. Most important to her is to be more functional and less symptomatic now; life prolongation is not her priority. Her care preferences are eliminating medications that affect her alertness, strength, tiredness, and appetite. She wants fewer blood tests, health care visits, and clinicians; she hopes to avoid conflicting recommendations. Based on the predominance of renal failure on her function and symptoms, her nephrologist agrees to be the primary decision maker. The primary care provider cares for her other conditions. Interactions with the endocrinologist and cardiologist is by electronic consultation as needed. Several medications are discontinued because they either do not target her outcome goals or impede alertness, strength, tiredness, or appetite, which she prioritizes. Her diet is changed to low salt without other restrictions. She does not start insulin. Mrs Smith and her nephrologist agree to forego dialysis given the treatment burden involved and the uncertainty that it will relieve her fatigue or improve her functioning. Understanding her high risk for stroke and its potential adverse effect on functioning, she switches to a newer anticoagulant despite uncertainty about bleeding risk. She wants to re-evaluate that decision as her health changes.

Compelling arguments can be made against patient priority–directed care. There is potential for chaos inherent in individually tailored decision making; neither patients nor clinicians are currently skilled in this approach; and much of the needed evidence is still lacking. Although concerns and complexities are real, the present siloed disease approach to patients with multiple chronic conditions is expensive, burdensome, of unclear benefit and potential harm, and unsustainable. The move from disease-based care to patient priority–directed care is a move in the right direction.

ACKNOWLEDGMENTS

The authors acknowledge and appreciate the outstanding administrative support of Denise Acampora and Eliza Kiwak and the time, efforts, and insights of the CareAlign steering committee and heads of the advisory and working groups, including Janet Austin, Chad Boult, Perry Cohen, Libby Hoy, Fred Masoudi, Gary Oftedahl, Michael Parchman, and Eileen Sullivan-Marx, as well as the members of the advisory and working groups and the stakeholder participants representing patients, caregivers, primary and specialty clinicians, payers, HIT, health system redesign, and health policy expertise.

REFERENCES

1. Carlos O, Weiss CO, Boyd CM, et al. Patterns of prevalent major chronic disease among older adults in the United States. JAMA 2007;298(10):1160–2.
2. Chamberlain AM, St Sauver JL, Gerber Y, et al. Multimorbidity in heart failure: a community perspective. Am J Med 2015;128(1):38–45.
3. Alecxih L, Shen S, Chan I, et al. Individuals living in the community with chronic conditions and functional limitations: a closer look. Available at: http://aspe.hhs.gov/daltcp/reports/2010/closerlook.pdf. Accessed February 9, 2016.
4. Yoon J, Zulman D, Scott JY, et al. Costs associated with multimorbidity among VA patients. Med Care 2014;52(Suppl 3):S31–6.
5. Stange KC. The problem of fragmentation and the need for integrative solutions. Ann Fam Med 2009;7:100–3.
6. Pham HH, Schrag D, O'Malley AS, et al. Care patterns in medicare and their implications for pay for performance. N Engl J Med 2007;356:1130–9.
7. Pham HH, O'Malley AS, Bach PB, et al. Primary care physicians' links to other physicians through medicare patients: the scope of care coordination. Ann Intern Med 2009;150(4):236–42.
8. Stange KC. In this issue: challenges of managing multimorbidity. Ann Fam Med 2012;10:2–3.
9. Cheung WY, Neville BA, Cameron DB, et al. Comparisons of patient and physician expectations for cancer survivorship care. J Clin Oncol 2009;27(15):2489–95.
10. Dhruva SS, Redberg RF. Variations between clinical trial participants and medicare beneficiaries in evidence used for medicare national coverage decisions. Arch Intern Med 2008;168(2):136–40.
11. Van Spall HG, Toren A, Kiss A. Eligibility criteria of randomized controlled trials published in high-impact general medical journals: a systematic sampling review. JAMA 2007;297(11):1233–40.

12. O'Hare AM, Hotchkiss JR, Kurella Tamura M, et al. Interpreting treatment effects from clinical trials in the context of real-world risk information: end-stage renal disease prevention in older adults. JAMA Intern Med 2014;174(3):391–7.
13. Tinetti ME. The Gap between clinical trials and the real world: extrapolating treatment effects from younger to older adults. JAMA Intern Med 2014;174(3): 397–8.
14. Guiding Principles for the Care of Older Adults with Multimorbidity: An Approach for Clinicians. Guiding.principles for the care of older adults with multimorbidity: an approach forclinicians: American Geriatrics Society Expert Panel on the Care of Older Adults withMultimorbidity. J Am Geriatr Soc 2012;60(10):E1–25. Available at. www.americangeriatrics.org/files/dlocuments/GuidingPrinciplesforMultimorbidity.pdf.
15. Uhlig K, Leff B, Kent D, et al. A framework for crafting clinical practice guidelines that are relevant to the care and management of people with multimorbidity. J Gen Intern Med 2014;29(4):670–9.
16. Kamerow D. How can we treat multiple chronic conditions? BMJ 2012;344:e1487.
17. Lorgunpai SJ, Grammas M, Lee DSH, et al. Potential therapeutic competition in community-living older adults in the U.S.: use of medications that may adversely affect a coexisting condition. PLoS One 2014;9(2):e89447.
18. Boyd CM, Wolff JL, Giovannetti E, et al. Healthcare task difficulty among older adults with multimorbidity. Med Care 2014;52:S118–25.
19. Montori VM, Brito JP, Murad MH. The optimal practice of evidence-based medicine: incorporating patient preferences in practice guidelines. JAMA 2013; 310(23):2503–4.
20. VT1 Tran, Harrington M, Montori VM, et al. Adaptation and validation of the Treatment Burden Questionnaire (TBQ) in English using an internet platform. BMC Med 2014;12:109.
21. Eton DT, Ramalho de Oliveira D, Egginton JS, et al. Building a measurement framework of burden of treatment in complex patients with chronic conditions: a qualitative study. Patient Relat Outcome Meas 2012;3:39–49.
22. Bayliss EA. Simplifying care for complex patients. Ann Fam Med 2012;10:3–5.
23. May CR, Eton DT, Boehmer K, et al. Rethinking the patient: using burden of treatment theory to understand the changing dynamics of illness. BMC Health Serv Res 2014;14:281. http://dx.doi.org/10.1186/1472-6963-14-281.
24. Naik AD, Martin LA, Moye, J, et al. Health values and treatment goals among older, multimorbid adults facing life-threatening illness. J Am Geriatr Soc, in press.
25. Naik AD, McCullough LB. Health intuitions inform patient-centered care. Am J Bioeth 2014;14(6):1–3.
26. Case SM, O'Leary J, Kim N, et al. Relationship between universal health outcome priorities and willingness to take medication for primary prevention of myocardial infarction. J Am Geriatr Soc 2014;62(9):1753–8.
27. Fried TR, Tinetti ME, Iannone L, et al. Health outcome prioritization as a tool for decision making among older persons with multiple chronic conditions. Arch Intern Med 2011;171:1854–6.
28. Fried TR, McGraw S, Agostini JV, et al. Views of older persons with multiple conditions on competing outcomes and clinical decision-making. J Am Geriatr Soc 2008;56:1839–44.
29. Tinetti ME, McAvay G, Fried TR, et al. Variable priorities in the face of competing outcomes: the tradeoff among cardiovascular events, medication symptoms, and fall injuries. J Am Geriatr Soc 2008;56:1409–16.

30. Tinetti ME, Naik AD, Dodson JA. Patient goals-directed care: value-based care from the Patient's perspective. JAMA Cardiol, in press.
31. NCQA National Committee for Quality Assurance Patient-Centered Medical Home standards. Available at: http://www.ncqa.org/Programs/Recognition/Practices/PatientCenteredMedicalHomePCMH.aspx.
32. The Medical Home's Impact on Cost & Quality. An Annual Update of the eEvidence, 2012-2013. Available at: https://www.pcpcc.org/resource/medical-homes-impact-cost-quality. Accessed February 2, 2016.
33. American College of Physicians. The Patient-Centered Medical Home Neighbor: the interface of the patient-centered medical home with specialty/subspecialty practices. Philadelphia: American College of Physicians; 2010. Policy Paper.
34. Tinetti ME, Fried TR, Boyd CM. Designing health care for the most common chronic condition—multimorbidity. JAMA 2012;307(23):2493–4.
35. Tinetti ME, McAvay G, Chang SS, et al. Contribution of multiple chronic diseases to universal health outcomes in older adults. J Am Geriatr Soc 2011;59:1686–91.
36. National Quality Forum. Multiple chronic conditions (MCC) measurement framework. Available at: http://www.qualityforum.org/Projects/Multiple_Chronic_Conditions_Measurement_Framework.aspx. Accessed February 2, 2016.
37. Institute of Medicine. Vital signs: core metrics for health and health care progress. 2015. Available at: http://iom.nationalacademies.org/Reports/2015/Vital-Signs-Core-Metrics.aspx. Accessed February 2, 2016.

Multimorbidity in Older Adults with Heart Failure

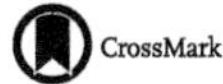

Kumar Dharmarajan, MD, MBA[a,b,*], Shannon M. Dunlay, MD, MS[c,d]

KEYWORDS

• Heart failure • Multimorbidity • Multiple chronic conditions • Geriatrics
• Quality of care • Health outcomes • Polypharmacy • Cognitive impairment

KEY POINTS

- Multimorbidity is a common feature of heart failure in older persons that impacts diagnosis, management, and outcomes.
- Diagnosis of heart failure may be difficult in patients with multimorbidity, as many diseases commonly found in older persons produce dyspnea, exercise intolerance, fatigue, and weakness.
- Treatment of heart failure is complicated by multimorbidity, which creates high potential for drug-disease and drug-drug interactions in the setting of polypharmacy.
- Treatment of complex older persons with multimorbidity and heart failure should be patient-focused rather than disease-focused.
- The care of older patients with multimorbidity and heart failure should prioritize universal rather than disease-specific health outcomes, cognitive assessment, provision of non-pharmacologic treatments, minimization of treatment burden for patients and caregivers, and care coordination by multidisciplinary teams.

Disclosure Statement: K. Dharmarajan works under contract with the Centers for Medicare & Medicaid Services to develop and maintain performance measures and is a member of a scientific advisory board for Clover Health.
Funding/Support: Dr K. Dharmarajan is supported by grant K23AG048331 from the National Institute on Aging and the American Federation for Aging Research through the Paul B. Beeson Career Development Award Program. Dr S. M. Dunlay is supported by grant K23HL116643 from the National Heart, Lung, and Blood Institute.
[a] Section of Cardiovascular Medicine, Department of Internal Medicine, Yale University School of Medicine, 1 Church Street, Suite 200, New Haven, CT 06510, USA; [b] Center for Outcomes Research and Evaluation, Yale-New Haven Hospital, 1 Church Street, Suite 200, New Haven, CT 06510, USA; [c] Division of Cardiovascular Diseases, Department of Internal Medicine, Mayo Clinic, 200 First Street Southwest, Rochester, MN 55905, USA; [d] Division of Health Care Policy and Research, Department of Health Sciences Research, Mayo Clinic, 200 First Street Southwest, Rochester, MN 55905, USA
* Corresponding author.
E-mail address: kumar.dharmarajan@yale.edu

Clin Geriatr Med 32 (2016) 277–289
http://dx.doi.org/10.1016/j.cger.2016.01.002 geriatric.theclinics.com

INTRODUCTION

Multimorbidity, or the presence of multiple chronic conditions (MCCs), is the rule and not the exception among older adults with heart failure (HF). Almost 90% of adults with HF have 2 or more additional chronic conditions,[1] and almost 60% have 5 or more.[2] Multimorbidity is especially common in persons with HF and preserved ejection fraction (HFPEF), the most common form of HF in the elderly.[3] In addition to this high comorbidity burden, older adults with HF are more likely to have common geriatric conditions that reduce life expectancy and quality of life, such as functional limitations, mobility disability, and cognitive impairment.[4,5]

Multimorbidity is also tightly linked to adverse outcomes. For example, chronic kidney disease and chronic obstructive pulmonary disease (COPD) predict a greater risk of hospitalization for HF, hospitalization for noncardiac conditions, and death among Medicare beneficiaries with HF.[6] Similarly, the presence of geriatric conditions, including mobility disability and dementia, is associated with both short-term and long-term mortality among persons with newly diagnosed[5] and longstanding[4] HF. The frequent presence of multimorbidity likely explains why most index hospitalizations and 30-day readmissions among older persons with HF are for conditions other than HF.[7,8]

Despite its importance, multimorbidity has only recently become a focus of research and clinical practice for cardiology specialty societies in the United States. In 2014, the American Heart Association (AHA), American College of Cardiology (ACC), and US Department of Health and Human Services jointly published "Strategies to Enhance Application of Clinical Practice Guidelines in Patients with Cardiovascular Disease and Comorbid Conditions."[9] This statement demonstrated a commitment by the AHA and ACC to have all future clinical practice guidelines explicitly discuss the applicability and quality of guideline recommendations for patients with common combinations of comorbidities. This initiative was followed by a joint workshop of the ACC, American Geriatrics Society, and National Institute on Aging to improve care for persons with MCCs by identifying their unmet needs, formulating a research agenda, and developing strategies to translate findings into improved care.[10]

In light of the increasing focus on MCCs in clinical research and guideline development, the aim in this review of multimorbidity in older adults with HF is to synthesize previous research to provide clinically useful information to improve patient outcomes. First described is the epidemiology of specific cardiovascular, noncardiovascular, and geriatric conditions among older patients with HF. Then, difficulties created by multimorbidity are described for the diagnosis and treatment of HF. Finally, specific recommendations are made for treating older patients with MCCs and HF. These recommendations are consistent with a patient-centered rather than a disease-centered framework for conceptualizing both treatment and outcomes.

EPIDEMIOLOGY OF MULTIMORBIDITY IN HEART FAILURE

Older patients with HF typically have MCCs. As might be expected, these persons frequently have other cardiovascular conditions in addition to HF, with exact estimates varying by the data source used and the study population. For example, administrative data have shown that among Medicare beneficiaries with HF who are 65 years of age and older, 86% have hypertension, 72% have ischemic heart disease, and 29% have atrial fibrillation.[9] Similarly, prospectively collected interview and examination data from the National Health and Nutrition Examination Survey (NHANES) found that among persons with HF across all ages, 73% have hypertension, 48% have had a myocardial infarction, 27% have angina, and 20% have had a stroke.[2] The co-occurrence of these cardiovascular diseases is common and is even more pronounced among older persons with HFPEF.[1]

HF is also frequently accompanied by coexisting noncardiac conditions, including metabolic disorders that promote cardiovascular disease, illnesses that result from shared risk factors such as smoking, and unrelated diseases. For example, recent data describing Medicare beneficiaries with HF have shown that 47% have diabetes, 63% have hyperlipidemia, 31% have COPD, 45% have chronic kidney disease, 51% have anemia, and 45% have osteoarthritis.[9] Consistent with these findings, NHANES data for patients with HF at all ages found that 38% have diabetes, 54% have hyperlipidemia, 47% have obesity, 31% have COPD, 46% have chronic kidney disease, 62% have osteoarthritis, and 24% have a history of cancer.[2] The frequency of these noncardiac conditions has increased with time among all age groups[2,11–14] and will likely further increase as the population ages, the prevalence of obesity increases, and treatments for chronic disease prolong life.

Although multimorbidity is common among adults with HF at all ages, older adults with HF are particularly likely to have concomitant geriatric conditions and syndromes.[14] Recent Medicare data found that 27% of older persons with HF have cognitive impairment[9] and 39% require assistance with walking.[4] These findings likely underestimate the prevalence of both cognitive impairment and mobility disability in older adults with HF, as the assessment of geriatric conditions in typical clinical practice and subsequent documentation in billing data is low.[15–17] Rigorous prospective evaluation has therefore found a greater prevalence of cognitive impairment in HF. For example, a recent study of hospitalized older patients with HF found that 25% had mild cognitive impairment and 22% had moderate to severe cognitive impairment based on Mini-Mental Status Examination score.[15] A second study found that 23% of hospitalized HF patients could not accurately complete the Mini-Cog, a short 3-item recall and clock-drawing test.[18] Similarly, prospective interview and physical examination of patients with HF found 57% to have difficulty walking 2 to 3 blocks or climbing one flight of stairs.[2] Another observational study of older persons newly diagnosed with HF found that approximately half had difficulty with at least one activity of daily living, including walking within the home, getting out of bed, eating, dressing, bathing, and toileting or at least one instrumental activity of daily living, including performing housework, shopping, preparing meals, paying bills, and using the phone.[5] Frailty is also common in this population, as approximately 1 in 4 older persons with HF have at least 3 of the following: weak grip strength, physical exhaustion, slowness, low activity, and unintentional weight loss of 10 or more pounds in the past year.[19,20] In addition, more than 1 in 3 suffer from urinary incontinence or overactive bladder,[21,22] and more than 1 in 10 have visual impairment significant enough to impair reading even with the help of contact lenses or glasses.[2]

In summary, multimorbidity is exceedingly common in HF, especially among older persons, who are more likely to have common geriatric conditions and syndromes, such as cognitive impairment, mobility disability, functional limitations, and frailty (**Fig. 1**). As a result, the diagnosis and management of HF in older persons present unique challenges that are further described in the next section.

IMPACT OF MULTIMORBIDITY ON DIAGNOSIS AND MANAGEMENT OF HEART FAILURE

Diagnostic Challenges

Multimorbidity increases the difficulty of diagnosing symptomatic HF. Many conditions commonly found in older persons with HF can produce dyspnea or exercise intolerance. These conditions include coronary artery disease, arrhythmias such as

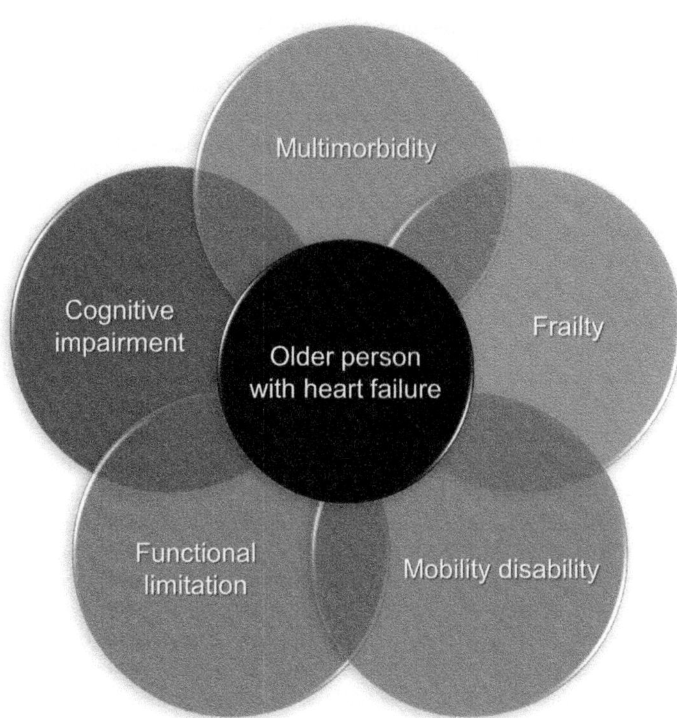

Fig. 1. Complex overlap of chronic medical conditions and geriatric syndromes in older adults with HF.

atrial fibrillation and flutter, valvular heart disease, COPD and asthma, pneumonia, pulmonary hypertension, obesity, anemia, and other acute or chronic conditions.[23,24] These conditions, as well as depression, obstructive sleep apnea, infections, various rheumatologic abnormalities, frailty, and sarcopenia, can also result in other common symptoms associated with HF, such as fatigue and weakness. There is no singular pathognomonic finding or diagnostic test that differentiates symptoms of HF from symptoms of these other conditions.[25] Although serum levels of brain natriuretic peptide (BNP) and N-terminal pro-BNP are elevated in persons with decompensated HF, the availability of test results does not necessarily improve accuracy of diagnosis in patients presenting with undifferentiated dyspnea.[26]

The diagnosis of HF is further complicated by the fact that most older persons with HF have HFPEF.[3] The diagnosis of this condition requires the simultaneous demonstration of symptoms consistent with HF, left ventricular ejection fraction greater than 50%, and evidence of diastolic dysfunction.[27,28] However, the risk of falsely diagnosing HFPEF can be considerable, because many older adults have preserved left ventricular systolic function and evidence of diastolic relaxation abnormalities by echocardiogram.[29,30] These findings are especially common among the oldest old.

Treatment Challenges

Multimorbidity also makes the management of HF more difficult. A critical limitation is the lack of high-quality data on treating acute and chronic illnesses in the setting of MCCs. Multimorbid patients have been largely excluded from the most pivotal randomized clinical trials. An analysis of randomized trials over a 15-year period from the highest impact general medical journals and subspecialty journals found that more than 90% used MCCs as a reason for exclusion.[31] Similarly, a study of phase 3 and 4 clinical trials from 5 of the highest impact medical journals found that almost one-half of trials excluded participants based on criteria that are highly associated with multimorbidity in the elderly, including physical disability, functional limitations, decreased life expectancy, cognitive impairment, living in a residential or nursing home, or concurrent serious illness.[32] Twenty percent of these trials had maximum age cutoffs.[32] Not surprisingly, the average age and comorbidity profile of clinical trial participants does not match that of Medicare beneficiaries in general, who are significantly older and more medically complex.[33]

The poor alignment between trial participants and the general older population is also present in the pivotal clinical trials for HFPEF, the quintessential form of HF among older persons. For example, the TOPCAT (Treatment of Preserved Cardiac Function Heart Failure with an Aldosterone Antagonist) trial of spironolactone in HFPEF excluded participants with a systolic blood pressure greater than 160 mm Hg, atrial fibrillation with a resting heart rate greater than 90 beats per minute, or a life expectancy of less than 3 years.[34] Similarly, the CHARM-Preserved (Candesartan in Heart Failure: Assessment of Reduction in Mortality and Morbidity-Preserved) trial excluded participants with persistent systolic or diastolic hypertension despite treatment or a life expectancy less than 2 years.[35] The I-PRESERVE (Irbesartan in Heart Failure with Preserved Ejection Fraction) trial excluded patients with a blood pressure more than 160/95 mm Hg, a hemoglobin less than 11 g/dL, or a life expectancy less than 3 years.[36] Only this last trial had a median age greater than 70 (72 years).

As a result, little data exist on the benefits and risks of common treatments for HF in the setting of multiple potential drug-disease and drug-drug interactions that accompany multimorbidity. For example, what are the effects of β-blocker use in the setting of chronotropic incompetence, a common condition in the elderly known to worsen exercise intolerance in HF?[37,38] Do β-blockers worsen common symptoms of dizziness and fatigue in the oldest old?[39] Do the lipophilic β-blockers approved for HF with reduced ejection fraction[13]—metoprolol succinate, carvedilol, and bisoprolol—worsen cognitive function and contribute to behavioral disturbances in persons with pre-existing cognitive impairment?[40,41] Analogously, to what extent do nitrates intensify feelings of disequilibrium and increase the incidence of syncope among multimorbid older persons with cardiovascular disease who have been shown to have a heightened blood pressure response to nitrate administration.[42,43] How can one characterize the net benefit or harm of common treatment regimens for older patients hospitalized with multifactorial dyspnea from HF as well as acute lung disease due to exacerbated COPD, acute asthma, or pneumonia? Many of these patients are treated for more than one acute cardiopulmonary condition with a wide range of agents, including intravenous diuretics, inhaled β-agonists, intravenous steroids, and antibiotics.[44]

Concerns about adverse effects from treatment are not simply academic. A prominent example followed the 1999 publication of the Randomized Aldactone Evaluation Study (RALES), which found that administration of spironolactone to persons with severe HF with reduced ejection fraction led to significant reductions in all-cause death, hospitalization for HF, and HF symptoms.[45] The average age at study enrollment was 65 years. Following publication of RALES, prescription of spironolactone to older persons hospitalized with HF increased greatly in North America, including in Ontario, Canada, where a 5-fold increase in hospitalization for hyperkalemia was identified.[46] Moreover, the additional use of spironolactone did not result in reduced death from all causes or readmissions for HF.[46] Unsurprisingly, the average age of patients with HF treated with spironolactone in real-world clinical practice was 13 years greater than in the pivotal RALES clinical trial. The possibility of drug-disease and drug-drug interactions arising from treatment of HF will only increase with time as society ages, chronic conditions become more prevalent, and polypharmacy increases.[2,47]

MANAGEMENT OF HEART FAILURE IN THE SETTING OF MULTIMORBIDITY

The authors suggest that the treatment of complex older persons with HF and MCCs be patient-focused rather than disease-focused. A holistic approach to treatment can help individual patients best meet their unique health goals while minimizing risk from either excessive or poorly coordinated treatments. They have the following specific recommendations (**Table 1**).

Focus on Universal Health Outcomes

The health status of patients with MCCs is affected by multiple disease processes and their treatments.[48] As a result, it is most sensible to seek improvement in "universal" health outcomes that transcend specific medical conditions.[49] These universal outcomes include (1) symptoms such as pain, fatigue, and dyspnea; (2) health-related quality of life; (3) functional status; (4) all-cause hospitalization and readmission; and (5) death.[48,50] As a result, in treating HF, stringent sodium restriction would not be advisable if it results in poor oral intake, impaired quality of life, and weight loss. Similarly, significant diuresis may be contraindicated if it results in either orthostasis or

Table 1
Recommendations for caring for older patients with multimorbidity and heart failure

Recommendation	Tools and Tips
1. Focus on universal health outcomes	• Identify symptoms including pain, dyspnea, fatigue, lightheadedness • Quantify health-related quality of life through validated tools such as the SF12[79] • Determine functional status including patient-reported difficulty with ADLs/IADLs and gait speed • Aim to reduce all-cause hospitalization rather than HF-only hospitalization • Discuss prognosis for survival and perform advance care planning
2. Formally assess cognitive function	• MOCA • Mini Mental Status Examination • Mini-Cog
3. Focus on nonpharmacologic treatments	• Exercise • If appropriate, pelvic floor training for urinary incontinence, physical countermeasures for orthostasis, and others
4. Minimize treatment burden	• Ask patients what aspects of care are most burdensome • Discontinue unnecessary medications • Reduce unnecessary medical appointments
5. Enhance care coordination	• Communicate with other clinicians involved in the patient's care • Develop an integrated multidisciplinary plan of care • Enlist community resources to provide additional support

Abbreviations: ADL, activity of daily living; IADL, instrumental activity of daily living; SF12, Short-Form 12.

hypotension that limits walking and overall functional status. Placement of an implantable cardioverter defibrillator that lowers the likelihood of sudden cardiac death may be harmful for older patients who prefer to die suddenly rather than experience suffering associated with a more prolonged death from advanced illness including end-stage HF, oxygen-dependent lung disease, or metastatic cancer.

Formally Assess Cognitive Function

The self-management of HF is complex and relies on intact memory and executive function. Unsurprisingly, older patients with HF and cognitive impairment experience worse outcomes than persons who are cognitively intact.[51] Nevertheless, the most vulnerable patients with HF may be those with mild cognitive impairment rather than those with moderate to severe dementia.[15] In many instances, mild cognitive impairment is not diagnosed,[15] and HF patients with this condition may not receive the same support given to patients with more severe cognitive deficits. It is therefore critical that cognitive function be systematically assessed in all older patients with HF. Validated assessment methods include the Montreal Cognitive Assessment (MOCA),[52] the Mini-Mental Status Examination,[53] and the Mini-Cog.[54] The MOCA is particularly well validated for detecting mild cognitive impairment, and the Mini-Cog is the least time consuming to perform.[55]

Prioritize Nonpharmacologic Treatments

Where possible, use nonpharmacologic interventions to improve patient outcomes with minimal side effects. For example, consensus guidelines recommend that multimorbid patients with HF regularly exercise to improve physical function, enhance health-related quality of life, reduce symptoms of breathlessness, and decrease likelihood of hospital admission.[13,56–59] Exercise may be particularly important for older persons with HFPEF who frequently have concomitant impairments in skeletal muscle perfusion and metabolism that contribute to exercise intolerance.[60,61] Regular physical activity can also improve symptoms primarily caused by other medical conditions commonly associated with HF in older persons, including coronary artery disease,[62] peripheral artery disease,[63] COPD,[64] and depression.[65] Nevertheless, exercise is not the only nonpharmacologic intervention that can help older patients with HF. Those with urinary incontinence that is exacerbated by diuretic use, for example, may benefit from pelvic floor training rather than using antispasmodic agents with anticholinergic effects that can worsen cognitive function.[66] Similarly, older persons with orthostasis may experience reduced symptoms if physical countermeasures like crossing and tensing legs are used before rising from a bed or chair.[67,68]

Minimize Treatment Burden

Older patients with HF and multimorbidity may be overwhelmed not only by their burden of illness but also by the burden associated with treating these conditions (**Box 1**). The work of being a patient with HF often includes (1) taking and managing complex medication regimens; (2) monitoring symptoms, physical findings, and results of point-of-care testing; (3) making changes to lifestyle; (4) arranging and attending visits with health care providers; (5) navigating health insurance and social service systems; and (6) assuming financial burdens associated with health care.[69,70] As a result, intensifying treatment may paradoxically add to a patient's problems, increase nonadherence to treatment recommendations, and worsen outcomes.[71] Although some treatment burden is to be expected, the chance of overtaxing patients and their caregivers can be minimized by first establishing the weight of this burden. Although few validated instruments to assess treatment burden

Box 1
Typical burden of an older person with heart failure and multimorbidity

- Has 4 other chronic conditions in addition to heart failure[1]
- Takes 10 or more medications a day[47]
- Spends about 2 hours per day on health-related activities[80]
- Attends 15 or more outpatient appointments with physicians each year[81]
- Needs assistance with at least one activity of daily living[5,82]
- Experiences hospitalizations for multiple conditions[7,8]

All are best estimates based on the available published literature, but burden is likely to vary widely across individual patients.
Data from Refs.[1,5,7,8,47,80–82]

exist, one can simply start by asking patients if they can do what is asked of them, and if so, at what cost?[70] Their responses should be used to prioritize the conditions worth addressing and the specific strategies used. Reducing polypharmacy is one relatively easy way to decrease treatment burden and may improve quality of life without other adverse effects.[72]

Enhance Care-Coordination

Care coordination and multidisciplinary team-based care has been shown to improve outcomes in older multimorbid patients at high risk for hospitalization. For example, Medicare demonstration projects successful in lowering preventable hospitalizations through improved care coordination had the following common features: (1) frequent in-person meetings between care coordinators and patients; (2) in-person meetings between care coordinators and health providers; (3) supplemental educational sessions for patients and caregivers; (4) medication management services; and (5) timely and comprehensive transitional care after hospitalization.[73] Similarly, reductions in readmission after hospitalization for HF have been achieved through use of multipronged strategies delivered by multidisciplinary teams of physicians, nurses, social workers, pharmacists, physical therapists, and care managers both during and after hospitalization.[74–76] The most successful hospitals have used a large number of strategies designed to integrate hospital and postacute care[77] and have successfully reduced readmissions from the full range of medical conditions to which older patients with HF are vulnerable after hospital discharge.[78]

SUMMARY

Multimorbidity is a common feature of HF that impacts diagnosis, management, and outcomes. It is therefore critical that providers caring for older patients with HF adopt broad patient-centered perspectives rather than focus exclusively on cardiovascular conditions. Treatment strategies should be closely aligned to patients' specific health goals and well-calibrated to the workload they wish to expend. With this perspective, benefits of treatment can be maximized while minimizing potentially harmful consequences.

REFERENCES

1. Chamberlain AM, St Sauver JL, Gerber Y, et al. Multimorbidity in heart failure: a community perspective. Am J Med 2015;128:38–45.

2. Wong CY, Chaudhry SI, Desai MM, et al. Trends in comorbidity, disability, and polypharmacy in heart failure. Am J Med 2011;124:136–43.
3. Owan TE, Hodge DO, Herges RM, et al. Trends in prevalence and outcome of heart failure with preserved ejection fraction. N Engl J Med 2006;355:251–9.
4. Chaudhry SI, Wang Y, Gill TM, et al. Geriatric conditions and subsequent mortality in older patients with heart failure. J Am Coll Cardiol 2010;55:309–16.
5. Murad K, Goff DC Jr, Morgan TM, et al. Burden of comorbidities and functional and cognitive impairments in elderly patients at the initial diagnosis of heart failure and their impact on total mortality: the cardiovascular health study. JACC Heart Fail 2015;3:542–50.
6. Braunstein JB, Anderson GF, Gerstenblith G, et al. Noncardiac comorbidity increases preventable hospitalizations and mortality among Medicare beneficiaries with chronic heart failure. J Am Coll Cardiol 2003;42:1226–33.
7. Dunlay SM, Redfield MM, Weston SA, et al. Hospitalizations after heart failure diagnosis a community perspective. J Am Coll Cardiol 2009;54:1695–702.
8. Dharmarajan K, Hsieh AF, Lin Z, et al. Diagnoses and timing of 30-day readmissions after hospitalization for heart failure, acute myocardial infarction, or pneumonia. JAMA 2013;309:355–63.
9. Arnett DK, Goodman RA, Halperin JL, et al. AHA/ACC/HHS strategies to enhance application of clinical practice guidelines in patients with cardiovascular disease and comorbid conditions: from the American Heart Association, American College of Cardiology, and US Department of Health and Human Services. Circulation 2014;130:1662–7.
10. ACC/AGS/NIA multimorbidity in older adults with CV disease workshop. 2015. Available at: http://www.accagsniamultimorbidityworkshop.com. Accessed 4 August 2015.
11. Bueno H, Ross JS, Wang Y, et al. Trends in length of stay and short-term outcomes among medicare patients hospitalized for heart failure, 1993-2006. JAMA 2010;303:2141–7.
12. Chen J, Normand SL, Wang Y, et al. National and regional trends in heart failure hospitalization and mortality rates for Medicare beneficiaries, 1998-2008. JAMA 2011;306:1669–78.
13. Yancy CW, Jessup M, Bozkurt B, et al. 2013 ACCF/AHA guideline for the management of heart failure: a report of the American College of Cardiology Foundation/American Heart Association Task Force on practice guidelines. Circulation 2013;128:e240–327.
14. Ahluwalia SC, Gross CP, Chaudhry SI, et al. Change in comorbidity prevalence with advancing age among persons with heart failure. J Gen Intern Med 2011; 26:1145–51.
15. Dodson JA, Truong TT, Towle VR, et al. Cognitive impairment in older adults with heart failure: prevalence, documentation, and impact on outcomes. Am J Med 2013;126:120–6.
16. Newcomer R, Clay T, Luxenberg JS, et al. Misclassification and selection bias when identifying Alzheimer's disease solely from Medicare claims records. J Am Geriatr Soc 1999;47:215–9.
17. Lin PJ, Kaufer DI, Maciejewski ML, et al. An examination of Alzheimer's disease case definitions using Medicare claims and survey data. Alzheimers Dement 2010;6:334–41.
18. Patel A, Parikh R, Howell EH, et al. Mini-cog performance: novel marker of post discharge risk among patients hospitalized for heart failure. Circ Heart Fail 2015;8:8–16.

19. Boxer RS, Wang Z, Walsh SJ, et al. The utility of the 6-minute walk test as a measure of frailty in older adults with heart failure. Am J Geriatr Cardiol 2008;17:7–12.
20. McNallan SM, Chamberlain AM, Gerber Y, et al. Measuring frailty in heart failure: a community perspective. Am Heart J 2013;166:768–74.
21. Palmer MH, Hardin SR, Behrend C, et al. Urinary incontinence and overactive bladder in patients with heart failure. J Urol 2009;182:196–202.
22. Hwang R, Chuan F, Peters R, et al. Frequency of urinary incontinence in people with chronic heart failure. Heart Lung 2013;42:26–31.
23. Ray P, Birolleau S, Lefort Y, et al. Acute respiratory failure in the elderly: etiology, emergency diagnosis and prognosis. Crit Care 2006;10:R82.
24. Wahls SA. Causes and evaluation of chronic dyspnea. Am Fam Physician 2012; 86:173–82.
25. Hawkins NM, Petrie MC, Jhund PS, et al. Heart failure and chronic obstructive pulmonary disease: diagnostic pitfalls and epidemiology. Eur J Heart Fail 2009; 11:130–9.
26. Lokuge A, Lam L, Cameron P, et al. B-type natriuretic peptide testing and the accuracy of heart failure diagnosis in the emergency department. Circ Heart Fail 2010;3:104–10.
27. Paulus WJ, Tschope C, Sanderson JE, et al. How to diagnose diastolic heart failure: a consensus statement on the diagnosis of heart failure with normal left ventricular ejection fraction by the Heart Failure and Echocardiography Associations of the European Society of Cardiology. Eur Heart J 2007;28:2539–50.
28. Borlaug BA, Paulus WJ. Heart failure with preserved ejection fraction: pathophysiology, diagnosis, and treatment. Eur Heart J 2011;32:670–9.
29. Fischer M, Baessler A, Hense HW, et al. Prevalence of left ventricular diastolic dysfunction in the community. Results from a Doppler echocardiographic-based survey of a population sample. Eur Heart J 2003;24:320–8.
30. Kuznetsova T, Herbots L, Lopez B, et al. Prevalence of left ventricular diastolic dysfunction in a general population. Circ Heart Fail 2009;2:105–12.
31. Jadad AR, To MJ, Emara M, et al. Consideration of multiple chronic diseases in randomized controlled trials. JAMA 2011;306:2670–2.
32. Zulman DM, Sussman JB, Chen X, et al. Examining the evidence: a systematic review of the inclusion and analysis of older adults in randomized controlled trials. J Gen Intern Med 2011;26:783–90.
33. Dhruva SS, Redberg RF. Variations between clinical trial participants and Medicare beneficiaries in evidence used for Medicare national coverage decisions. Arch Intern Med 2008;168:136–40.
34. Pitt B, Pfeffer MA, Assmann SF, et al. Spironolactone for heart failure with preserved ejection fraction. N Engl J Med 2014;370:1383–92.
35. Yusuf S, Pfeffer MA, Swedberg K, et al. Effects of candesartan in patients with chronic heart failure and preserved left-ventricular ejection fraction: the CHARM-preserved trial. Lancet 2003;362:777–81.
36. Massie BM, Carson PE, McMurray JJ, et al. Irbesartan in patients with heart failure and preserved ejection fraction. N Engl J Med 2008;359:2456–67.
37. Brubaker PH, Joo KC, Stewart KP, et al. Chronotropic incompetence and its contribution to exercise intolerance in older heart failure patients. J Cardiopulm Rehabil 2006;26:86–9.
38. Borlaug BA, Olson TP, Lam CS, et al. Global cardiovascular reserve dysfunction in heart failure with preserved ejection fraction. J Am Coll Cardiol 2010;56: 845–54.

39. Jonsson R, Sixt E, Landahl S, et al. Prevalence of dizziness and vertigo in an urban elderly population. J Vestib Res 2004;14:47–52.
40. Neil-Dwyer G, Bartlett J, McAinsh J, et al. Beta-adrenoceptor blockers and the blood-brain barrier. Br J Clin Pharmacol 1981;11:549–53.
41. Westerlund A. Central nervous system side-effects with hydrophilic and lipophilic beta-blockers. Eur J Clin Pharmacol 1985;28(Suppl):73–6.
42. Del Rosso A, Ungar A, Bartoli P, et al. Usefulness and safety of shortened head-up tilt testing potentiated with sublingual glyceryl trinitrate in older patients with recurrent unexplained syncope. J Am Geriatr Soc 2002;50:1324–8.
43. Thadani U, Ripley TL. Side effects of using nitrates to treat heart failure and the acute coronary syndromes, unstable angina and acute myocardial infarction. Expert Opin Drug Saf 2007;6:385–96.
44. Dharmarajan K, Strait KM, Lagu T, et al. Acute decompensated heart failure is routinely treated as a cardiopulmonary syndrome. PLoS One 2013;8:e78222.
45. Pitt B, Zannad F, Remme WJ, et al. The effect of spironolactone on morbidity and mortality in patients with severe heart failure. Randomized Aldactone Evaluation Study Investigators. N Engl J Med 1999;341:709–17.
46. Juurlink DN, Mamdani MM, Lee DS, et al. Rates of hyperkalemia after publication of the Randomized Aldactone Evaluation Study. N Engl J Med 2004;351:543–51.
47. Dunlay SM, Eveleth JM, Shah ND, et al. Medication adherence among community-dwelling patients with heart failure. Mayo Clin Proc 2011;86:273–81.
48. Working Group on Health Outcomes for Older Persons with Multiple Chronic Conditions, Adams K, Bayliss E, Permanente K, et al. Universal health outcome measures for older persons with multiple chronic conditions. J Am Geriatr Soc 2012; 60:2333–41.
49. Tinetti ME, Studenski SA. Comparative effectiveness research and patients with multiple chronic conditions. N Engl J Med 2011;364:2478–81.
50. Reuben DB, Tinetti ME. Goal-oriented patient care–an alternative health outcomes paradigm. N Engl J Med 2012;366:777–9.
51. Dodson JA, Chaudhry SI. Geriatric conditions in heart failure. Curr Cardiovasc Risk Rep 2012;6:404–10.
52. Nasreddine ZS, Phillips NA, Bedirian V, et al. The Montreal Cognitive Assessment, MoCA: a brief screening tool for mild cognitive impairment. J Am Geriatr Soc 2005;53:695–9.
53. Folstein MF, Folstein SE, McHugh PR. "Mini-mental state". A practical method for grading the cognitive state of patients for the clinician. J Psychiatr Res 1975;12: 189–98.
54. Borson S, Scanlan J, Brush M, et al. The mini-cog: a cognitive 'vital signs' measure for dementia screening in multi-lingual elderly. Int J Geriatr Psychiatry 2000; 15:1021–7.
55. Tsoi KK, Chan JY, Hirai HW, et al. Cognitive tests to detect dementia: a systematic review and meta-analysis. JAMA Intern Med 2015;175(9):1450–8.
56. Taylor RS, Sagar VA, Davies EJ, et al. Exercise-based rehabilitation for heart failure. Cochrane Database Syst Rev 2014;(4):CD003331.
57. Edelmann F, Gelbrich G, Dungen HD, et al. Exercise training improves exercise capacity and diastolic function in patients with heart failure with preserved ejection fraction: results of the Ex-DHF (Exercise training in Diastolic Heart Failure) pilot study. J Am Coll Cardiol 2011;58:1780–91.
58. Kitzman DW, Brubaker PH, Morgan TM, et al. Exercise training in older patients with heart failure and preserved ejection fraction: a randomized, controlled, single-blind trial. Circ Heart Fail 2010;3:659–67.

59. Haykowsky M, Brubaker P, Kitzman D. Role of physical training in heart failure with preserved ejection fraction. Curr Heart Fail Rep 2012;9:101–6.
60. Haykowsky MJ, Brubaker PH, John JM, et al. Determinants of exercise intolerance in elderly heart failure patients with preserved ejection fraction. J Am Coll Cardiol 2011;58:265–74.
61. Haykowsky MJ, Brubaker PH, Morgan TM, et al. Impaired aerobic capacity and physical functional performance in older heart failure patients with preserved ejection fraction: role of lean body mass. J Gerontol A Biol Sci Med Sci 2013; 68:968–75.
62. Fihn SD, Gardin JM, Abrams J, et al. 2012 ACCF/AHA/ACP/AATS/PCNA/SCAI/STS Guideline for the diagnosis and management of patients with stable ischemic heart disease: a report of the American College of Cardiology Foundation/American Heart Association Task Force on Practice Guidelines, and the American College of Physicians, American Association for Thoracic Surgery, Preventive Cardiovascular Nurses Association, Society for Cardiovascular Angiography and Interventions, and Society of Thoracic Surgeons. J Am Coll Cardiol 2012;60:e44–164.
63. Hirsch AT, Haskal ZJ, Hertzer NR, et al. ACC/AHA 2005 Practice Guidelines for the management of patients with peripheral arterial disease (lower extremity, renal, mesenteric, and abdominal aortic): a collaborative report from the American Association for Vascular Surgery/Society for Vascular Surgery, Society for Cardiovascular Angiography and Interventions, Society for Vascular Medicine and Biology, Society of Interventional Radiology, and the ACC/AHA Task Force on Practice Guidelines (Writing Committee to Develop Guidelines for the Management of Patients With Peripheral Arterial Disease): endorsed by the American Association of Cardiovascular and Pulmonary Rehabilitation; National Heart, Lung, and Blood Institute; Society for Vascular Nursing; TransAtlantic Inter-Society Consensus; and Vascular Disease Foundation. Circulation 2006;113: e463–654.
64. Global Initiative for Chronic Obstructive Lung Disease (GOLD) 2015. Global strategy for the diagnosis, management and prevention of COPD. Available at: http://www.goldcopd.org/guidelines-global-strategy-for-diagnosis-management.html. Accessed August 7, 2015.
65. Blumenthal JA, Babyak MA, O'Connor C, et al. Effects of exercise training on depressive symptoms in patients with chronic heart failure: the HF-ACTION randomized trial. JAMA 2012;308:465–74.
66. Shamliyan T, Wyman J, Kane RL. Nonsurgical treatments for urinary incontinence in adult women: diagnosis and comparative effectiveness. Rockville (MD): Agency for Healthcare Research and Quality; 2012.
67. Krediet CT, van Dijk N, Linzer M, et al. Management of vasovagal syncope: controlling or aborting faints by leg crossing and muscle tensing. Circulation 2002; 106:1684–9.
68. van Dijk N, Quartieri F, Blanc JJ, et al. Effectiveness of physical counterpressure maneuvers in preventing vasovagal syncope: the Physical Counterpressure Manoeuvres Trial (PC-Trial). J Am Coll Cardiol 2006;48:1652–7.
69. May C, Montori VM, Mair FS. We need minimally disruptive medicine. BMJ 2009; 339:b2803.
70. Mair FS, May CR. Thinking about the burden of treatment. BMJ 2014;349:g6680.
71. Eton DT, Ramalho de Oliveira D, Egginton JS, et al. Building a measurement framework of burden of treatment in complex patients with chronic conditions: a qualitative study. Patient Relat Outcome Meas 2012;3:39–49.

72. Kutner JS, Blatchford PJ, Taylor DH Jr, et al. Safety and benefit of discontinuing statin therapy in the setting of advanced, life-limiting illness: a randomized clinical trial. JAMA Intern Med 2015;175:691–700.
73. Brown RS, Peikes D, Peterson G, et al. Six features of Medicare coordinated care demonstration programs that cut hospital admissions of high-risk patients. Health Aff (Millwood) 2012;31:1156–66.
74. Rich MW, Beckham V, Wittenberg C, et al. A multidisciplinary intervention to prevent the readmission of elderly patients with congestive heart failure. N Engl J Med 1995;333:1190–5.
75. Feltner C, Jones CD, Cene CW, et al. Transitional care interventions to prevent readmissions for persons with heart failure: a systematic review and meta-analysis. Ann Intern Med 2014;160:774–84.
76. Dharmarajan K, Krumholz HM. Strategies to reduce 30-day readmissions in older patients hospitalized with heart failure and acute myocardial infarction. Curr Geriatr Rep 2014;3:306–15.
77. Bradley EH, Curry L, Horwitz LI, et al. Hospital strategies associated with 30-day readmission rates for patients with heart failure. Circ Cardiovasc Qual Outcomes 2013;6:444–50.
78. Dharmarajan K, Hsieh AF, Lin Z, et al. Hospital readmission performance and patterns of readmission: retrospective cohort study of Medicare admissions. BMJ 2013;347:f6571.
79. Ware J Jr, Kosinski M, Keller SD. A 12-item Short-Form Health Survey: construction of scales and preliminary tests of reliability and validity. Med Care 1996;34:220–33.
80. Jowsey T, Yen L, W PM. Time spent on health related activities associated with chronic illness: a scoping literature review. BMC Public Health 2012;12:1044.
81. Bahler C, Huber CA, Brungger B, et al. Multimorbidity, health care utilization and costs in an elderly community-dwelling population: a claims data based observational study. BMC Health Serv Res 2015;15:23.
82. Dunlay SM, Manemann SM, Chamberlain AM, et al. Activities of daily living and outcomes in heart failure. Circ Heart Fail 2015;8:261–7.

Multiple Chronic Conditions in Older Adults with Acute Coronary Syndromes

Joakim Alfredsson, MD, PhD[a,b,c], Karen P. Alexander, MD[c,*]

KEYWORDS

- Acute coronary syndrome • Myocardial infarction (MI) • Older adults
- Multiple chronic conditions • Type 2 MI

KEY POINTS

- Multimorbidity is increasingly prevalent among older adults presenting with acute myocardial infarction, and includes both cardiovascular (CV) (heart failure, hypertension, and arrhythmias) and non-CV (anemia, chronic kidney disease, and depression) conditions.
- Hospital mortality and length of stay increase in a dose-dependent fashion with the number of CV and non-CV comorbidities.
- Evidence-based recommendations for patients with multiple chronic conditions (MCCs) are not available, as such patients are often excluded from randomized clinical trial populations.
- Type 2 myocardial infarctions (MIs), due to mismatch in oxygen supply and demand, are common with comorbid disease presentations (eg, chronic obstructive pulmonary disease, pneumonia, atrial fibrillation) and carry a twofold higher mortality rate than other MI types.
- Individualized decision making is recommended, as the presence of MCC may shift risk-benefit ratios of standard treatments.

INTRODUCTION

Multimorbidity (≥2 conditions) is present in up to 70% of older (age ≥65 years) community-dwelling populations.[1,2] With older age, comorbidity dyads (2 conditions) and triads (3 conditions) more often include cardiovascular (CV) risk factors, and the risk for an acute coronary syndrome (ACS) rises commensurately. As the age of the population with myocardial infarction (MI) increases, so too does the accompanying comorbidity burden.[3] Comorbid conditions in ACS populations can be classified as

Disclosure Statement: The authors have nothing to disclose.

[a] Department of Cardiology, Linköping University, Linköping, Sweden; [b] Department of Medical and Health Sciences, Linköping University, Linköping, Sweden; [c] Duke Clinical Research Institute, Duke University Medical Center, Durham, NC 27710, USA

* Corresponding author.

E-mail address: Karen.alexander@duke.edu

Clin Geriatr Med 32 (2016) 291–303

http://dx.doi.org/10.1016/j.cger.2016.01.009 **geriatric.theclinics.com**

concordant or discordant to the CV disease causal pathway.[4] Concordant comorbidities include CV risk factors, stroke, and peripheral vascular disease, whereas discordant comorbidities include anemia, chronic kidney disease (CKD), chronic obstructive pulmonary disease (COPD), and cancer.

ACSs include non–ST-elevation MI (NSTEMI), ST-elevation MI (STEMI), and unstable angina, with diagnosis based on biomarker elevation along with symptoms or electrocardiogram (ECG) changes indicating ischemia. With increasingly sensitive biomarker assays, elevation of troponins above the MI detection limit is frequently found among those presenting for cardiac conditions other than ACS, such as heart failure (HF) or arrhythmias. Troponin also may be elevated in patients presenting with noncardiac illnesses, such as COPD, anemia, or severe infections, especially if septicemia is present. The universal definition of MI distinguishes between 2 primary MI presentations: type 1 MI caused by plaque rupture with thrombus formation, and type 2 MI caused by oxygen supply and demand mismatch.[5] Clinically distinguishing between these MI types may be challenging.

Almost 50% of patients with troponin elevations in the emergency room have presenting diagnoses other than ACS.[6] Also among MI populations, approximately 26% of all MIs are type 2 MIs.[7] Patients with type 2 MIs are older and have more comorbidity (anemia, COPD, and renal failure) compared with those with type 1 MIs. These patients also have lower peak troponins, receive less invasive care, and are discharged on fewer cardiac medications. Importantly, mortality with type 2 MIs was nearly 50% at 2 years, and twofold higher than with type 1 MIs[8] (**Fig. 1**). Understanding the significance and typical patterns of troponin elevations in the setting of comorbid illness is of utmost important. This will better inform the treatment of an ACS in the context of comorbid diseases. It will also help clarify which troponin elevations reflect an MI, and which are present only due to underlying coronary disease and represent myocardial injury instead of myocardial infarction.

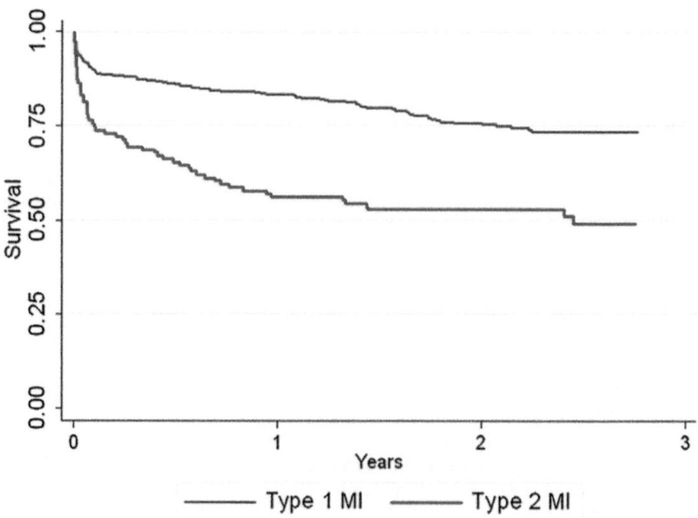

Fig. 1. Kaplan-Meier survival curves according to classification of myocardial infarction as type 1 and type 2. (*From* Saaby L, Poulsen TS, Diederichsen AC, et al. Mortality rate in type 2 myocardial infarction: observations from an unselected hospital cohort. Am J Med 2014;127:299; with permission.)

CARDIOVASCULAR COMORBIDITIES IN ACUTE CORONARY SYNDROME POPULATIONS

CV comorbidities have been increasing over time, as shown in a report from the National Heart, Lung and Blood Institute Dynamic Registry of Percutaneous Coronary Intervention.[9] There is also a strong correlation between older age and CV comorbidity in ACS populations.[10] The prevalence of more than one CV comorbidity is also increasing[11] (**Fig. 2**). Comorbidity prevalence rates differ by geographic region, time period, study type (randomized clinical trial [RCT] or registry), type of ACS, as well as definitions used and method of data collection (claims data or questionnaire). Patients in RCTs are younger, more often men, and have fewer comorbid conditions compared with patients in clinical registries.[12,13] Still, registries may leave out those with greatest comorbid burden and not include all patients hospitalized for ACS.[14] Nonetheless, the best available information about CV comorbidity in patients with ACS comes from registries. The reported prevalence of CV risk factors varies widely; for example, hypertension varies from 29% to 76%, hyperlipidemia from 11% to 80%, and diabetes from 15% to 35% (**Table 1**). The prevalence of other CV comorbidities in patients with ACS varies more narrowly; for example, HF from 4% to 25%, stroke from 4% to 15%, and peripheral arterial disease (PAD) from 3% to 10%.

Atrial Fibrillation

In the Global Registry of Acute Coronary Events (GRACE), a history of atrial fibrillation (AF) was present in 8%, and 5% developed new AF during hospitalization.[15] Higher prevalence has been reported in 2 smaller trials.[16,17] After adjustment, new-onset AF is associated with increased in-hospital mortality and preexisting AF is significantly associated with in-hospital and 30-day mortality.[15,18] Management of patients with ACS with AF is challenging, as they usually have indications for both oral anticoagulation (OAC) and antiplatelet treatment. This dual and sometimes triple (OAC + dual antiplatelet therapy) antithrombotic treatment increases bleeding complications, particularly in the presence of comorbidities such as anemia and CKD.[19,20]

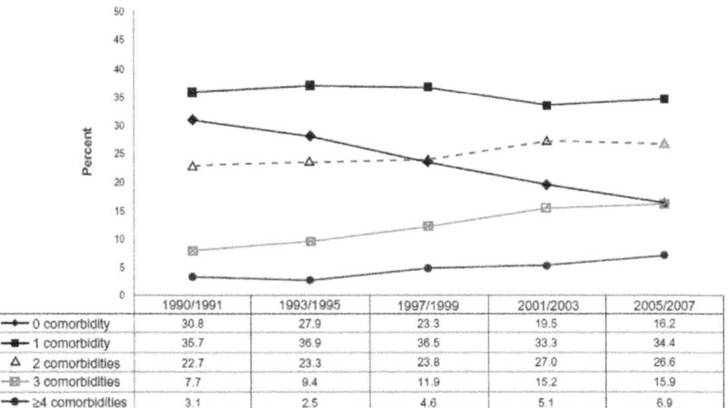

	1990/1991	1993/1995	1997/1999	2001/2003	2005/2007
0 comorbidity	30.8	27.9	23.3	19.5	16.2
1 comorbidity	35.7	36.9	36.5	33.3	34.4
2 comorbidities	22.7	23.3	23.8	27.0	26.6
3 comorbidities	7.7	9.4	11.9	15.2	15.9
≥4 comorbidities	3.1	2.5	4.6	5.1	6.9

Fig. 2. Prevalence of previously diagnosed multimorbidity among patients hospitalized with acute MI according to study period. (*From* McManus DD, Nguyen HL, Saczynski JS, et al. Multiple cardiovascular comorbidities and acute myocardial infarction: temporal trends (1990-2007) and impact on death rates at 30 days and 1 year. Clin Epidemiol 2012;4:118; with permission.)

Table 1
Prevalence of CV comorbid conditions in ACS populations

Population (n)	Age, Average, y	HTN, %	HF, %	Stroke, %	PAD, %	DM, %	HL, %
MI (US 2007–2013; n = 443,117)[64]	63	71	—	5[a]	5	31	37[c]
MI (US 1999–2008[d]; n = 46,086)[65]	67–69[d]	45–76[d]	6–8[d]	4	3–5[d]	27–32[d]	46–80[d]
MI (US 2003, 2005 and 2007; n = 2972)[22]	71	75	25	12	19	35	—
ACS (Switzerland 2002–2012;n = 29,620)[29]	72 vs 64[e]	62	4	6[a]	5	15	57
ACS/PCI (Canada 1995–2000; n = 10,500)[66]	30% ≥70	51	14	—	—	20	55
STEMI (women vs men)[e] (Sweden 1995–2006; n = 18,876)[21]	73 vs 66	40 vs 29	10 vs 5	10 vs 8	4 vs 3	21 vs 17	—
STEMI (Korea 2006–13; n = 22,514)[67]	64	49	—	—	—	26	11
NSTEMI (Korea 2006–13;n = 17,464)[67]	67	58	—	—	—	34	14
NSTE ACS (Canada 1999–2008; n = 6711)[68]	68	63	12	10[b]	10	29	54
NSTE ACS (Sweden 2006–10; n = 40,616)[23]	73	56	17	15	7	26	32[c]

Abbreviations: ACS, acute coronary syndromes; CV, cardiovascular; DM, diabetes mellitus; HF, heart failure; HL, hyperlipidemia; HTN, hypertension; MI, myocardial infarction; NSTEMI, non-ST-elevation MI; NSTE ACS, non-ST-elevation ACS; PAD, peripheral artery disease; PCI, percutaneous coronary intervention; STEMI, ST-elevation MI.

[a] Defined as prior cerebrovascular disease.
[b] Defined as stroke or transient ischemic attack.
[c] Defined as treated with a statin.
[d] Values relate to 1999 and 2008, respectively.
[e] Values relate to women and men, respectively.
Data from Refs.[21–23,29,64–68]

NONCARDIOVASCULAR COMORBIDITIES IN ACUTE CORONARY SYNDROME POPULATIONS

Non-CV comorbidity is less well described in older ACS populations, but frequent conditions include CKD, anemia, COPD, and cognitive impairment/depression.[10,21]

Chronic Kidney Disease

CKD may be captured along the estimated glomerular filtration rate (eGFR) continuum and stratified into stages or simply reported as present or absent. In the Worcester Heart Attack Study, the prevalence of CKD was 21.7%.[22] In 2 large STEMI and non-STEMI cohorts, CKD (defined as eGFR <60 mL/min) was present in approximately 30%.[21,23] In-hospital and long-term mortality increase with CKD. CKD also increases risk for ischemic and bleeding outcomes across CKD stages and as a continuous inverse function of eGFR.[24] For antithrombotic medications that undergo clearance by the kidney, dosage adjustment based on renal function is particularly important to avoid excess dosing and associated bleeding complications.[25]

Cancer

Within 90 days of cancer diagnosis, there is an increased incidence of MI.[26] Cancer treatments, particularly radiation therapy, also increase risk of coronary artery disease up to 15 years later.[27] In a large registry of patients with NSTEMI, the prevalence of malignant disease (within the past 3 years) was 3% to 5%.[23,28] Similar prevalence was reported from the Acute Myocardial Infarction in Switzerland (AMIS) Plus registry (4.3%).[29] However, most ACS datasets do not collect cancer history. Cardio-oncology is emerging as a research and clinical care discipline that focuses on the overlap of cancer and CV disease.[30] This will facilitate the expansion of knowledge about intersections between these 2 common conditions.

Anemia

Anemia is often the result of multimorbidity, inflammation, kidney disease, or subacute bleeding. In an analysis of more than 70,000 patients with ACS from The Acute Coronary Treatment and Intervention Outcomes Network-Get With The Guidelines (ACTION-GWTG), 3.3% had a hemoglobin less than 10 g/dL and 13.6% had a hemoglobin of 10 to 12 g/dL. Anemic patients were older, with a higher prevalence of comorbid conditions.[31,32] Anemia is a significant predictor of bleeding in established bleeding risk scores from ACS populations.[33–35] Although the pathophysiological mechanism is not well understood, there is an association between bleeding and mortality during longer term follow-up.[32,36–38] Hospital-acquired anemia is common in ACS populations, and is also associated with worse outcomes during follow-up.[39]

Chronic Lung Disease

Prevalence of chronic lung disease (CLD) in patients with ACS, although not well defined or graded in severity, ranges from 6% to 25% in different reports.[3,4,6,8,10] A recent meta-analysis showed risk of MI increased with COPD (hazard ratio [HR] 1.72, 95% confidence interval [CI] 1.22–2.42) but causality for both may be related to smoking status.[40] This meta-analysis showed weak evidence for increased in-hospital mortality after MI among patients with CLD (odds ratio [OR] 1.13, 0.97–1.31), but did support an increased risk of death during follow-up (HR 1.26, 1.13–1.40). In the SWEDEHEART registry, the 6% of patients with NSTEMI and with a diagnosis of COPD had almost twice the mortality at 1 year (24.6% vs 13.8%) compared with those without COPD. Patients with COPD also received less revascularization and guideline-recommended treatment.[41]

Dementia and Depression

Cognitive disorders and psychiatric conditions are seldom reported among ACS populations despite their high prevalence in older adults. Although the gold standard for cognitive impairment is neuropsychiatric testing, this is limited by time and resource constraints. Therefore, screening with cognitive function surveys (for example, Mini-Mental Status Examination or Telephone Inventory of Cognition- Modified) or using diagnostic codes for dementia is required to assess prevalence. The risk of progressive cognitive decline is higher among those with coronary artery disease, as noted in the longitudinal cohort from the Whitehall II study.[42] In a large ACS cohort from Taiwan and another from Switzerland, only 2.1% of patients carried a diagnosis of dementia.[29,43] Yet, among an older (age $\geq$65 years) ACS population, only 45% had normal cognition on a screening test, and 25% had moderate to severe cognitive impairment.[44] Patients with cognitive impairment or dementia have higher in-hospital mortality and are less likely to receive guideline-recommended treatment after an MI.[43,45]

Depression increases the risk of having an MI and is a predictor of worse prognosis after an MI.[46,47] Approximately 20% of patients with ACS meet the diagnostic criteria for major depression. Depressive symptoms are more prevalent among patients with lower socioeconomic profiles and greater CV risk factor burden.[48] Also, women more often have a history of depression and have more depressive symptoms at the time of ACS admission. Regardless of age, gender, or socioeconomic profile, patients with depressive symptoms have worse quality of life following ACS. Both dementia and depression are associated with increased risk of hospital readmission after an ACS event.[49] This underscores the importance of screening for cognitive dysfunction and depression when assessing the health status of patients with coronary artery disease.[50]

MULTIPLE CHRONIC CONDITIONS IN ACUTE CORONARY SYNDROME POPULATIONS

Although having multiple chronic conditions (MCCs) is the norm, few studies focus on MCCs in elderly ACS populations. One study of 2972 patients with acute MI examined 7 CV conditions (AF, hypertension, coronary heart disease [CHD], diabetes, HF, PAD, and stroke) along with 5 non-CV conditions (anemia, depression, cancer, COPD, and CKD).[22] Hypertension was the most common CV comorbidity (77%), and CKD was the most common noncardiovascular comorbid condition (22%).[22] The most common CV dyad was CHD + hypertension, whereas the most common non-CV dyad was anemia + CKD. Almost 25% had 4 or more CV conditions, and 8% had 3 or more non-CV conditions. Another study of 9518 hospitalized patients with MI at 11 centers from 1990 to 2007 assessed the prevalence and prognostic impact of 5 CV comorbidities (AF, diabetes, HF, hypertension, and stroke).[11] A single CV comorbidity was found in 35%, 2 in 25%, 3 in 12%, and 4 or more in 5% of the population. The proportion of patients with 4 or more comorbidities doubled (from 3% to 7%), whereas the proportion of patients with no comorbid conditions declined (from 31% to 16%) over the study period. Age and sex were associated with multiple comorbid conditions, with women having more CV comorbidity than men.[11] Women with ACS are older, which accounts for much of the difference, but even after adjustment for age, most CV comorbid conditions are more frequent in women.[21,28]

The presence of multiple CV comorbidities was associated with increased 30-day and 1-year mortality after adjustment for other factors, and there was increased risk for each additional comorbid condition.[11] Another study demonstrated that multiple CV or non-CV conditions were associated with significantly higher in-hospital mortality, after adjustment for age, sex race, MI type, and other CV and non-CV comorbidities[22] (**Fig. 3**). Mortality increased from 3.7% to 14.2% as the number of CV conditions increased from 0 to 4 or more. Mortality increased from 6.9% to 15.9% as non-CV conditions increased from 0 to 3 or more. Both CV and non-CV conditions were also associated with prolonged length of stay.

The Swiss AMIS Plus registry of 29,620 patients with ACS studied comorbidity assessed by the Charlson Comorbidity index (CCI), which combines 20 CV and non-CV conditions weighted in a summary score.[51] More than half had no comorbidity (CCI = 0), whereas 12.9% had a CCI $\geq$ 3. Risk of in-hospital mortality increased with higher CCI (adjusted OR for CCI1 1.36 [95% CI 1.16–1.60], CCI2 1.65 [95% CI 1.38–1.97], and CCI3 2.20 [95% CI 1.86–2.57] with CCI = 0 as reference).[29] Adding multimorbidity assessed with CCI to a conventional ACS risk score (GRACE score) has also been shown to improve risk prediction of mortality,[52] which highlights the importance of MCC in determining outcomes.

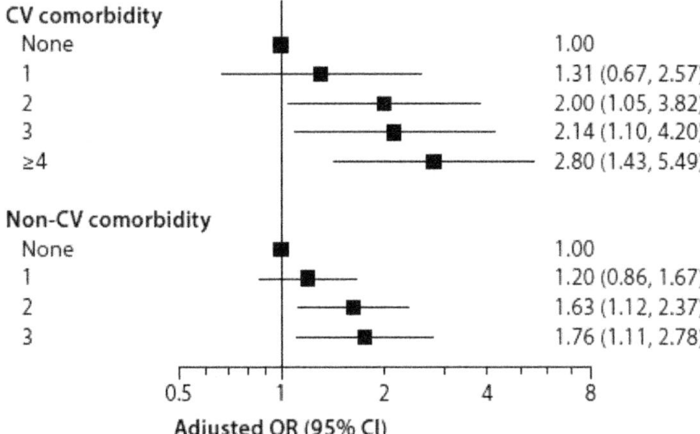

Fig. 3. Multivariable adjusted association between presence of cardiac and noncardiac comorbidities and hospital mortality. (*Data from* Chen HY, Saczynski JS, McManus DD, et al. The impact of cardiac and noncardiac comorbidities on the short-term outcomes of patients hospitalized with acute myocardial infarction: a population-based perspective. Clin Epidemiol 2013;5:439–48.)

MULTIPLE CHRONIC CONDITIONS AND EVIDENCE-BASED MEDICINE

Patients with MCCs are disproportionately excluded from RCTs, so applicability of trial results is uncertain for this group. Clinical guidelines focus recommendations primarily from the perspective of a single condition. Therefore, evidence-based recommendations for patients with MCCs are not available, as the heterogeneity of the population limits the applicability of most trials and guidelines.[53–55] A cautionary note from observational studies suggests that patients with ACS and comorbid conditions such as diabetes, CKD, or COPD are less often treated with evidence-based medicine, which could contribute to worse outcomes.[41,56–58] Clinical guidelines acknowledge the deficiency of evidence for this challenging group. Clinical guidelines on NSTE ACS from the American College of Cardiology/American Heart Association (ACC/AHA) and European Society of Cardiology (ESC) recognize the complexity of patients with MCCs, and recommend that comorbidities and preferences be an integral part of the decision-making process[59,60] (**Box 1**). The presence of MCCs may shift the risk-benefit ratio of standard treatments, which is why a more individualized approach is necessary, even if this inevitably means that decisions are based on less high-quality evidence.[53,54]

CLINICAL IMPLICATIONS

Patients with ACS with MCCs are vulnerable to adverse outcomes and clinical circumstances are often unique. Patients' preferences are particularly important for this group, as individual risk-benefit ratios may vary considerably. Clinical care of these patients should incorporate preferences, recognize limitations of evidence, frame the clinical decision in the context of risk, benefit, and prognosis, and choose therapies that optimize patient-centered benefits.[61] Despite an increased age and comorbidity burden of ACS populations, survival after an MI has increased substantially.[62] Furthermore, even as the prevalence of comorbidity has increased, hospital mortality following ACS has decreased, indicating that prognosis has improved for patients with

Box 1
2012 guidelines for non ST-elevation acute coronary syndromes (NSTE ACS): recommendations for older patients

Class 1 Recommendations

1. Older patients with NSTE ACS should be treated with guideline-directed medical therapy, an early invasive strategy, and revascularization as appropriate. (*Level of Evidence: A*)
2. Pharmacotherapy in older patients with NSTE ACS should be individualized and dose adjusted by weight and/or creatinine clearance to reduce adverse events caused by age-related changes in pharmacokinetics/dynamics, volume of distribution, comorbidities, drug interactions, and increased drug sensitivity. (*Level of Evidence: A*)
3. Management decisions for older patients with NSTE ACS should be patient centered and consider patient preferences/goals, comorbidities, functional and cognitive status, and life expectancy. (*Level of Evidence: B*)

Data from Amsterdam EA, Wenger NK, Brindis RG, et al. 2014 AHA/ACC guideline for the management of patients with non-ST-elevation acute coronary syndromes: a report of the American College of Cardiology/American Heart Association task force on practice guidelines. J Am Coll Cardiol 2014;64:23; and Roffi M, Patrono C, Collet JP, et al. 2015 ESC guidelines for the management of acute coronary syndromes in patients presenting without persistent ST-segment elevation: task force for the management of acute coronary syndromes in patients presenting without persistent ST-segment elevation of the European Society of Cardiology (ESC). Eur Heart J 2016;37(3):267–315.

MCCs.[63] Hence, MCCs should not prompt a nihilistic approach but rather recognition of the limited evidence base for guideline-recommended treatments and the importance of individualizing clinical decision making.

SUMMARY AND FUTURE PERSPECTIVE

Patients with MCCs have worse prognosis after an ACS compared with patients without comorbid conditions, and mortality increases incrementally with each comorbid condition. Although recognition of the importance of comorbidity among ACS populations is increasing, short-term and long-term outcomes are determined by the severity of the ACS coupled with the severity of the comorbid conditions and the patient's physiologic reserve. Randomized trials should include patients with MCCs by enrolling representative older adults. Disease-based registries should collect data on an expanded list of comorbid conditions to augment information on multimorbidity in ACS populations. In addition, data on the severity of comorbidities is needed, as most studies only identify comorbidities as dichotomous variables. Long-term studies also need to incorporate new comorbidities that accrue during follow-up. With declining mortality rates from ACS, a growing number of older adults will add "prior MI" to their list of comorbid conditions. These patients will require an individualized treatment approach to optimize patient-centered outcomes for both CV and non-CV diseases.

REFERENCES

1. Barnett K, Mercer SW, Norbury M, et al. Epidemiology of multimorbidity and implications for health care, research, and medical education: a cross-sectional study. Lancet 2012;380:37–43.
2. Rocca WA, Boyd CM, Grossardt BR, et al. Prevalence of multimorbidity in a geographically defined American population: patterns by age, sex, and race/ethnicity. Mayo Clin Proc 2014;89:1336–49.

3. Koopman C, Bots ML, van Dis I, et al. Shifts in the age distribution and from acute to chronic coronary heart disease hospitalizations. Eur J Prev Cardiol 2016;23(2): 170–7.
4. Piette JD, Kerr EA. The impact of comorbid chronic conditions on diabetes care. Diabetes Care 2006;29:725–31.
5. Thygesen K, Alpert JS, Jaffe AS, et al. Third universal definition of myocardial infarction. Eur Heart J 2012;33:2551–67.
6. Alcalai R, Planer D, Culhaoglu A, et al. Acute coronary syndrome vs nonspecific troponin elevation: clinical predictors and survival analysis. Arch Intern Med 2007;167:276–81.
7. Baron T, Hambraeus K, Sundstrom J, et al. Type 2 myocardial infarction in clinical practice. Heart 2015;101:101–6.
8. Saaby L, Poulsen TS, Diederichsen AC, et al. Mortality rate in type 2 myocardial infarction: observations from an unselected hospital cohort. Am J Med 2014;127: 295–302.
9. Bortnick AE, Epps KC, Selzer F, et al. Five-year follow-up of patients treated for coronary artery disease in the face of an increasing burden of co-morbidity and disease complexity (from the NHLBI dynamic registry). Am J Cardiol 2014;113:573–9.
10. Forman DE, Chen AY, Wiviott SD, et al. Comparison of outcomes in patients aged <75, 75 to 84, and >/= 85 years with ST-elevation myocardial infarction (from the action registry-GWTG). Am J Cardiol 2010;106:1382–8.
11. McManus DD, Nguyen HL, Saczynski JS, et al. Multiple cardiovascular comorbidities and acute myocardial infarction: temporal trends (1990-2007) and impact on death rates at 30 days and 1 year. Clin Epidemiol 2012;4:115–23.
12. Alexander KP, Newby LK, Cannon CP, et al. Acute coronary care in the elderly, part i: non-ST-segment-elevation acute coronary syndromes: a scientific statement for healthcare professionals from the American Heart Association Council on Clinical Cardiology: in collaboration with the society of geriatric cardiology. Circulation 2007;115:2549–69.
13. Hutchinson-Jaffe AB, Goodman SG, Yan RT, et al. Comparison of baseline characteristics, management and outcome of patients with non-ST-segment elevation acute coronary syndrome in versus not in clinical trials. Am J Cardiol 2010;106: 1389–96.
14. Aspberg S, Stenestrand U, Koster M, et al. Large differences between patients with acute myocardial infarction included in two Swedish health registers. Scand J Public Health 2013;41:637–43.
15. McManus DD, Huang W, Domakonda KV, et al. Trends in atrial fibrillation in patients hospitalized with an acute coronary syndrome. Am J Med 2012;125: 1076–84.
16. Chamberlain AM, Gersh BJ, Mills RM, et al. Antithrombotic strategies and outcomes in acute coronary syndrome with atrial fibrillation. Am J Cardiol 2015; 115:1042–8.
17. Poci D, Hartford M, Karlsson T, et al. Effect of new versus known versus no atrial fibrillation on 30-day and 10-year mortality in patients with acute coronary syndrome. Am J Cardiol 2012;110:217–21.
18. Lopes RD, White JA, Atar D, et al. Incidence, treatment, and outcomes of atrial fibrillation complicating non-ST-segment elevation acute coronary syndromes. Int J Cardiol 2013;168:2510–7.
19. Hess CN, Peterson ED, Peng SA, et al. Use and outcomes of triple therapy among older patients with acute myocardial infarction and atrial fibrillation. J Am Coll Cardiol 2015;66:616–27.

20. Paikin JS, Wright DS, Crowther MA, et al. Triple antithrombotic therapy in patients with atrial fibrillation and coronary artery stents. Circulation 2010;121:2067–70.
21. Lawesson SS, Alfredsson J, Fredrikson M, et al. A gender perspective on short- and long term mortality in ST-elevation myocardial infarction–a report from the Swedeheart register. Int J Cardiol 2013;168:1041–7.
22. Chen HY, Saczynski JS, McManus DD, et al. The impact of cardiac and noncardiac comorbidities on the short-term outcomes of patients hospitalized with acute myocardial infarction: a population-based perspective. Clin Epidemiol 2013;5: 439–48.
23. Szummer K, Oldgren J, Lindhagen L, et al. Association between the use of fondaparinux vs low-molecular-weight heparin and clinical outcomes in patients with non-ST-segment elevation myocardial infarction. JAMA 2015;313:707–16.
24. Melloni C, Cornel JH, Hafley G, et al. Impact of chronic kidney disease on long-term ischemic and bleeding outcomes in medically managed patients with acute coronary syndromes: insights from the trilogy ACS trial. Eur Heart J Acute Cardiovasc Care 2015 [pii: 2048872615598631].
25. Alexander KP, Chen AY, Roe MT, et al. Excess dosing of antiplatelet and antithrombin agents in the treatment of non-ST-segment elevation acute coronary syndromes. JAMA 2005;294:3108–16.
26. Zhu J, Fang F, Sjolander A, et al. Myocardial infarction or mental disorders after cancer diagnosis and cancer-specific survival. Psychoneuroendocrinology 2015;61:8.
27. Mulrooney DA, Yeazel MW, Kawashima T, et al. Cardiac outcomes in a cohort of adult survivors of childhood and adolescent cancer: retrospective analysis of the childhood cancer survivor study cohort. BMJ 2009;339:b4606.
28. Alfredsson J, Stenestrand U, Wallentin L, et al. Gender differences in management and outcome in non-ST-elevation acute coronary syndrome. Heart 2007;93: 1357–62.
29. Radovanovic D, Seifert B, Urban P, et al. Validity of Charlson Comorbidity Index in patients hospitalised with acute coronary syndrome. Insights from the nationwide AMIS plus registry 2002-2012. Heart 2014;100:288–94.
30. Herrmann J, Lerman A, Sandhu NP, et al. Evaluation and management of patients with heart disease and cancer: cardio-oncology. Mayo Clin Proc 2014;89: 1287–306.
31. Hanna EB, Alexander KP, Chen AY, et al. Characteristics and in-hospital outcomes of patients with non-ST-segment elevation myocardial infarction undergoing an invasive strategy according to hemoglobin levels. Am J Cardiol 2013; 111:1099–103.
32. Lawler PR, Filion KB, Dourian T, et al. Anemia and mortality in acute coronary syndromes: a systematic review and meta-analysis. Am Heart J 2013;165: 143–53.
33. Mathews R, Peterson ED, Chen AY, et al. In-hospital major bleeding during ST-elevation and non-ST-elevation myocardial infarction care: derivation and validation of a model from the action registry(r)-GWTG. Am J Cardiol 2011;107: 1136–43.
34. Mehran R, Pocock SJ, Nikolsky E, et al. A risk score to predict bleeding in patients with acute coronary syndromes. J Am Coll Cardiol 2010;55:2556–66.
35. Subherwal S, Bach RG, Chen AY, et al. Baseline risk of major bleeding in non-ST-segment-elevation myocardial infarction: the crusade (can rapid risk stratification of unstable angina patients suppress adverse outcomes with early

implementation of the ACC/AHA guidelines) bleeding score. Circulation 2009; 119:1873–82.

36. Eikelboom JW, Mehta SR, Anand SS, et al. Adverse impact of bleeding on prognosis in patients with acute coronary syndromes. Circulation 2006;114:774–82.
37. Lopes RD, Subherwal S, Holmes DN, et al. The association of in-hospital major bleeding with short-, intermediate-, and long-term mortality among older patients with non-ST-segment elevation myocardial infarction. Eur Heart J 2012;33: 2044–53.
38. Rao SV, O'Grady K, Pieper KS, et al. Impact of bleeding severity on clinical outcomes among patients with acute coronary syndromes. Am J Cardiol 2005; 96:1200–6.
39. Salisbury AC, Alexander KP, Reid KJ, et al. Incidence, correlates, and outcomes of acute, hospital-acquired anemia in patients with acute myocardial infarction. Circ Cardiovasc Qual Outcomes 2010;3:337–46.
40. Rothnie KJ, Yan R, Smeeth L, et al. Risk of myocardial infarction (MI) and death following MI in people with chronic obstructive pulmonary disease (COPD): a systematic review and meta-analysis. BMJ Open 2015;5:e007824.
41. Andell P, Koul S, Martinsson A, et al. Impact of chronic obstructive pulmonary disease on morbidity and mortality after myocardial infarction. Open Heart 2014;1: e000002.
42. Singh-Manoux A, Sabia S, Lajnef M, et al. History of coronary heart disease and cognitive performance in midlife: the Whitehall II study. Eur Heart J 2008;29: 2100–7.
43. Lin CF, Wu FL, Lin SW, et al. Age, dementia and care patterns after admission for acute coronary syndrome: an analysis from a nationwide cohort under the national health insurance coverage. Drugs Aging 2012;29:819–28.
44. Gharacholou SM, Reid KJ, Arnold SV, et al. Cognitive impairment and outcomes in older adult survivors of acute myocardial infarction: findings from the translational research investigating underlying disparities in acute myocardial infarction patients' health status registry. Am Heart J 2011;162:860–9.
45. Tehrani DM, Darki L, Erande A, et al. In-hospital mortality and coronary procedure use for individuals with dementia with acute myocardial infarction in the United States. J Am Geriatr Soc 2013;61:1932–6.
46. Lichtman JH, Froelicher ES, Blumenthal JA, et al. Depression as a risk factor for poor prognosis among patients with acute coronary syndrome: systematic review and recommendations: a scientific statement from the American Heart Association. Circulation 2014;129:1350–69.
47. Radholm K, Wirehn AB, Chalmers J, et al. Use of antidiabetic and antidepressant drugs is associated with increased risk of myocardial infarction: a nationwide register study. Diabet Med 2015;2:12822.
48. Smolderen KG, Strait KM, Dreyer RP, et al. Depressive symptoms in younger women and men with acute myocardial infarction: insights from the VIRGO study. J Am Heart Assoc 2015;4:e001424.
49. Ahmedani BK, Solberg LI, Copeland LA, et al. Psychiatric comorbidity and 30-day readmissions after hospitalization for heart failure, AMI, and pneumonia. Psychiatr Serv 2015;66:134–40.
50. Rumsfeld JS, Alexander KP, Goff DC Jr, et al. Cardiovascular health: the importance of measuring patient-reported health status: a scientific statement from the American Heart Association. Circulation 2013;127:2233–49.

51. Charlson ME, Pompei P, Ales KL, et al. A new method of classifying prognostic comorbidity in longitudinal studies: development and validation. J Chronic Dis 1987;40:373–83.
52. Erickson SR, Cole E, Kline-Rogers E, et al. The addition of the Charlson Comorbidity Index to the grace risk prediction index improves prediction of outcomes in acute coronary syndrome. Popul Health Manag 2014;17:54–9.
53. Boyd CM, Darer J, Boult C, et al. Clinical practice guidelines and quality of care for older patients with multiple comorbid diseases: implications for pay for performance. JAMA 2005;294:716–24.
54. Boyd CM, Leff B, Wolff JL, et al. Informing clinical practice guideline development and implementation: prevalence of coexisting conditions among adults with coronary heart disease. J Am Geriatr Soc 2011;59:797–805.
55. Parekh AK, Barton MB. The challenge of multiple comorbidity for the US health care system. JAMA 2010;303:1303–4.
56. Blicher TM, Hommel K, Olesen JB, et al. Less use of standard guideline-based treatment of myocardial infarction in patients with chronic kidney disease: a Danish nation-wide cohort study. Eur Heart J 2013;34:2916–23.
57. Bursi F, Vassallo R, Weston SA, et al. Chronic obstructive pulmonary disease after myocardial infarction in the community. Am Heart J 2010;160:95–101.
58. Norhammar A, Lindback J, Ryden L, et al. Improved but still high short- and long-term mortality rates after myocardial infarction in patients with diabetes mellitus: a time-trend report from the Swedish register of information and knowledge about Swedish heart intensive care admission. Heart 2007;93:1577–83.
59. Amsterdam EA, Wenger NK, Brindis RG, et al. 2014 AHA/ACC guideline for the management of patients with non-ST-elevation acute coronary syndromes: a report of the American College of Cardiology/American Heart Association task force on practice guidelines. J Am Coll Cardiol 2014;64:23.
60. Roffi M, Patrono C, Collet JP, et al. 2015 ESC guidelines for the management of acute coronary syndromes in patients presenting without persistent ST-segment elevation: task force for the management of acute coronary syndromes in patients presenting without persistent ST-segment elevation of the European Society of Cardiology (ESC). Eur Heart J 2016;37(3):267–315.
61. Guiding principles for the care of older adults with multimorbidity: an approach for clinicians. Guiding principles for the care of older adults with multimorbidity: an approach for clinicians: American Geriatrics Society expert panel on the care of older adults with multimorbidity. J Am Geriatr Soc 2012;60:E1–25.
62. Rosamond WD, Chambless LE, Heiss G, et al. Twenty-two-year trends in incidence of myocardial infarction, coronary heart disease mortality, and case fatality in 4 US communities, 1987-2008. Circulation 2012;125:1848–57.
63. Gili M, Sala J, Lopez J, et al. Impact of comorbidities on in-hospital mortality from acute myocardial infarction, 2003-2009. Rev Esp Cardiol 2011;64:1130–7 [in Spanish].
64. Paixao AR, Enriquez JR, Wang TY, et al. Risk factor burden and control at the time of admission in patients with acute myocardial infarction: results from the NCDR. Am Heart J 2015;170:173–9.
65. Yeh RW, Sidney S, Chandra M, et al. Population trends in the incidence and outcomes of acute myocardial infarction. N Engl J Med 2010;362:2155–65.
66. Hubacek J, Galbraith PD, Gao M, et al. External validation of a percutaneous coronary intervention mortality prediction model in patients with acute coronary syndromes. Am Heart J 2006;151:308–15.

67. Kook HY, Jeong MH, Oh S, et al. Current trend of acute myocardial infarction in Korea (from the Korea Acute Myocardial Infarction Registry from 2006 to 2013). Am J Cardiol 2014;114:1817–22.
68. Gyenes GT, Yan AT, Tan M, et al. Use and timing of coronary angiography and associated in-hospital outcomes in Canadian non-ST-segment elevation myocardial infarction patients: insights from the Canadian Global Registry of acute coronary events. Can J Cardiol 2013;29:1429–35.

Multimorbidity in Older Adults with Aortic Stenosis

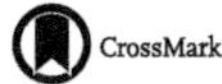

Brian R. Lindman, MD, MS[a,*], Jay N. Patel, MD[b]

KEYWORDS

- Aortic stenosis • Multimorbidity • Comorbidity • Geriatrics • Frailty
- Cardiovascular disease • Transcatheter aortic valve replacement • Cardiac surgery

KEY POINTS

- Medical and aging-related comorbidities are very common in older patients with calcific aortic stenosis.
- Clinicians increasingly face challenging scenarios that result from the intersection of aortic stenosis and multiple comorbidities.
- Medical and aging-related comorbidities influence health status, interpretation of the presence and etiology of symptoms, estimates of procedural risk, and anticipated benefit from valve replacement.
- The number, type, and severity of comorbidities substantially influence the evaluation, management, and treatment of patients with aortic stenosis.
- Awareness and incorporation of the influence of comorbidities on outcomes after valve replacement is critical to treating the patient and not just fixing the valve.

INTRODUCTION

Calcific aortic stenosis (AS) is generally a disease of older adults. A recent metaanalysis of 7 population-based studies from Europe and North America found that the prevalence of AS in persons greater than 75 years of age was 12.4% and the prevalence of severe AS was 3.4%.[1] As the population ages, the absolute number of patients with significant AS will increase substantially.

Within the aortic valve leaflets, an active biological process occurs to cause fibrosis and calcification, leading to restricted leaflet motion.[2] As the aortic valve becomes progressively obstructed, maintenance of cardiac output imposes a chronic increase in left ventricular pressure that leads to hypertrophic ventricular remodeling and

Disclosures: Dr B.R. Lindman has received a research grant and serves on the scientific advisory board for Roche Diagnostics. This work was supported by NIH K23 HL116660.

[a] Cardiovascular Division, Washington University School of Medicine, Campus Box 8086, 660 South Euclid Avenue, St Louis, MO 63110, USA; [b] Department of Medicine, Washington University School of Medicine, 660 South Euclid Avenue, Campus Box 8121, St Louis, MO 63110, USA

* Corresponding author.

E-mail address: blindman@dom.wustl.edu

Clin Geriatr Med 32 (2016) 305–314

http://dx.doi.org/10.1016/j.cger.2016.01.006 geriatric.theclinics.com

eventually diastolic and systolic dysfunction.[3,4] Symptoms such as shortness of breath and chest pain can be disabling, markedly reduce quality of life, and are associated with an average life expectancy of 2 to 3 years.[5–7] The only effective treatment for symptomatic severe AS is valve replacement.[3,8] However, surgery has significant risks, including stroke and death, and at least one-third of patients do not undergo surgery owing largely to advanced age, left ventricular dysfunction, or associated comorbidities.[5,9,10]

Recently, a less invasive approach to valve replacement using balloons and catheters—transcatheter aortic valve replacement (TAVR)—has been introduced as a viable alternative for patients at high or prohibitive risk for surgery.[11–14] TAVR has been a transformative innovation, allowing for the treatment of many patients who previously did not have a therapeutic option. Based on current regulatory approval indications, recent estimates indicate that there are approximately 300,000 TAVR candidates in Europe and North America and almost 30,000 new TAVR candidates annually.[1] As indications for TAVR (based mostly on estimates of operative risk) are lowered, this number will increase substantially.

Primarily because of 2 forces—the aging of the population and the emergence of TAVR as a therapeutic option—clinicians increasingly face challenging scenarios that result from the intersection of AS and multiple comorbidities. These include multiple medical comorbidities as well as numerous aging-related, or geriatric, comorbidities. AS is often conceptualized as a mechanical problem (valve obstruction) requiring a mechanical solution (valve replacement). There can be a myopic focus on the valve as the singular cause of the patient's impairments (eg, shortness of breath); accordingly, it is often assumed that once the valve is fixed, the patient's symptoms will resolve and quality of life improve. The frequent occurrence of multiple, often severe, comorbidities influences—sometimes dramatically—this linear, simple diagnostic and treatment framework. Indeed, among patients with AS, medical and aging-related comorbidities influence health status, the determination of whether symptoms related to AS are present, estimates of procedural risk, and anticipated benefit from valve replacement. In short, these comorbidities are common and introduce a significant degree of complexity into the evaluation, management, and treatment of patients with AS.

Herein, we review the aging-related and medical comorbidities commonly coexistent in patients with AS (**Table 1**). Their prevalence and impact on clinical outcomes

Table 1
Prevalence of geriatric and medical comorbidities in aortic stenosis

Condition	Prevalence (%)[a]
Disability	5–76
Frailty	20–84
Cognitive impairment	28–45
Chronic obstructive pulmonary disease	8–59
Pulmonary hypertension	47–65
Chronic kidney disease	3–57
End-stage renal disease	2–4
Chronic liver disease	2–3
Anemia	49–64
Diabetes	20–42

[a] Prevalence is highly dependent on the population examined and the definition used for the condition, particularly for disability and frailty.

depends on the population of patients with AS examined. Specifically, studies examining patients evaluated for and treated with TAVR include older patients with more numerous and more severe comorbidities. In that regard, where possible, we tried to include data from multiple different AS populations to provide perspective on the range of comorbidity prevalence and clinical effects.

GERIATRIC OR AGING-RELATED COMORBIDITIES

Frailty

Frailty is a geriatric syndrome characterized by an increased vulnerability to stressors owing to impairments in multiple organ systems, particularly the cardiovascular and musculoskeletal systems.[15,16] Although frailty is a "system-wide" syndrome, there is mounting evidence for a bidirectional relationship between cardiovascular disease and frailty.[17] As such, frailty is not necessarily separate and distinct from AS. Rather, the heart failure that results from severe AS may impair functionality, mobility, eating habits, and so on in ways that contribute to the development or progression of frailty. Conversely, frailty may influence the timing of symptom onset, the severity of the clinical presentation, and the response to valve replacement in a patient with significant AS. These issues remain to be elucidated.

Until the emergence of TAVR, frailty was largely incorporated into clinical decision making in the form of a subjective "eye-ball test." Owing to the general recognition that frailty is common and likely affects clinical outcomes, there is rapidly growing interest in how to incorporate the concept of frailty into risk assessment and treatment decisions for patients with AS.[8,18,19] Based on different definitions of frailty and the population examined, the prevalence of frailty in patients with severe AS ranges from approximately 20% to 84%.[13,20–23]

Some studies suggest that a single test, most commonly the 5-m gait speed, provides the best prediction of clinical events after valve replacement, whereas others suggest that an integrated frailty score has greater prognostic utility.[20,24] In patients greater than 70 years of age referred for cardiac surgery, including valve surgery, a 5-m gait time of greater than 6 seconds (46% of patients) was associated with a 3-fold increased hazard of in-hospital morbidity and mortality after adjustment for the Society of Thoracic Surgeons Predicted Risk of Mortality or Major Morbidity (STS-PROMM).[25] In a recent TAVR trial enrolling patients at prohibitive risk for surgery, 84% of patients had a 5-m gait time of greater than 6 seconds.[13] A slower timed get up and go test and worse nutrition have also been associated with worse 30-day and 1-year mortality and cardiovascular event rates.[23] Among patients treated with TAVR, frailty as determined by an integrative score was associated with a 2.5-fold increased adjusted hazard of 1-year mortality and a higher 1-year rate of "poor outcome" (integrating mortality and quality of life).[26]

Beyond predicting increased mortality and cardiovascular event rates, frailty before TAVR predicts greater functional decline and loss of independence after TAVR.[22] Among patients greater than 70 years of age undergoing TAVR, functional decline at 6 months after TAVR (defined as dependence for $\geq$1 basic activities of daily living compared with before TAVR) occurred in 21% of patients. A multidimensional frailty score was able to predict this functional decline, whereas clinical risk scores such as the STS and EuroSCORE were not. This has important implications for predicting outcomes that matter to patients.

Across varying definitions of frailty, there is a consistent association between frailty and worse clinical outcomes after TAVR, including procedural morbidity and mortality, longer term mortality, and progressive loss of independence. Frailty is generally not correlated with other clinical risk scores, so it adds new information to risk prediction.[23,25] Elucidating how frailty should be incorporated into risk stratification and treatment decisions is an active area of ongoing research.[18,19]

Disability

The prevalence of disability in patients with AS also depends on the definition or instrument used and the population assessed. Among patients greater than 70 years of age referred for cardiac surgery, the rate of having any disability was 5% using the basic activities of daily living scale, 32% using the instrumental activities of daily living scale, and 76% using the more sensitive Nagi scale.[20] Three or more disabilities (out of 7) on the Nagi scale was associated with a 3-fold higher unadjusted hazard of in-hospital morbidity or mortality. Among patients treated with TAVR, 23% to 29% were dependent for 1 or more basic activities of daily living.[22,24,26] In an inoperable TAVR trial cohort, 21% were dependent for 2 or more and 14% were dependent for 3 or more basic activities of daily living.[13] Among patients treated with TAVR, an increasing degree of dependence for basic activities of daily living is associated with increased 30-day and 1-year mortality.[23] Patients with AS undergoing TAVR also have a relatively high rate of mobility impairment. In 1 study, 25% of patients could not perform a 6-minute walk test.[26] In an inoperable cohort of patients, 18% had experienced a fall in the last 6 months.[13]

Cognitive Impairment

The prevalence of cognitive impairment in patients with AS undergoing TAVR has been reported to be 28% to 45%.[13,22,23,27] In a large cohort of 2137 patients from the Placement of Aortic Transcatheter Valve (PARTNER) trial, each 1-point decrease in the Mini-Mental Status Examination score was associated with higher odds of poor 6-month and 1-year clinical outcomes.[28] Other studies also show an association between cognitive impairment and increased mortality after TAVR and surgical aortic valve replacement (AVR).[23,29] Schoenenberger and colleagues[22] showed an association between cognitive impairment before TAVR and greater dependence in basic activities of daily living 6 months after TAVR. Whether transcatheter versus surgical AVR has a differential impact on postprocedure cognitive function and whether embolic protection devices during TAVR can decrease postprocedure cognitive decline remain to be determined.

MEDICAL COMORBIDITIES

Chronic Obstructive Pulmonary Disease

The presence and severity of associated lung disease influences the management, treatment, and outcomes of patients with AS.[3] In patients with significant lung disease, it can be difficult to discern whether symptoms of shortness of breath are owing to the AS, lung disease, or a combination of both. The prevalence of lung disease ranges from less than 10% in those undergoing surgical AVR to almost 60% in inoperable patients undergoing TAVR.[11,13,30,31] Among patients treated with TAVR, up to 30% have oxygen-dependent lung disease.[13]

In a study of 2553 patients included in the PARTNER trial, chronic obstructive pulmonary disease (COPD) was present in 43% and was associated with increased 1-year mortality (23.4% vs 19.6%; $P = .02$).[31] Among those with COPD, oxygen dependence and poor mobility were each associated independently with increased mortality. These findings are supported by large TAVR registry studies from the United States, United Kingdom, and France.[32–34] COPD has also been shown to be an independent risk factor for mortality among patients treated with surgical AVR.[35]

Pulmonary Hypertension

Pulmonary hypertension (PH) is present in 50% to 65% of patients with severe AS and is classified as severe in up to 15% to 25%.[30,36–38] In patients treated with surgical AVR or TAVR, PH has been associated with increased mortality, morbidity, and resource use after valve replacement.[30,37–40] Among patients with moderate or severe PH treated with TAVR, oxygen-dependent lung disease, inability to perform a 6-minute walk, impaired renal function, and lower aortic valve mean gradient were independently associated with increased 1-year mortality.[38] A risk score including these factors was able to identify patients with a 15% versus 59% 1-year mortality. There are somewhat conflicting data as to whether an increased pulmonary vascular resistance exacerbates the risk associated with an increased pulmonary artery systolic pressure.[38,41] In asymptomatic patients with severe AS, exercise-induced PH is associated with increased cardiac event rates during follow-up.[42]

Chronic Kidney Disease

The prevalence of chronic kidney disease depends on the definition used and specific AS population studied, but ranges from less than 10% to greater than 50%.[12,34,43,44] Chronic kidney disease is associated with increased mortality after TAVR and surgical AVR.[33,45,46] End-stage renal disease is less common but occurs in 2% of surgical AVRs and up to 4% of patients in the US TAVR registry, where it is associated with a 66% increase in the hazard of 1-year mortality.[34,46] Acute kidney injury after valve replacement is also associated with increased mortality and may occur less commonly after TAVR compared with surgical AVR.[14,47]

Chronic Liver Disease

Chronic liver disease is relatively uncommon in patients treated for AS; in the recent PARTNER and CoreValve trials, it was 2% to 3%.[12,13] Nevertheless, it was associated with a 2-fold greater adjusted hazard of mortality in the overall study cohort treated with surgical AVR or TAVR.[45] Other studies have demonstrated that liver disease is associated with increased risk of early mortality after TAVR.[48] Larger studies are needed to elucidate how the severity of liver disease affects periprocedural morbidity and early and late mortality.

Anemia

The prevalence of anemia in many TAVR-treated populations is greater than 50%.[49–51] In a multicenter study of 1696 TAVR patients, preoperative anemia was independently associated with increased 1-year mortality, particularly in those with preoperative hemoglobin less than 10 g/dL (hazard ratio, 2.78; 95% CI, 1.60–4.82).[50] Anemia is also associated with worse functional status and quality of life before and after TAVR.[51]

Diabetes Mellitus

The prevalence of diabetes mellitus in patients with AS has increased over time and is as high as 42% in recent, older, higher risk cohorts.[13,14,46,52] Many studies have demonstrated that diabetes is associated with increased mortality after surgical AVR or TAVR.[33,53,54] According to a post hoc analysis of PARTNER trial patients, there was a survival benefit, no increase in stroke, and less renal failure in diabetic patients treated with TAVR compared with surgical AVR.[52] However, this survival benefit with TAVR among diabetic patients was not observed in the CoreValve subgroup analysis.[14]

Cardiac and Vascular Comorbidities

There is a very high prevalence of associated cardiac and vascular comorbidities in patients with AS, including heart failure, atrial arrhythmias, hypertension, coronary artery disease, cerebrovascular disease, and peripheral vascular disease. A detailed treatment of these comorbidities is beyond the scope of this paper. The presence and severity of each of them contributes to the procedural and long-term risk of patients treated with surgical or transcatheter valve replacement. Coronary disease, in particular, adds complexity to management decisions regarding whether, when, and how to revascularize a patient with severe AS.[55]

COMORBIDITIES AND THE EVALUATION AND TREATMENT OF AORTIC STENOSIS

The number, type, and severity of comorbidities substantially influence the evaluation, management, and treatment of patients with AS. As documented, comorbidities—and often many of them together—are common in patients with AS. They can make it difficult to distinguish the "asymptomatic" from the "symptomatic" patient. An older adult may curtail certain activities and attribute developing limitations to "normal aging" when in fact they are signs of new-onset heart failure. In contrast, a patient with limited mobility, deconditioning, and oxygen-dependent lung disease may be short of breath for several reasons, making it difficult to ascribe symptoms to the AS. Moreover, the relative contribution of AS versus associated comorbidities to a patient's health status can be difficult to discern. This is important and relevant because it likely has implications for the anticipated benefit that will accrue from valve replacement. Thus, patients whose symptoms are largely unrelated to AS are unlikely to derive significant benefit from valve replacement. Finally, the number and severity of associated comorbidities has implications for procedural risk from valve replacement and for whether a transcatheter or surgical approach is most appropriate.

The emergence of TAVR as a treatment option for patients with AS at increased surgical risk has coincided with the emergence of multidisciplinary heart valve teams as the centerpiece for making these complex and challenging management and treatment decisions.[8,56,57] Relevant to our focus here, it is clear that the number and severity of medical and geriatric comorbidities must be incorporated into the decision-making process about whether and how the valve should be replaced.[8,18,56] We have moved beyond the "eye-ball test" to incorporate aging-related comorbidities into our decision-making process; multiple objective tests of frailty and disability have been shown to improve risk prediction estimates beyond clinical factors alone.[19,23,25] Nonetheless, further studies are needed to elucidate how these factors should be considered in our treatment decisions.

TAVR has been a life-saving therapy for many who were previously not treated for their AS. However, even after TAVR, up to 30% of these patients are dead by 1 year and 20% survive but have no significant improvement in their quality of life.[11,18,58] Further, it is clear that medical and aging-related comorbidities substantially influence these outcomes. Moving forward, we need to develop new and better ways to incorporate comorbidities not only into our procedural risk estimates, but into our assessment of the likelihood for longer term benefit (defined holistically) from valve replacement.[18] How and to what extent various comorbidities influence survival after valve replacement, quality of life, repeat hospitalizations, and functionality requires further study. Ultimately, we need to consider how to treat the whole patient, not just a mechanical problem with a mechanical solution.

SUMMARY

AS is a disease of older adults, most of whom have associated medical and aging-related comorbidities. With the aging of the population and the emergence of TAVR as a treatment option, clinicians will increasingly be confronted with the intersection of AS and multimorbidity. This convergence makes the evaluation, management, and treatment of AS more complex in multiple ways. To optimize patient-centered clinical outcomes, new treatment paradigms are needed that recognize the import and influence of multimorbidity on patients with AS. The simplistic framework of a mechanical solution for a mechanical problem must be replaced by a more refined, nuanced, and holistic treatment paradigm.

REFERENCES

1. Osnabrugge RL, Mylotte D, Head SJ, et al. Aortic stenosis in the elderly: disease prevalence and number of candidates for transcatheter aortic valve replacement: a meta-analysis and modeling study. J Am Coll Cardiol 2013;62:1002–12.
2. Miller JD, Weiss RM, Heistad DD. Calcific aortic valve stenosis: methods, models, and mechanisms. Circ Res 2011;108:1392–412.
3. Lindman BR, Bonow RO, Otto CM. Current management of calcific aortic stenosis. Circ Res 2013;113:223–37.
4. Otto CM, Prendergast B. Aortic-valve stenosis–from patients at risk to severe valve obstruction. N Engl J Med 2014;371:744–56.
5. Bach DS, Siao D, Girard SE, et al. Evaluation of patients with severe symptomatic aortic stenosis who do not undergo aortic valve replacement: the potential role of subjectively overestimated operative risk. Circ Cardiovasc Qual Outcomes 2009; 2:533–9.
6. Ross J Jr, Braunwald E. Aortic stenosis. Circulation 1968;38:61–7.
7. Schwarz F, Baumann P, Manthey J, et al. The effect of aortic valve replacement on survival. Circulation 1982;66:1105–10.
8. Nishimura RA, Otto CM, Bonow RO, et al. 2014 AHA/ACC guideline for the management of patients with valvular heart disease: a Report of the American College of Cardiology/American Heart Association Task force on Practice Guidelines. Circulation 2014;129:e521–643.
9. Iung B, Baron G, Butchart EG, et al. A prospective survey of patients with valvular heart disease in Europe: the Euro Heart Survey on Valvular Heart Disease. Eur Heart J 2003;24:1231–43.
10. Iung B, Cachier A, Baron G, et al. Decision-making in elderly patients with severe aortic stenosis: why are so many denied surgery? Eur Heart J 2005;26:2714–20.
11. Leon MB, Smith CR, Mack M, et al. Transcatheter aortic-valve implantation for aortic stenosis in patients who cannot undergo surgery. N Engl J Med 2010; 363:1597–607.
12. Smith CR, Leon MB, Mack MJ, et al. Transcatheter versus surgical aortic-valve replacement in high-risk patients. N Engl J Med 2011;364:2187–98.
13. Popma JJ, Adams DH, Reardon MJ, et al. Transcatheter aortic valve replacement using a self-expanding bioprosthesis in patients with severe aortic stenosis at extreme risk for surgery. J Am Coll Cardiol 2014;63:1972–81.
14. Adams DH, Popma JJ, Reardon MJ, et al. Transcatheter aortic-valve replacement with a self-expanding prosthesis. N Engl J Med 2014;370:1790–8.
15. Bergman H, Ferrucci L, Guralnik J, et al. Frailty: an emerging research and clinical paradigm–issues and controversies. J Gerontol A Biol Sci Med Sci 2007;62:731–7.

16. Fried LP, Tangen CM, Walston J, et al. Frailty in older adults: evidence for a phenotype. J Gerontol A Biol Sci Med Sci 2001;56:M146–56.
17. Flint K. Which came first, the frailty or the heart disease? Exploring the vicious cycle. J Am Coll Cardiol 2015;65:984–6.
18. Lindman BR, Alexander KP, O'Gara PT, et al. Futility, benefit, and transcatheter aortic valve replacement. JACC Cardiovasc Interv 2014;7:707–16.
19. Afilalo J, Alexander KP, Mack MJ, et al. Frailty assessment in the cardiovascular care of older adults. J Am Coll Cardiol 2014;63:747–62.
20. Afilalo J, Mottillo S, Eisenberg MJ, et al. Addition of frailty and disability to cardiac surgery risk scores identifies elderly patients at high risk of mortality or major morbidity. Circ Cardiovasc Qual Outcomes 2012;5:222–8.
21. Ewe SH, Ajmone Marsan N, Pepi M, et al. Impact of left ventricular systolic function on clinical and echocardiographic outcomes following transcatheter aortic valve implantation for severe aortic stenosis. Am Heart J 2010;160:1113–20.
22. Schoenenberger AW, Stortecky S, Neumann S, et al. Predictors of functional decline in elderly patients undergoing transcatheter aortic valve implantation (TAVI). Eur Heart J 2013;34:684–92.
23. Stortecky S, Schoenenberger AW, Moser A, et al. Evaluation of multidimensional geriatric assessment as a predictor of mortality and cardiovascular events after transcatheter aortic valve implantation. JACC Cardiovasc Interv 2012;5:489–96.
24. Green P, Woglom AE, Genereux P, et al. The impact of frailty status on survival after transcatheter aortic valve replacement in older adults with severe aortic stenosis: a single-center experience. JACC Cardiovasc Interv 2012;5:974–81.
25. Afilalo J, Eisenberg MJ, Morin JF, et al. Gait speed as an incremental predictor of mortality and major morbidity in elderly patients undergoing cardiac surgery. J Am Coll Cardiol 2010;56:1668–76.
26. Green P, Arnold SV, Cohen DJ, et al. Relation of frailty to outcomes after transcatheter aortic valve replacement (from the PARTNER trial). Am J Cardiol 2015; 116:264–9.
27. Zanettini R, Gatto G, Mori I, et al. Cardiac rehabilitation and mid-term follow-up after transcatheter aortic valve implantation. J Geriatr Cardiol 2014;11:279–85.
28. Arnold SV, Reynolds MR, Lei Y, et al. Predictors of poor outcomes after transcatheter aortic valve replacement: results from the PARTNER (Placement of Aortic Transcatheter Valve) trial. Circulation 2014;129:2682–90.
29. Eleid MF, Michelena HI, Nkomo VT, et al. Causes of death and predictors of survival after aortic valve replacement in low flow vs. normal flow severe aortic stenosis with preserved ejection fraction. Eur Heart J Cardiovasc Imaging 2015;16(11):1270–5.
30. Melby SJ, Moon MR, Lindman BR, et al. Impact of pulmonary hypertension on outcomes after aortic valve replacement for aortic valve stenosis. J Thorac Cardiovasc Surg 2011;141:1424–30.
31. Dvir D, Waksman R, Barbash IM, et al. Outcomes of patients with chronic lung disease and severe aortic stenosis treated with transcatheter versus surgical aortic valve replacement or standard therapy: insights from the PARTNER trial (placement of AoRTic TraNscathetER Valve). J Am Coll Cardiol 2014;63:269–79.
32. Chopard R, Meneveau N, Chocron S, et al. Impact of chronic obstructive pulmonary disease on Valve Academic Research Consortium-defined outcomes after transcatheter aortic valve implantation (from the FRANCE 2 Registry). Am J Cardiol 2014;113:1543–9.
33. Ludman PF, Moat N, de Belder MA, et al. Transcatheter aortic valve implantation in the United Kingdom: temporal trends, predictors of outcome, and 6-year

follow-up: a report from the UK Transcatheter Aortic Valve Implantation (TAVI) registry, 2007 to 2012. Circulation 2015;131:1181–90.

34. Holmes DR Jr, Brennan JM, Rumsfeld JS, et al. Clinical outcomes at 1 year following transcatheter aortic valve replacement. JAMA 2015;313:1019–28.
35. Iturra SA, Suri RM, Greason KL, et al. Outcomes of surgical aortic valve replacement in moderate risk patients: implications for determination of equipoise in the transcatheter era. J Thorac Cardiovasc Surg 2014;147:127–32.
36. Faggiano P, Antonini-Canterin F, Ribichini F, et al. Pulmonary artery hypertension in adult patients with symptomatic valvular aortic stenosis. Am J Cardiol 2000;85: 204–8.
37. Roselli EE, Abdel Azim A, Houghtaling PL, et al. Pulmonary hypertension is associated with worse early and late outcomes after aortic valve replacement: implications for transcatheter aortic valve replacement. J Thorac Cardiovasc Surg 2012;144:1067–74.e2.
38. Lindman BR, Zajarias A, Maniar HS, et al. Risk stratification in patients with pulmonary hypertension undergoing transcatheter aortic valve replacement. Heart 2015;101:1656–64.
39. Lucon A, Oger E, Bedossa M, et al. Prognostic implications of pulmonary hypertension in patients with severe aortic stenosis undergoing transcatheter aortic valve implantation: study from the FRANCE 2 registry. Circ Cardiovasc Interv 2014;7:240–7.
40. Rodes-Cabau J, Webb JG, Cheung A, et al. Transcatheter aortic valve implantation for the treatment of severe symptomatic aortic stenosis in patients at very high or prohibitive surgical risk: acute and late outcomes of the multicenter Canadian experience. J Am Coll Cardiol 2010;55:1080–90.
41. O'Sullivan CJ, Wenaweser P, Ceylan O, et al. Effect of pulmonary hypertension hemodynamic presentation on clinical outcomes in patients with severe symptomatic aortic valve stenosis undergoing transcatheter aortic valve implantation: insights from the new proposed pulmonary hypertension classification. Circ Cardiovasc Interv 2015;8:e002358.
42. Lancellotti P, Magne J, Donal E, et al. Determinants and prognostic significance of exercise pulmonary hypertension in asymptomatic severe aortic stenosis. Circulation 2012;126:851–9.
43. Faggiano P, Frattini S, Zilioli V, et al. Prevalence of comorbidities and associated cardiac diseases in patients with valve aortic stenosis. Potential implications for the decision-making process. Int J Cardiol 2012;159:94–9.
44. Di Eusanio M, Fortuna D, De Palma R, et al. Aortic valve replacement: results and predictors of mortality from a contemporary series of 2256 patients. J Thorac Cardiovasc Surg 2011;141:940–7.
45. Mack MJ, Leon MB, Smith CR, et al. 5-year outcomes of transcatheter aortic valve replacement or surgical aortic valve replacement for high surgical risk patients with aortic stenosis (PARTNER 1): a randomised controlled trial. Lancet 2015; 385(9986):2477–84.
46. Brown JM, O'Brien SM, Wu C, et al. Isolated aortic valve replacement in North America comprising 108,687 patients in 10 years: changes in risks, valve types, and outcomes in the Society of Thoracic Surgeons National Database. J Thorac Cardiovasc Surg 2009;137:82–90.
47. Bagur R, Webb JG, Nietlispach F, et al. Acute kidney injury following transcatheter aortic valve implantation: predictive factors, prognostic value, and comparison with surgical aortic valve replacement. Eur Heart J 2010;31:865–74.

48. Beohar N, Zajarias A, Thourani VH, et al. Analysis of early out-of hospital mortality after transcatheter aortic valve implantation among patients with aortic stenosis successfully discharged from the hospital and alive at 30 days (from the placement of aortic transcatheter valves trial). Am J Cardiol 2014;114:1550–5.
49. Capodanno D, Barbanti M, Tamburino C, et al. A simple risk tool (the OBSERVANT score) for prediction of 30-day mortality after transcatheter aortic valve replacement. Am J Cardiol 2014;113:1851–8.
50. Nuis RJ, Sinning JM, Rodes-Cabau J, et al. Prevalence, factors associated with, and prognostic effects of preoperative anemia on short- and long-term mortality in patients undergoing transcatheter aortic valve implantation. Circ Cardiovasc Interv 2013;6:625–34.
51. DeLarochelliere H, Urena M, Amat-Santos IJ, et al. Effect on outcomes and exercise performance of anemia in patients with aortic stenosis who underwent transcatheter aortic valve replacement. Am J Cardiol 2015;115:472–9.
52. Lindman BR, Pibarot P, Arnold SV, et al. Transcatheter versus surgical aortic valve replacement in patients with diabetes and severe aortic stenosis at high risk for surgery: an analysis of the PARTNER trial (placement of aortic transcatheter valve). J Am Coll Cardiol 2014;63:1090–9.
53. Halkos ME, Kilgo P, Lattouf OM, et al. The effect of diabetes mellitus on in-hospital and long-term outcomes after heart valve operations. Ann Thorac Surg 2010;90: 124–30.
54. Tamburino C, Capodanno D, Ramondo A, et al. Incidence and predictors of early and late mortality after transcatheter aortic valve implantation in 663 patients with severe aortic stenosis. Circulation 2011;123:299–308.
55. Goel SS, Ige M, Tuzcu EM, et al. Severe aortic stenosis and coronary artery disease–implications for management in the transcatheter aortic valve replacement era: a comprehensive review. J Am Coll Cardiol 2013;62:1–10.
56. Holmes DR Jr, Mack MJ, Kaul S, et al. 2012 ACCF/AATS/SCAI/STS expert consensus document on transcatheter aortic valve replacement. J Am Coll Cardiol 2012;59:1200–54.
57. Holmes DR Jr, Rich JB, Zoghbi WA, et al. The heart team of cardiovascular care. J Am Coll Cardiol 2013;61:903–7.
58. Reynolds MR, Magnuson EA, Lei Y, et al. Health-related quality of life after transcatheter aortic valve replacement in inoperable patients with severe aortic stenosis. Circulation 2011;124:1964–72.

Multimorbidity in Older Adults with Atrial Fibrillation

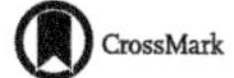

Michael A. Chen, MD, PhD

KEYWORDS

• Older adults • Multimorbidity • Atrial fibrillation • Rate control • Rhythm control • Shared decision-making • Polypharmacy • Geriatric syndromes

KEY POINTS

- Older adults with atrial fibrillation often have multiple comorbid conditions, including geriatric syndromes.
- Although management issues, such as rate versus rhythm control and anticoagulation, are similar for young and older adults, patients with multiple chronic conditions require special attention.
- Shared decision-making is necessary, but may be challenging, in order to properly balance the risks and benefits of interventions (medical and procedural) in the management of atrial fibrillation in older adults with multimorbidity.

INTRODUCTION

The increase in the aging population and advances in treatment of acute medical problems have resulted in a growing number of older adults with multiple chronic conditions. Specifically, "multimorbidity" is defined as being present when a patient has at least 2 chronic medical or psychiatric conditions that may or may not interact. "Comorbidity" is defined as one or more conditions that coexist in the context of a primary disease. Older adults are also at risk for having common "geriatric syndromes," such as cognitive impairment, polypharmacy, incontinence, and falls. All of these entities add to the complexity of caring for older adults. This article addresses how these conditions impact the care of patients with atrial fibrillation.

Multimorbidity is present in more than two-thirds of Medicare beneficiaries over the age of 65, with about one-third having 4 or more conditions. Approximately 83% of those 85 years and older have 2 or more chronic conditions.[1] The associated burden to patients and to the health care system is high. For example, in 2010 there were 1.9

No commercial or financial conflicts of interest or funding sources apply to my work on this article.

Cardiology, Harborview Medical Center, University of Washington School of Medicine, 325 9th Avenue, Box 359748, Seattle, WA 98104, USA
E-mail address: michen@u.washington.edu

Clin Geriatr Med 32 (2016) 315–329
http://dx.doi.org/10.1016/j.cger.2016.01.001 geriatric.theclinics.com
0749-0690/16/$ – see front matter

million Medicare hospital readmissions, and beneficiaries with 2 or more chronic conditions accounted for 98% of those readmissions.

EPIDEMIOLOGY OF ATRIAL FIBRILLATION AND MULTIMORBIDITY

The incidence and prevalence of atrial fibrillation increase markedly with increasing age (**Figs. 1** and **2**). Risk factors for atrial fibrillation include multiple conditions that are also increasingly common with age (**Table 1**). In Medicare patients with atrial fibrillation, the vast majority have multiple conditions (**Fig. 3**). In one study using a national sample of 1297 respondents with atrial fibrillation, 98% reported at least one other comorbid condition with 90% reporting cardiovascular conditions (hypertension [66%], hyperlipidemia [57%], arrhythmia [other than atrial fibrillation] [37%], diabetes [29%], prior myocardial infarction [21%], congestive heart failure [19%], stroke [13%], and transient ischemic attack [TIA] [9%]).[2] Overall, 45% had Charlson Comorbidity Index (CCI) scores of 1 to 2, and 21% had scores of at least 3 (**Fig. 4**). Apart from cardiovascular conditions, the most common comorbidities in that study were urologic (62%), pain-related (61%), respiratory (42%), and gastrointestinal conditions (41%) (**Table 2**). Another analysis of Medicare beneficiaries noted the 10 most common chronic comorbid conditions stratified by age greater than or less than 65 years (**Table 3**). The lists are quite similar, although arthritis appears 2 places higher in the older age group and diabetes 2 places higher in the younger age group.

The impact of age on hospitalizations for atrial fibrillation was examined in a recent study of 192,846 such admissions from 1051 hospitals in the 2009 to 2010 Nationwide

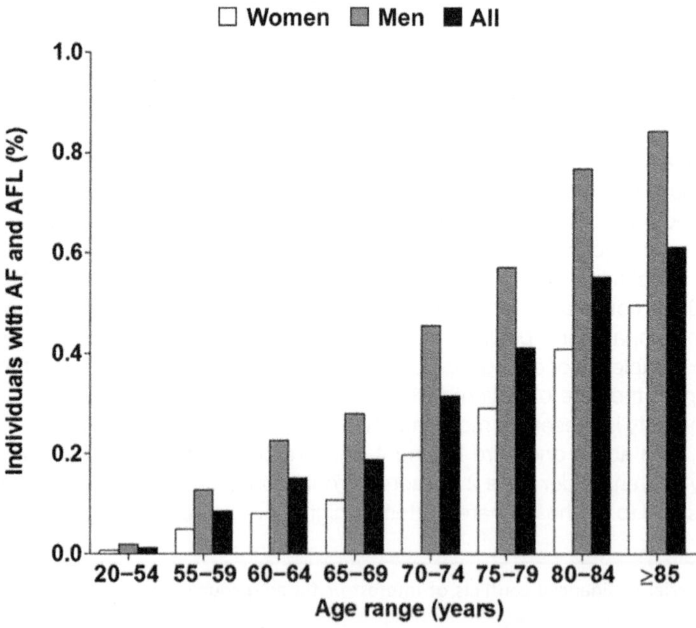

Fig. 1. Prevalence of atrial fibrillation and atrial flutter stratified by age and gender. Data were abstracted from the MarketScan Commercial Claims and Encounters database and Medicare Supplemental database from Thomson Reuters (Cambridge, MA), July 1, 2004–December 31, 2005. AF, atrial fibrillation; AFL, atrial flutter. (*From* Naccarelli GV, Varker H, Lin J, et al. Increasing prevalence of atrial fibrillation and flutter in the United States. Am J Cardiol 2009;104:1537; with permission.)

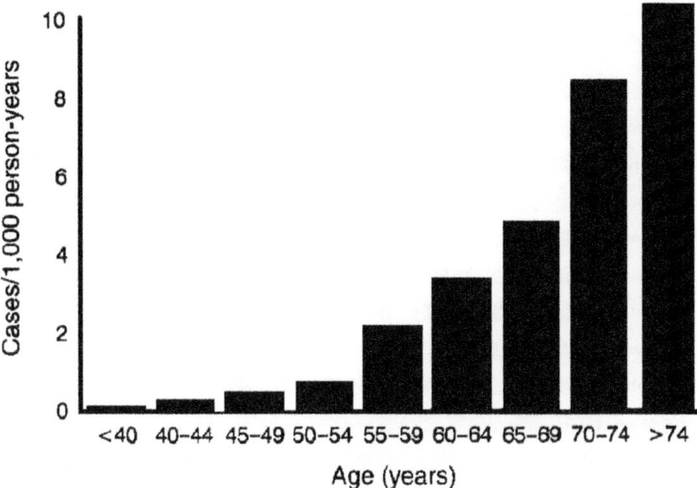

Fig. 2. Incidence of atrial fibrillation in the Manitoba follow-up study, 1948 to 1992. This was a study of 3983 men in pilot training in the Royal Canadian Air Force during and after World War II who were followed for 44 years. (*From* Krahn AD, Manfreda J, Tate RB, et al. The natural history of atrial fibrillation: incidence, risk factors, and prognosis in the Manitoba follow-up study. Am J Med 1995;98(5):478; with permission.)

Table 1
Risk factors for atrial fibrillation, stroke, and stroke in patients with atrial fibrillation

Risk Factors for Atrial Fibrillation[5]	Risk Factors for Stroke[14]	Risk Factors for Stroke in Patients with Atrial Fibrillation[14]
Increasing age	Increasing age	Increasing age
Hypertension	Hypertension	Hypertension
Diabetes mellitus	Diabetes mellitus	Diabetes mellitus
Heart failure	Atrial fibrillation/flutter	Heart failure
Valvular heart disease	Dyslipidemia	Prior stroke or TIA
Myocardial infarction	Smoking	Vascular disease
Obesity	Physical inactivity	Female sex
Obstructive sleep apnea	Diet	—
Cardiothoracic surgery	Family history	—
Smoking	Chronic kidney disease	—
Exercise	Sleep apnea	—
Alcohol use	Psychosocial factors	—
Hyperthyroidism	—	—
Increased pulse pressure	—	—
European ancestry	—	—
Family history	—	—
Genetic variants	—	—

Note the marked overlap in the risk factor profiles.

Data from January CT, Wann LS, Alpert JS, et al. 2014 AHA/ACC/HRS guideline for the management of patients with atrial fibrillation: a report of the American College of Cardiology/American Heart Association Task Force on Practice Guidelines and the Heart Rhythm Society. J Am Coll Cardiol 2014;64(21):e1–76; and Mozaffarian D, Benjamin EJ, Go AS, et al. Heart disease and stroke statistics—2015 update: a report from the American Heart Association. Circulation 2015;131(4):e29–322.

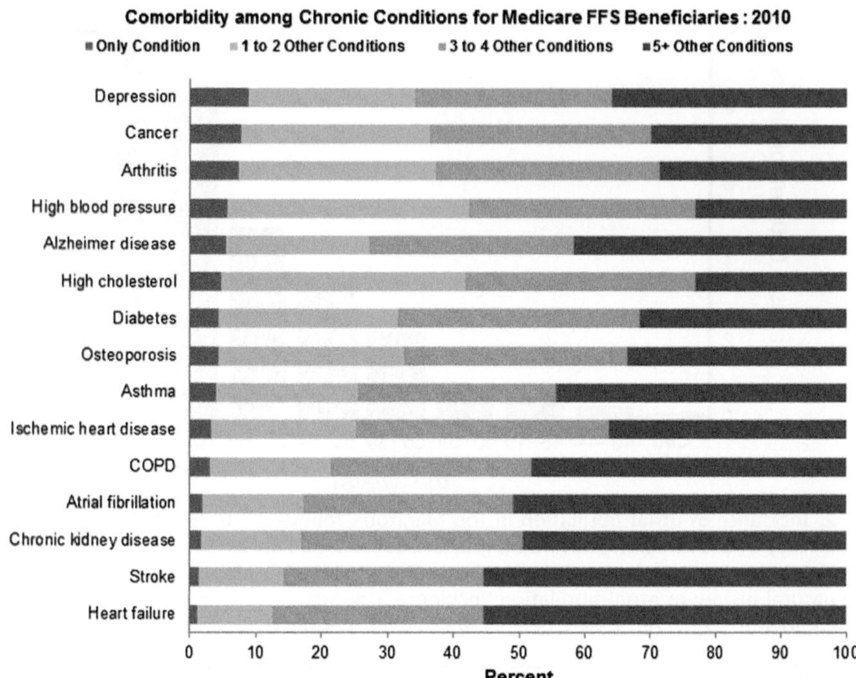

Fig. 3. Comorbidity among chronic conditions for Medicare beneficiaries: 2010. FFS, Fee For Service. (*From* Centers for Medicare and Medicaid Services. Chronic conditions among Medicare beneficiaries, Chartbook, 2012 edition. Baltimore (MD): Thomson Reuters; 2012.)

Inpatient Sample.[3] In this analysis, there was a marked increase in hospitalizations with increasing age (**Fig. 5**). The most common comorbidities in younger patients (defined as being <65 years of age) were hypertension (57%), diabetes mellitus (23%), obesity (21%), chronic obstructive pulmonary disease (COPD; 17%), and alcohol abuse (8%), whereas for older patients (those ≥65 years), the most common comorbidities were hypertension (70%), diabetes mellitus (25%), COPD (23%), chronic kidney disease (14%), and obesity (8%). Notable differences were that younger patients had higher rates of obesity and alcohol use, whereas older patients were more likely to have kidney disease. There was also a longer average length of stay (3.7 vs 2.9 days; $P<.001$) and higher in-hospital mortality (1% vs 0.3%; $P<.001$) for older vs younger patients. Older patients were less likely to be discharged home (74% vs 84%) and more likely to be discharged to a skilled or intermediate-care facility (10% vs 1%), indicating increasing disability/loss of functional independence. This finding is a particularly important adverse outcome in multimorbid older adults.

TREATMENT OF ATRIAL FIBRILLATION

The fundamental management issues are similar in all patients with atrial fibrillation and include rate control versus rhythm control and anticoagulation. However, multimorbidity and geriatric syndromes often complicate management in elderly patients.

Rate Control Versus Rhythm Control

Central to the management of atrial fibrillation is the choice of main treatment strategy of rate versus rhythm control. A rate control strategy focuses on control of the

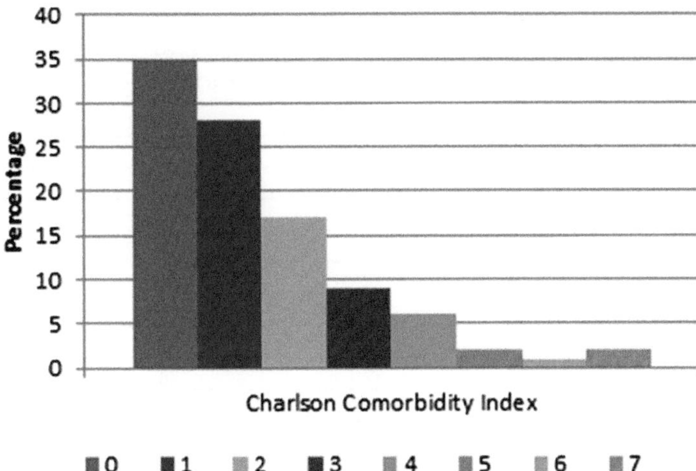

Fig. 4. Distribution of Charlson Comorbidity Index from the 1297 respondents to the 2009 National Health and Wellness survey who reported a diagnosis of atrial fibrillation. CCI was calculated as the weighted presence of the summed result of reports of the following conditions: human immunodeficiency virus or AIDS, metastatic tumor, lymphoma, leukemia, any tumor, moderate or severe renal disease, hemiplegia, diabetes, mild liver disease, ulcer disease, connective tissue disease, chronic pulmonary disease, dementia, cerebrovascular disease, peripheral vascular disease, myocardial infarction, and congestive heart failure; note that the adjusted CCI does not include diabetes with end organ damage and moderate or severe liver disease, which appear in the original CCI. The greater the total index score, the greater the comorbidity burden. Percentages were rounded to the nearest whole number. (*Data from* LaMori JC, Mody SH, Gross HJ, et al. Burden of comorbidities among patients with atrial fibrillation. Ther Adv Cardiovasc Dis 2013;7(2):53–62.)

ventricular rate, typically using atrioventricular (AV)-nodal blocking medications, such as β-blockers, calcium channel blockers, or digoxin. A rhythm control strategy, on the other hand, aims to maintain patients in sinus rhythm and may include cardioversion, antiarrhythmic medications, ablation, or a combination of these. Adequate rate control can reduce symptoms of atrial fibrillation (eg, palpitations, dyspnea, and other heart failure symptoms) as well as reduce the risk of developing tachycardia-mediated cardiomyopathy. Several clinical trials comparing rate control and rhythm control in patients eligible for both strategies suggest that rate control and anticoagulation are associated with fewer hospitalizations and no difference in mortality (rhythm control in these trials rarely included catheter ablation).[4] Because multimorbidity and atrial fibrillation both increase with age, a rate control strategy is often preferred in those older than 80 years, who have been underrepresented in clinical trials, may be more sensitive to drug side effects including proarrhythmia, and are more likely to have permanent atrial fibrillation (which reduces the likelihood of success with a rhythm control strategy).[5]

Because of age-related changes in the sympathetic nervous system, many elderly patients will not require medications for rate control (so-called auto rate control). If medications are needed, the most commonly used agents are AV-nodal blockers, including β-blockers, non-dihydropyridine calcium channel blockers (diltiazem, verapamil), and digoxin. β-Blockers may be problematic for patients with COPD or asthma. Calcium channel blockers may cause lower extremity swelling, which can exacerbate pre-existing venous insufficiency and complicate heart failure diagnosis and

Table 2
Prevalence of comorbidities by organ system from 1297 respondents to the 2009 National Health and Wellness survey who reported a diagnosis of atrial fibrillation

Comorbidity	Population Prevalence (%)
Cardiovascular	90
Urologic	62
Pain	61
Other	49
Respiratory	42
Gastrointestinal	41
Sleep condition	29
Psychological	28
Cancer	26
Dermatologic	26
Neurologic	22
Ophthalmic	20
Musculoskeletal	12
Autoimmune	5
Infectious	4

Data from LaMori JC, Mody SH, Gross HJ, et al. Burden of comorbidities among patients with atrial fibrillation. Ther Adv Cardiovasc Dis 2013;7(2):53–62.

Table 3
Ten most common comorbid chronic conditions among Medicare beneficiaries with atrial fibrillation

Beneficiaries ≥65 y of Age (N = 2,426,865) (Mean Number of Conditions 5.8; Median 6)			Beneficiaries <65 y of Age (N = 105,876) (Mean Number of Conditions = 5.8; Median = 6)		
	N	%		N	%
Hypertension	2,015,235	83.0	Hypertension	85,908	81.1
Ischemic heart disease	1,549,125	63.8	Ischemic heart disease	68,289	64.5
Hyperlipidemia	1,507,395	62.1	Hyperlipidemia	64,153	60.6
HF	1,247,748	51.4	HF	62,764	59.3
Anemia	1,027,135	42.3	Diabetes mellitus	56,246	53.1
Arthritis	965,472	39.8	Anemia	48,252	45.6
Diabetes mellitus	885,443	36.5	CKD	42,637	40.3
CKD	784,631	32.3	Arthritis	34,949	33.0
COPD	561,826	23.2	Depression	34,900	33.0
Cataracts	546,421	22.5	COPD	33,218	31.4

Abbreviations: CKD, chronic kidney disease; HF, heart failure.

From January CT, Wann LS, Alpert JS, et al. 2014 AHA/ACC/HRS guideline for the management of patients with atrial fibrillation: a report of the American College of Cardiology/American Heart Association task force on practice guidelines and the Heart Rhythm Society. J Am Coll Cardiol 2014;64:e1–76; with permission; and *Courtesy of* the Centers for Medicare and Medicaid Services, Office of Information Products and Data Analytics CMMS. CMS administrative claims data, January 2011 - December 2011, From the Chronic Condition Warehouse. 2012. Available at: www.ccwdata.org. Accessed July 15, 2014.

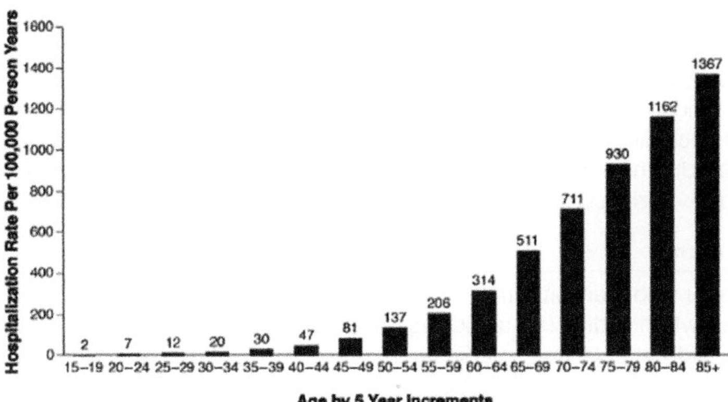

Fig. 5. Atrial fibrillation hospitalization rates per 100,000 person-years by age group. Data from 129,846 hospitalizations at 1051 hospitals (2009–2010) in the Nationwide Inpatient Sample. Results based on calculating the proportion of the US population in each age group hospitalized with atrial fibrillation. US population based on US census data for each age group. (*From* Naderi S, Wang Y, Miller AL, et al. The impact of age on the epidemiology of atrial fibrillation hospitalizations. Am J Med 2014;127:158.e3; with permission.)

management. Diltiazem and verapamil are commonly associated with constipation in older adults. Older patients are at increased risk for digoxin toxicity because of declines in renal function and muscle mass, volume depletion, and susceptibility to electrolyte abnormalities (particularly hypokalemia and hypomagnesemia). Digoxin also interacts with numerous medications, including antiarrhythmic agents such as amiodarone and propafenone, thereby increasing the risk for adverse events. Digoxin toxicity accounts for the third highest number of hospitalizations for adverse drug events in older adults.[6] Unrecognized toxicity is common because the early clinical signs and symptoms are nonspecific, including fatigue, malaise, weakness, nausea, and anorexia.

Apart from these considerations, both calcium channel blockers and β-blockers can lower blood pressure and impair an older adult's ability to increase cardiac output in response to a decrease in blood pressure (eg, on standing). Orthostatic hypotension is common in older adults and can be exacerbated by almost all antihypertensive medications. Age-associated declines in baroreceptor responsiveness can further contribute to an increased risk for falls and syncope.

Rate control targets have been studied, most recently in the RACE-II (Rate Control Efficacy in Permanent Atrial Fibrillation) trial, in which a lenient rate control strategy to maintain resting heart rate less than 110 bpm was compared with a strict rate control strategy aimed at a resting rate less than 80 bpm.[7] The composite endpoint for the trial comprised cardiovascular death, hospitalization for heart failure, stroke, systemic embolism, bleeding, and life-threatening arrhythmic events. After 3 years of follow-up, the lenient strategy was noninferior to the strict strategy (event rate 12.9% vs 14.9%, respectively; hazard ratio 0.84; 90% confidence interval [CI] 0.58–1.21). Of note, the difference in achieved resting heart rates in the 2 groups differed by only 10 bpm (about 75 bpm vs about 85 bpm), and nearly 80% of the lenient group had resting rates less than 100 bpm. The benefits of lenient rate control in minimally symptomatic or asymptomatic patients could include fewer medications and/or lower doses and fewer office visits. For example, in the trial there were nearly 9 times as many visits needed in the strict rate control group. A more lenient strategy might also put patients at lower risk for symptomatic bradycardia and the need for a pacemaker.

Tachy-brady syndrome

"Tachy-brady syndrome" is an age-associated condition in which patients have resting bradycardia (usually sinus bradycardia) with paroxysmal supraventricular tachyarrhythmias, most commonly atrial fibrillation. Medications used to treat the tachyarrhythmias, including AV-nodal blockers and antiarrhythmic agents, often exacerbate the bradycardia. In some cases, the bradycardia may be severe enough to cause symptoms (fatigue, dizziness, falls, syncope), prompting referral for pacemaker implantation.

Rhythm Control

In patients for whom an initial rate control strategy fails because of ongoing symptoms from the arrhythmia, difficulty achieving rate control, tachycardia-mediated cardiomyopathy, or side effects from medications, a rhythm control strategy may be undertaken. This rhythm control strategy can entail a combination of electrical or chemical cardioversion, antiarrhythmic medication, and ablation therapy. Use of antiarrhythmic drugs in older patients may be complicated by age-associated alterations in pharmacokinetics and pharmacodynamics, changes in renal and hepatic clearance, and a multitude of drug-drug and drug-disease interactions.[5,8]

Catheter ablation involves delivery of radiofrequency energy to regions of the left atrium with the objective of preventing propagation of atrial fibrillation. Two randomized trials have compared ablation with antiarrhythmic therapy as first-line rhythm control treatment. Both showed higher rates of freedom from atrial fibrillation in the ablation arm at the end of follow-up (1 year and 2 years).[9,10] Based on these findings, current guidelines suggest considering catheter ablation as first-line therapy in selected patients before a trial of antiarrhythmic drug treatment when a rhythm control strategy is desired. However, data on the efficacy of catheter ablation in elderly patients are limited. Factors associated with higher complication rates include older age, female sex, and a CHADS2 score 2 or greater (CHADS2 assigns 1 point for congestive heart failure, hypertension, age ≥75 years, and diabetes, and 2 points for prior stroke or TIA; see Anna L. Parks, Margaret C. Fang: Anticoagulation in Older Adults with Multimorbidity, in this issue).[5]

An important point is that in most older adults, selection of a rhythm control strategy does not obviate anticoagulation. Of the strokes that occurred during the AFFIRM (Atrial Fibrillation Follow-up Investigation of Rhythm Management) trial (of rate vs rhythm control), the majority occurred after warfarin had been stopped or when the international normalized ratio was subtherapeutic.[11]

An alternative rhythm control strategy in selected patients is the surgical MAZE procedure, which involves making incisions and/or creating radiofrequency or cryoablation lesions in the atria to extinguish the re-entrant circuits. The MAZE procedure is typically performed in conjunction with other open heart surgery, but can be done as an isolated procedure in highly symptomatic patients (only 5.3% in one review from 2005 to 2010).[12] The Atrial Fibrillation Catheter Ablation versus Surgical Ablation Treatment randomized trial compared outcomes of catheter versus surgical ablation and showed greater freedom from atrial fibrillation following surgical ablation, but at the cost of a higher complication rate.[13]

Prevention of Stroke and Systemic Embolization

Among patients with atrial fibrillation, increasing age is a potent risk factor for stroke or systemic embolization. In the Framingham Heart Study, only 1.5% of strokes were attributed to atrial fibrillation in patients 50 to 59 years of age, but the proportion increased more than 15-fold to 23.5% among patients 80 to 89 years of age.[14] In another analysis, it was estimated that 30% to 36% of strokes were due to atrial fibrillation in patients aged 80 to 89 years.[15] Thus, prevention of stroke and systemic embolization is a primary objective of managing atrial fibrillation. Assessment of stroke risk, the role of anticoagulation, and balancing stroke risk versus bleeding risk in older patients with multimorbidity are reviewed in the article by Anna L. Parks, Margaret C. Fang: Anticoagulation in Older Adults with Multimorbidity, in this issue and are not discussed here. For patients who are poor candidates for anticoagulation, for example, due to high risk for life-threatening hemorrhage, percutaneous and surgical approaches to reducing stroke risk may be viable options in selected cases.

Because the left atrial appendage is the most common site of thrombus formation in patients with atrial fibrillation, techniques for excluding the left atrial appendage from the circulation have been developed. One approach involves transcatheter deployment of a plug that occludes the appendage, exemplified by the WATCHMAN device (Boston Scientific, Marlborough, MA) and the Amplatzer Cardiac Plug (St. Jude Medical, St. Paul, MN). A second approach is to tie off the left atrial appendage using an epicardial snare, called an LARIAT device (Sentre-Heart, Inc., Redwood City, CA), via a subxiphoid pericardial access. In a 2011 series of 143 patients who underwent placement of the Amplatzer device, there were 3 ischemic strokes, 2 device embolizations, and 5 pericardial effusions.[16] The WATCHMAN device has been evaluated in clinical trials, suggesting noninferiority when compared with warfarin.[17] Safety and efficacy have also been evaluated in patients ineligible for warfarin.[18] The device is US Food and Drug Administration approved for use in the United States to reduce the risk of thromboembolism in patients with nonvalvular atrial fibrillation. How these devices will fit into the armamentarium of thromboembolic risk reduction is uncertain, and recommendations for their use are not provided in the most recent American Heart Association/American College of Cardiology (AHA/ACC) guidelines. The 2012 European Society of Cardiology guidelines for the management of atrial fibrillation give a weak recommendation for their use in high-stroke-risk patients with a contraindication to long-term anticoagulation.[19] Exclusion of the appendage at the time of an MAZE procedure in conjunction with mitral valve surgery is recommended in the AHA/ACC guidelines.

COMMON COMORBID CONDITIONS AND GERIATRIC SYNDROMES

Heart Failure

Clinical trials and registry data have shown that 20% to 30% of patients with clinical heart failure also have atrial fibrillation,[20] and the prevalence of atrial fibrillation increases from 4% to 50% as the New York Heart Association functional class increases from class I to class IV.[21] The relationship between these 2 entities is complex. In some patients, atrial fibrillation can lead to heart failure. For example, patients with atrial fibrillation and poor heart rate control can develop tachycardia-mediated cardiomyopathy and associated heart failure. In older adults with diastolic dysfunction, often in association with longstanding hypertension, new onset atrial fibrillation can precipitate clinical heart failure. Conversely, in patients with heart failure, elevated left atrial pressure and/or atrial myopathy can lead to atrial fibrillation. Heart failure and multimorbidity are discussed in detail in Kumar Dharmarajan, Shannon Marie Dunlay: Multimorbidity in Older Adults with Heart Failure, in this issue, but the combination of heart failure and atrial fibrillation in particular complicates management. For example, evidence-based therapy for heart failure with reduced ejection fraction includes multiple medications and the possibility of devices such as implanted defibrillators and cardiac resynchronization therapy. Comorbid atrial fibrillation often requires additional medications, such as anticoagulants, or higher doses (for rate control).

Of particular importance in older adults is the relationship between atrial fibrillation and heart failure with preserved ejection fraction (HFpEF) because the prevalence of both conditions is strongly associated with advancing age. Both are also associated with other comorbidities common in aging, such as hypertension and diabetes. In a community-based study of more than 900 patients with newly diagnosed HFpEF (age 77 $\pm$ 12 years, 61% women), two-thirds had atrial fibrillation at some point in their disease course.[22] Overall, 29% had prior atrial fibrillation, 23% had concurrent atrial fibrillation, and among subjects who were in sinus rhythm at the time of HFpEF diagnosis, 32% developed atrial fibrillation during a mean follow-up of 3.7 years. In this study, older age and diastolic dysfunction were associated with incident atrial fibrillation, whereas statin use was protective. Compared with those without atrial fibrillation, prior, concurrent, and incident atrial fibrillation were independently associated with a 2-fold increase in mortality (hazard ratio 2.1; 95% CI, 1.4–3.0; *P*<.001). In patients with symptoms of HFpEF that are difficult to manage despite adequate ventricular rate control, a rhythm control strategy, which may include ablation, may be preferred, as recommended by national guidelines.[5,23]

Prior Stroke

Age is one of the most potent risk factors for stroke in patients with or without atrial fibrillation (**Fig. 6**). In addition, stroke and atrial fibrillation share many common risk factors (see **Table 1**). As noted above, the percentage of strokes attributable to atrial fibrillation increases sharply with age[14]; consequently, nearly 50% of atrial fibrillation–related strokes occur in patients over the age of 75. Thus, stroke is a frequent comorbidity in older adults with atrial fibrillation. Prior stroke places patients in the highest risk category for future stroke, and prior stroke or TIA warrants a class I recommendation for anticoagulation in patients with atrial fibrillation.[5] Furthermore, patients with stroke may have cognitive or motor impairments that make the management of atrial fibrillation challenging. Balance and mobility problems may make practitioners wary of

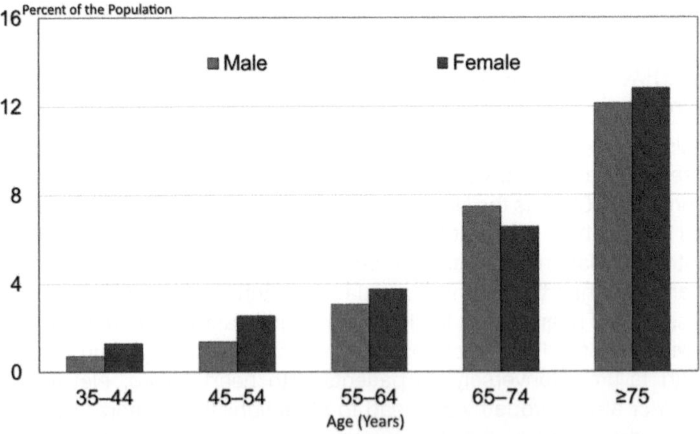

Fig. 6. Prevalence of stroke by age and sex, US, 1999 to 2008. Prevalence increased markedly with age and was higher in women than in men for all age groups except one. (*Data from* National Heart, Lung, and Blood Institute. Unpublished tabulation of the National Health and Nutrition Examination Survey, 1971–1975, 1976–1980, 1988–1994,1999–2004, and 2005–2008 and Extrapolation to the US Population, 2008; and Morbidity and Mortality: 2012 Chart Book on Cardiovascular, Lung, and Blood Diseases, National Institutes of Health: National Heart, Lung, and Blood Institute.)

prescribing anticoagulation in these very high-risk patients. These same issues may also make older individuals more susceptible to iatrogenic hypotension and other adverse drug effects. Expressive difficulties can make it difficult for patients to report or describe symptoms. Depending on the severity of after-stroke deficits, individual patient's goals of care may limit the appropriateness of referrals for aggressive therapies such as ablation.

Geriatric Syndromes

Geriatric syndromes are common in older patients with atrial fibrillation and complicate its management. The most prominent of these are discussed below.

Cognitive impairment

Cognitive dysfunction is common in aging and can range in severity from mild cognitive impairment to severe dementia. Among individuals more than 70 years of age, up to 20% have mild cognitive impairment and up to 14% have dementia.[24,25] Cognitive impairment complicates the management of atrial fibrillation because of problems with adherence to complex medication regimens, difficulty attending follow-up appointments, and challenges in decision-making. Oftentimes, surrogate decision-makers are needed to guide management.

Recent studies implicate atrial fibrillation as a risk factor for cognitive decline even in the absence of stroke.[26–28] In an analysis of 5150 participants in the Cardiovascular Health Study, 552 of whom developed atrial fibrillation during 7 years of follow-up, mean scores on the 100-point Modified Mini-Mental State Examination declined faster in patients after incident atrial fibrillation than in those who did not develop atrial fibrillation (in the absence of clinical stroke).[29] For example, the predicted 5-year decline in mean scores from age 80 to age 85 was 6.4 points (95% CI: 5.9–7.0) for patients without atrial fibrillation, but it was 10.3 points (95% CI: 8.9–11.8) for patients experiencing incident atrial fibrillation at age 80. Potential reasons for these findings include subclinical embolic ischemic events and cerebral hypoperfusion from reduced cardiac output during atrial fibrillation (notably, removing patients with heart failure from the analysis did attenuate the relationship). In addition, atrial fibrillation may be a marker for other factors affecting cognition, although in this study adjustment was performed for demographic, behavioral, and traditional clinical risk factors for cognitive decline.[29]

Falls

Approximately one-third of community-dwelling adults at least 65 years of age experiences a fall each year.[30] Nonaccidental falls, defined as those without a mitigating circumstance (such as being tripped by a dog leash), can be instigated by neurologic or orthopedic problems, sensory impairment, orthostatic hypotension, other cardiovascular disorders such as arrhythmias, or medication side effects. An analysis of 442 consecutive patients more than 65 years of age presenting to a university hospital Emergency Department after a fall revealed a higher prevalence of atrial fibrillation in those with nonaccidental falls (26% vs 15%; $P = .003$).[31] Furthermore, atrial fibrillation was an independent risk factor for nonaccidental falls in a multivariable model. Among patients 81 years of age or younger, the risk of nonaccidental falls was 2.5 times greater in patients with a history of atrial fibrillation compared with those without such a history (odds ratio = 2.53; 95% CI 1.3–5, $P = .007$). The mechanistic links between atrial fibrillation and falls may include reduced cardiac output, impaired baroreceptor responsiveness, bradycardia, orthostatic hypotension, or medication side effects superimposed on other predisposing conditions such as gait or balance problems.[31] Understanding the relationship between falls and atrial fibrillation is important because a high risk of falls is frequently cited as a reason to withhold anticoagulation. Nonetheless, as discussed in Anna L. Parks, Margaret C. Fang: Anticoagulation in Older Adults with Multimorbidity, in this issue, the benefits of anticoagulation often outweigh the risks in older adults who are prone to falls.[32]

Polypharmacy

Polypharmacy, usually defined as regular use of 5 or more prescription drugs, can result in significant morbidity and even mortality. Adverse drug reactions are implicated in 6.5% of all hospitalizations, and the rate is up to 4 times higher in older adults. About half of these admissions involve cardiovascular medications, with warfarin being the most frequently implicated drug. Warfarin has significant drug interactions with cardiac and noncardiac medications (including antibiotics), and it is still the most commonly prescribed anticoagulant. In one study of patients 70 years of age or older (mean age 79.2 ± 5.5 years) admitted to an inpatient cardiology service, 50% of whom had atrial fibrillation, the mean number of medications on admission was 8.2, the mean number on discharge was 9, 95% were taking 4 or more medications, and 19% were discharged on 12 or more medications.[33] Evaluation for polypharmacy with discontinuation of nonessential medications should be a prominent goal in the care of older adults.

Sensory impairment

Sensory impairment, especially visual and hearing loss, can complicate medication use and increase risk of falls. Hearing loss may also interfere with communication and patients' understanding of management.

Incontinence

Incontinence can be exacerbated by diuretics used to treat comorbid hypertension or heart failure, and urinary urgency may place patients at risk for falls when rushing to the bathroom.

EVIDENCE AND GUIDELINES

Although more evidence is needed to support treatment recommendations for older, multimorbid adults, who have rarely been included in randomized trials, some guidance does exist. The American Geriatrics Society (AGS) expert panel on the care of older adults with multimorbidity places a strong focus on patient preferences, assessing risks and benefits (and the timelines for these), and shared decision-making (see Hillary D. Lum, Rebecca L. Sudore: Advance Care Planning and Goals of Care Communication in Older Adults with Cardiovascular Disease and Multi-Morbidity and Mary E. Tinetti, Jessica Esterson, Rosie Ferris, et al: Patient Priority–Directed Decision Making and Care for Older Adults with Multiple Chronic Conditions, in this issue). The AGS has also published a 2-page guide to the Management of Atrial Fibrillation in Older Adults (https://s3.amazonaws.com/ALTC-CG/altc0414AGS_Tip_crop-1.pdf). This document can be accessed via the smartphone application iGeriatrics. The US and European guidelines on the management of atrial fibrillation include short sections devoted to the care of older adults and make reference to multimorbidity or comorbidity but provide few specific recommendations.[5,34]

Shared Decision-Making

Shared decision-making is discussed in the articles by Hillary D. Lum, Rebecca L. Sudore: Advance Care Planning and Goals of Care Communication in Older Adults with Cardiovascular Disease and Multi-Morbidity and Mary E. Tinetti, Jessica Esterson, Rosie Ferris, et al: Patient Priority–Directed Decision Making and Care for Older Adults

Table 4
Balancing the risks and benefits of treatments

Risks	Treatment	Benefits
Bradycardia Orthostatic hypotension Fatigue	Rate control	Reduced symptoms (palpitations, dyspnea) Reduced risk of tachycardia-mediated cardiomyopathy
Medication side effects and interactions Higher rates of hospitalizations	Rhythm control	Reduced symptoms
Procedural complications	Ablation	Reduced symptoms
Procedural complications Risk of pacemaker-mediated cardiomyopathy/heart failure (RV pacing)	AV-nodal ablation and permanent pacemaker placement	Reduced symptoms Reduced risk of tachycardia mediated cardiomyopathy
Increased risk of bleeding	Anticoagulation	Reduced risk of stroke
Procedural complications	Left atrial appendage closure device	Reduced risk of stroke

These factors highlight a need for shared decision-making.
Abbreviation: RV, right ventricular.

with Multiple Chronic Conditions, in this issue. Because there are tradeoffs involved in the management of atrial fibrillation (**Table 4**), shared decision-making is essential. For example, variability in patients' values regarding the importance of avoiding bleeding complications versus reducing stroke risk may influence the decision about anticoagulation. Conversely, shared decision-making may be complicated by the presence of comorbidities such as cognitive dysfunction.

SUMMARY

Older adults with atrial fibrillation often have multiple comorbid conditions, including common geriatric syndromes. In a national sample of nearly 1300 patients with atrial fibrillation, 98% reported having at least one other medical condition. Although the principal management issues, such as rate control versus rhythm control and anticoagulation, are similar for younger and older adults, patients with multiple chronic conditions require special attention. Pharmacologic therapy, whether for rate or rhythm control, can result in complications in patients who are taking multiple medications for other conditions. Polypharmacy puts patients at risk for medication interactions and adverse drug events in part due to renal or hepatic dysfunction. Because the risks and benefits of therapy are complex and vary from patient to patient in large part due to the comorbidity burden, shared decision-making is mandatory, although it may also be challenging.

REFERENCES

1. Centers for Medicare and Medicaid Services. Chronic conditions among Medicare beneficiaries. In: Lochner K, editor. Baltimore (MD): United States Department of Health and Human Services; 2012. p. 11.
2. LaMori JC, Mody SH, Gross HJ, et al. Burden of comorbidities among patients with atrial fibrillation. Ther Adv Cardiovasc Dis 2013;7(2):53–62.
3. Naderi S, Wang Y, Miller AL, et al. The impact of age on the epidemiology of atrial fibrillation hospitalizations. Am J Med 2014;127(2):158.e1–7.

4. Olshansky B, Rosenfeld LE, Warner AL, et al. The Atrial Fibrillation Follow-up Investigation of Rhythm Management (AFFIRM) study: approaches to control rate in atrial fibrillation. J Am Coll Cardiol 2004;43(7):1201–8.
5. January CT, Wann LS, Alpert JS, et al. 2014 AHA/ACC/HRS guideline for the management of patients with atrial fibrillation: a report of the American College of Cardiology/American Heart Association Task Force on practice guidelines and the Heart Rhythm Society. J Am Coll Cardiol 2014;64(21):e1–76.
6. Budnitz DS, Lovegrove MC, Shehab N, et al. Emergency hospitalizations for adverse drug events in older Americans. N Engl J Med 2011;365(21):2002–12.
7. Van Gelder IC, Groenveld HF, Crijns HJ, et al. Lenient versus strict rate control in patients with atrial fibrillation. N Engl J Med 2010;362(15):1363–73.
8. Lee HC, TI Huang K, Shen WK. Use of antiarrhythmic drugs in elderly patients. J Geriatr Cardiol 2011;8(3):184–94.
9. Cosedis Nielsen J, Johannessen A, Raatikainen P, et al. Radiofrequency ablation as initial therapy in paroxysmal atrial fibrillation. N Engl J Med 2012;367(17): 1587–95.
10. Wazni OM, Marrouche NF, Martin DO, et al. Radiofrequency ablation vs antiarrhythmic drugs as first-line treatment of symptomatic atrial fibrillation: a randomized trial. JAMA 2005;293(21):2634–40.
11. Wyse DG, Waldo AL, DiMarco JP, et al. A comparison of rate control and rhythm control in patients with atrial fibrillation. N Engl J Med 2002;347(23):1825–33.
12. Ad N, Suri RM, Gammie JS, et al. Surgical ablation of atrial fibrillation trends and outcomes in North America. J Thorac Cardiovasc Surg 2012;144(5):1051–60.
13. Boersma LV, Castella M, van Boven W, et al. Atrial fibrillation catheter ablation versus surgical ablation treatment (FAST): a 2-center randomized clinical trial. Circulation 2012;125(1):23–30.
14. Mozaffarian D, Benjamin EJ, Go AS, et al. Heart disease and stroke statistics–2015 update: a report from the American Heart Association. Circulation 2015; 131(4):e29–322.
15. Wolf PA, Singer DE. Preventing stroke in atrial fibrillation. Am Fam Physician 1997; 56(9):2242–50.
16. Park JW, Bethencourt A, Sievert H, et al. Left atrial appendage closure with Amplatzer cardiac plug in atrial fibrillation: initial European experience. Catheter Cardiovasc Interv 2011;77(5):700–6.
17. Reddy VY, Doshi SK, Sievert H, et al. Percutaneous left atrial appendage closure for stroke prophylaxis in patients with atrial fibrillation: 2.3-year follow-up of the PROTECT AF (Watchman left atrial appendage system for embolic protection in patients with atrial fibrillation) trial. Circulation 2013;127(6):720–9.
18. Reddy VY, Mobius-Winkler S, Miller MA, et al. Left atrial appendage closure with the Watchman device in patients with a contraindication for oral anticoagulation: the ASAP study (ASA Plavix Feasibility Study with Watchman Left Atrial Appendage Closure Technology). J Am Coll Cardiol 2013;61(25):2551–6.
19. Camm AJ, Lip GY, De Caterina R, et al. 2012 focused update of the ESC Guidelines for the management of atrial fibrillation: an update of the 2010 ESC Guidelines for the Management of Atrial Fibrillation. Developed with the special contribution of the European Heart Rhythm Association. Eur Heart J 2012; 33(21):2719–47.
20. Darby AE, Dimarco JP. Management of atrial fibrillation in patients with structural heart disease. Circulation 2012;125(7):945–57.
21. Maisel WH, Stevenson LW. Atrial fibrillation in heart failure: epidemiology, pathophysiology, and rationale for therapy. Am J Cardiol 2003;91(6A):2D–8D.

22. Zakeri R, Chamberlain AM, Roger VL, et al. Temporal relationship and prognostic significance of atrial fibrillation in heart failure patients with preserved ejection fraction: a community-based study. Circulation 2013;128(10):1085–93.
23. Heart Failure Society of America, Lindenfeld J, Albert NM, et al. HFSA 2010 Comprehensive Heart Failure Practice Guideline. J Card Fail 2010;16(6):e1–194.
24. Plassman BL, Langa KM, Fisher GG, et al. Prevalence of dementia in the United States: the aging, demographics, and memory study. Neuroepidemiology 2007; 29(1–2):125–32.
25. Ritchie K, Artero S, Touchon J. Classification criteria for mild cognitive impairment: a population-based validation study. Neurology 2001;56(1):37–42.
26. Kwok CS, Loke YK, Hale R, et al. Atrial fibrillation and incidence of dementia: a systematic review and meta-analysis. Neurology 2011;76(10):914–22.
27. Dublin S, Anderson ML, Haneuse SJ, et al. Atrial fibrillation and risk of dementia: a prospective cohort study. J Am Geriatr Soc 2011;59(8):1369–75.
28. Marzona I, O'Donnell M, Teo K, et al. Increased risk of cognitive and functional decline in patients with atrial fibrillation: results of the ONTARGET and TRANSCEND studies. CMAJ 2012;184(6):E329–36.
29. Thacker EL, McKnight B, Psaty BM, et al. Atrial fibrillation and cognitive decline: a longitudinal cohort study. Neurology 2013;81(2):119–25.
30. Centers for Disease Control and Prevention. Important facts about falls. Home and recreational safety. 2015. Available at: http://www.cdc.gov/homeandrecreationalsafety/falls/adultfalls.html. Accessed November 20, 2015.
31. Sanders NA, Ganguly JA, Jetter TL, et al. Atrial fibrillation: an independent risk factor for nonaccidental falls in older patients. Pacing Clin Electrophysiol 2012; 35(8):973–9.
32. Man-Son-Hing M, Nichol G, Lau A, et al. Choosing antithrombotic therapy for elderly patients with atrial fibrillation who are at risk for falls. Arch Intern Med 1999;159(7):677–85.
33. Flood KL, Rohlfing A, Le CV, et al. Geriatric syndromes in elderly patients admitted to an inpatient cardiology ward. J Hosp Med 2007;2(6):394–400.
34. European Heart Rhythm Association, European Association for Cardio-Thoracic Surgery, Camm AJ, et al. Guidelines for the management of atrial fibrillation: the Task Force for the Management of Atrial Fibrillation of the European Society of Cardiology (ESC). Eur Heart J 2010;31(19):2369–429.

Anticoagulation in Older Adults with Multimorbidity

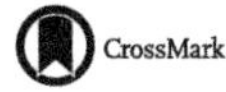

Anna L. Parks, MD[a], Margaret C. Fang, MD, MPH[b,*]

KEYWORDS

- Multimorbidity • Atrial fibrillation • Anticoagulation • Warfarin
- New oral anticoagulants • Polypharmacy • Bleeding risk

KEY POINTS

- Multimorbidity affects most older adults with atrial fibrillation (AF) and increases the risk of AF-associated ischemic stroke; most older AF patients will derive net benefit from anticoagulation.
- The newer target-specific oral anticoagulants have become viable alternatives to warfarin.
- Physicians must weigh the benefit of stroke prevention against the risks and burdens of anticoagulation, which increase with age and comorbidities.
- In selecting among available anticoagulant agents, physicians should consider a patient's coexisting medical conditions, medications, adherence, cost, ability to participate in monitoring, and preferences.

INTRODUCTION

Older individuals are at greatly increased risk of atrial fibrillation (AF) and AF-associated ischemic stroke. Although anticoagulant therapy can diminish stroke risk, the risks and burdens of therapy, combined with older patients' concomitant physical and medical problems, must be weighed when considering prescription of anticoagulants. Multimorbidity, or the coexistence of 2 or more chronic conditions, complicates the anticoagulation decision and the universal application of evidence-based guidelines to complex older patients with AF. This article reviews the appropriate use and challenges of anticoagulation in multimorbid patients with AF.

MULTIMORBIDITY AND ATRIAL FIBRILLATION

AF is the most common clinically significant cardiac arrhythmia, and the burden of disease falls disproportionately on older adults.[1] In the United States, the prevalence of

---

Disclosures: The authors have no relevant financial disclosures to report.
[a] Department of Medicine, University of California, San Francisco, 505 Parnassus Avenue, San Francisco, CA 94143, USA; [b] Division of Hospital Medicine, University of California, San Francisco, 533 Parnassus Avenue, Box 0131, San Francisco, CA 94143, USA
* Corresponding author.
E-mail address: Margaret.fang@ucsf.edu

Clin Geriatr Med 32 (2016) 331–346
http://dx.doi.org/10.1016/j.cger.2016.01.003 geriatric.theclinics.com
0749-0690/16/$ – see front matter

AF increases from 0.1% among those younger than age 55 to 9.0% among those 80 or older. AF prevalence is projected to increase alongside the aging of the US population; by 2050, an estimated 5.6 million adults will have AF, and more than 50% of these patients will be aged 80 or older (**Fig. 1**).[1] A more recent study projected an even greater disease burden, with a projected prevalence in 2050 of 7.56 million.[2]

The aging of the US population increases the likelihood not only of specific conditions like AF, but also of multimorbidity. More than two-thirds of Medicare beneficiaries—equivalent to 21.4 million adults—have 2 or more chronic diseases. The median number of conditions is 6 and AF is the 11th most common among these.[3] Accordingly, AF coexists frequently with other comorbidities, including hypertension, ischemic heart disease, and heart failure (**Fig. 2**). One-third of AF patients have concomitant chronic kidney disease, which has important implications for treatment, not only because of its association with increased risk of stroke and hemorrhage, but also because many new anticoagulants are at least partially cleared renally. Comorbidities like cataracts and arthritis are common among elderly AF patients and can greatly impact the logistics of anticoagulation. Multimorbidity, therefore, affects the majority of AF patients and should be a central consideration in its management.

In AF patients, multimorbidity is associated with increased stroke risk and worse outcomes after stroke.[4] An estimated 36% of strokes in patients 80 to 89 years old in the United States are due to AF[5] and a large percentage of patients who suffer cryptogenic strokes (strokes without a clear underlying cause) are later found to have AF on cardiac monitoring.[5] Multimorbid patients have a 37% increased risk of poor functional outcomes after ischemic stroke[6] and AF-associated strokes are associated with longer duration of stay, higher rates of disability, and increased mortality.[7] Multimorbidity is associated with a 2.5-fold increase in 30-day and 5-year mortality for patients with ischemic stroke. Thus, stroke prevention is a cornerstone of decreasing the morbidity and mortality associated with AF.

STROKE PREVENTION IN MULTIMORBID ADULTS WITH ATRIAL FIBRILLATION

Assessing Stroke Risk

Multimorbid older adults virtually always exceed the thresholds for stroke risk that warrant anticoagulation as established by current risk schemes. Stroke prediction scores, such as the $CHADS_2$ and CHA_2DS_2-VASc scores,[8,9] have been incorporated

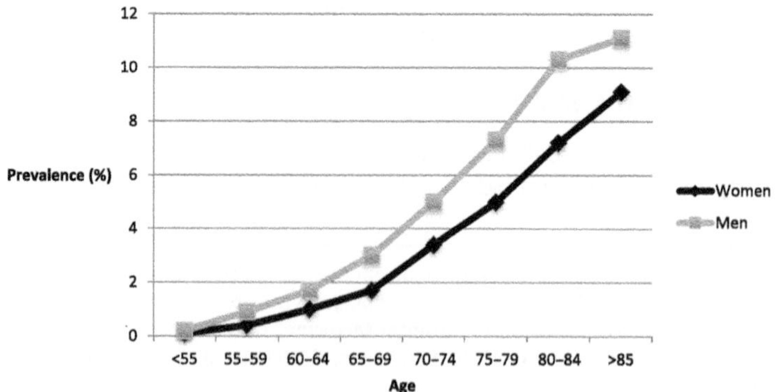

Fig. 1. Prevalence of diagnosed atrial fibrillation by age. (*Data from* Go AS, Hylek EM, Phillips KA, et al. Prevalence of diagnosed atrial fibrillation in adults: national implications for rhythm management and stroke prevention: the anticoagulation and risk factors in atrial fibrillation (ATRIA) study. JAMA 2001;285(18):2370–5.)

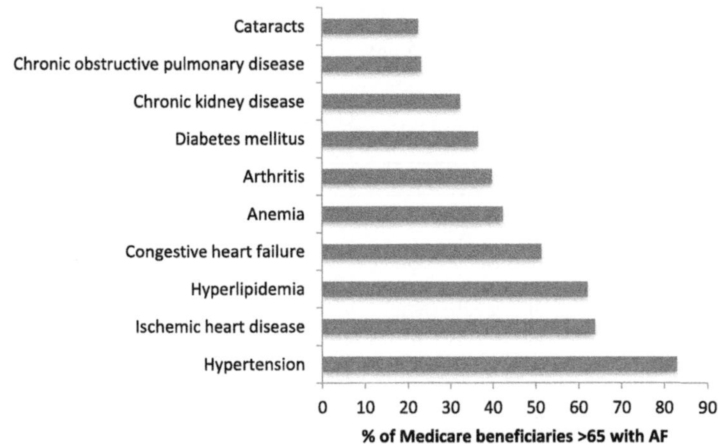

Fig. 2. The 10 most common comorbid chronic conditions among Medicare beneficiaries greater than 65 years of age with atrial fibrillation (AF). (*Data from* January CT, Wann LS, Alpert JS, et al. 2014 AHA/ACC/HRS guideline for the management of patients with atrial fibrillation: a report of the American college of cardiology/American heart association task force on practice guidelines and the heart rhythm society. J Am Coll Cardiol 2014;64(21):e1–76.)

into clinical guidelines to help guide which patients should receive anticoagulants[10–12] (**Table 1**). Risk scores use the presence of risk factors for stroke, such as prior stroke, hypertension, and other cardiovascular conditions, to estimate a person's annual risk for thromboembolism. Thresholds for anticoagulation have been lowered in recent years,[13,14] and the 2014 American Heart Association/American College of Cardiology/Heart Rhythm Society Guidelines for the management of AF now use a CHA_2DS_2-VASc score of 2 or greater to support prescribing anticoagulants, resulting in near universal anticoagulation for multimorbid older adults.

Understanding that anticoagulation will most likely be recommended, it is still worth using a risk score to estimate an individual's annual stroke risk. The estimate can be integrated with a person's risk for complications and personal preference for treatment to develop a shared decision regarding anticoagulation. For example, patients with CHA_2DS_2-VASc scores of 0 have only a 0.2% annual stroke risk, compared with scores of 6 or higher, which are associated with risks of 11% to 12%.[15] Understanding the range of stroke risks may help clinicians and patients to establish an informed decision that best balances the benefits of stroke prevention with complications and burdens of therapy.

ANTICOAGULATION OPTIONS

For many decades, vitamin K antagonists like warfarin represented the only option for chronic oral anticoagulation. In recent years, non–vitamin K oral anticoagulants, also called the "target-specific oral anticoagulants" (TSOACs), have become available and have significantly expanded the options for clinicians and patients.

Vitamin K Antagonists

Vitamin K antagonists remain the most widely used oral anticoagulants worldwide. Their efficacy has been well-established through multiple clinical trials. Warfarin reduces the risk of AF-related ischemic stroke by 68% and overall mortality by 33%;

Table 1
Comparison of the CHADS2 and CHA2DS2-VASc risk stratification scores for subjects with nonvalvular atrial fibrillation

CHADS2 Variable	Score	CHADS2VASC Variable	Score
Congestive heart failure	1	Congestive heart failure	1
Hypertension	1	Hypertension	1
Age >75	1	Age >75	2
Diabetes mellitus	1	Diabetes mellitus	1
Stroke/TIA	2	Stroke/TIA	2
CHADS2 Score	*Stroke rate (%/yr)*	Vascular disease	1
0	0.6	Age 65–74	1
1	3	Sex category female	1
2	4.2	*CHADS2VASC Score*	*Stroke rate (%/yr)*
3	7.1	0	0.2
4	11.1	1	0.6
5	12.5	2	2.2
6	13	3	3.2
—	—	4	4.8
—	—	5	7.2
—	—	6	9.7
—	—	7	11.2
—	—	8	10.8
—	—	9	12.2

Data from Friberg L, Rosenqvist M, Lip GY. Evaluation of risk stratification schemes for ischaemic stroke and bleeding in 182 678 patients with atrial fibrillation: the Swedish atrial fibrillation cohort study. Eur Heart J 2012;33(12):1500–10.

treatment of just 32 patients with AF prevents 1 stroke.[16] Not only are strokes less common in anticoagulated patients, warfarin also decreases the severity of strokes that do occur.[10] However, warfarin's efficacy in preventing stroke and minimizing bleeding risk requires a consistent international normalized ratio (INR) between 2.0 and 3.0.[17] Achieving and maintaining this narrow INR window is often quite difficult, particularly in complex older patients with multiple factors affecting INR control, including polypharmacy, inconsistent dietary vitamin K intake, and comorbidities. As a consequence, patients treated with warfarin require frequent INR monitoring, redosing, and dietary counseling. The delicate balance of managing warfarin is highlighted by studies showing patients remain in the therapeutic range only 50% of the time, and more than 1 in 4 patients newly started on warfarin therapy for AF discontinue therapy within 1 year.[18] Frail or multimorbid adults may have additional factors that increase the risk for discontinuation, such as declining cognitive function, poverty, polypharmacy, depression, and lack of social support.[19] Likewise, warfarin is the most common cause of emergency hospitalizations for adverse drug events among older Americans, accounting for more than 30,000 hospitalizations per year.[20]

Target-specific Oral Anticoagulants: Direct Thrombin Inhibitors and Factor Xa Inhibitors

The many challenges of safely using vitamin K antagonists led to the development of agents with fewer drug–drug interactions and easier administration. As of 2015, the currently available TSOACs are the direct thrombin inhibitor dabigatran etexilate and 3 factor Xa inhibitors: rivaroxaban, apixaban, and edoxaban. All TSOACs offer the advantages of fixed oral dosing (daily or twice daily), fewer drug–drug and dietary interactions, and no need for routine monitoring and dose adjustment. However, there are several disadvantages, including cost, the need for strict adherence to the medications, and variable renal clearance. There are also concerns about reversibility, although reversal agents are beginning to become available. TSOACs are currently approved for AF, acute treatment and prevention of venous thromboembolism (VTE), and prevention of VTE after arthroplasty.

Each TSOAC agent differs with regard to renal clearance, dosing, and drug interactions. Dabigatran at 150 mg twice daily was shown to be superior to warfarin in the Randomized Evaluation of Long-Term Anticoagulation Therapy (RE-LY) trial in terms of stroke prevention and intracranial hemorrhage risk.[21] Early anecdotal reports suggested increased bleeding compared with warfarin among elderly users of dabigatran, but a mini-sentinel study sponsored by the US Food and Drug Administration did not confirm this risk.[22] The next TSOAC to be approved was rivaroxaban, which at 20 mg daily was found to be noninferior to warfarin in the Rivaroxaban Once Daily Oral Direct Factor Xa Inhibition Compared with Vitamin K Antagonism for Prevention of Stroke and Embolism Trial in AF (ROCKET AF) study.[23] Another factor Xa inhibitor, apixaban, in the Apixaban for Reduction in Stroke and Other Thromboembolic Events in Atrial Fibrillation (ARISTOTLE) trial, showed a statistically significant mortality benefit compared with warfarin.[24] And finally, edoxaban, in the Effective aNticoaGulation with factor xA next GEneration in Atrial Fibrillation–Thrombolysis In Myocardial Infarction study 48 (ENGAGE AF–TIMI 48), was approved for use in AF based on noninferiority to warfarin, except in patients with a creatinine clearances of greater than 95 mL/min owing to lower efficacy in this subpopulation.[25]

A metaanalysis of the 4 TSOAC trials showed that relative to warfarin, TSOACs were associated with lower stroke risk (relative risk [RR], 0.81; 95% CI, 0.73–0.91) and a lower risk for intracranial hemorrhage (RR, 0.48; 95% CI, 0.39–0.59) but at the expense of an increased risk for gastrointestinal hemorrhage (RR, 1.25; 95% CI, 1.01–1.55). All-cause mortality was also lower with TSOACs (RR, 0.90; 95% CI, 0.85–0.95)[26] (**Table 2**).

Comparing Warfarin and Target-specific Oral Anticoagulants

For the multimorbid patient, clinicians must weigh the comparative efficacy and safety of this expanded array of therapeutic options (**Table 3**). In contrast with warfarin, the TSOACs' simpler pharmacokinetic properties relieve much of the burden associated with warfarin control. TSOACs produce a predictable anticoagulant response and have fewer drug–drug and dietary interactions and thus do not require monitoring. These drugs have a fast onset and shorter offset, simplifying initiation and periprocedural management. The TSOACs' predominantly positive attributes have resulted in recent guidelines recommending these new therapies over warfarin for AF.[10–12]

TSOACs also have several key drawbacks. Fewer long-term safety data are available for TSOACs than for warfarin, particularly for multimorbid adults who are often excluded from clinical trials, and new risks could emerge as usage grows. Their duration of action is shorter than warfarin, so some require twice daily dosing. The short duration of action also means that missing 1 dose can lead to insufficient anticoagulation and potentially devastating consequences. Although some estimates suggest that TSOACs may be more cost-effective from a public health perspective, the direct cost to individual patients may be greater than with warfarin.[27] Clearance is affected significantly by renal function, and unlike with warfarin, there are no validated ways to titrate dosing based on blood test measurements. Finally, there is no accepted way to

Table 2
Clinical trials comparing TSOACs to warfarin in AF and VTE

TSOAC	Trial (Year)	Indication	Dose	Dose in Renal Impairment	Dose in Hepatic Impairment
Dabigatran (direct thrombin inhibitor)	RE-LY (2009)	AF	150 mg twice daily	If CrCl is 15–30 mL/min: 75 mg twice daily	Administration in Child-Pugh B showed no change in exposure or pharmacodynamics
	RE-COVER (2009)	Acute VTE	150 mg twice daily after 5–10 d of parenteral anticoagulation	—	—
Rivaroxaban (factor Xa inhibitor)	ROCKET-AF (2011)	AF	20 mg daily with evening meal	If CrCl is 15–50 mL/min: 15 mg with evening meal	Avoid use in Child-Pugh B/C
	EINSTEIN-DVT (2010) EINSTEIN-PE (2012)	Acute PE or DVT	15 mg twice daily for 3 weeks followed by 20 mg once daily	—	—
Apixaban (factor Xa inhibitor)	ARISTOTLE (2011)	AF	5 mg twice daily	If patient has ≥2 of following: age >80, weight <60, SCr >1.5 mg/dL: 2.5 mg twice daily	Mild impairment: no change recommended. Moderate impairment: no dosing recommendation available; severe impairment: avoid use
	AMPLIFY (2013)	Acute VTE	10 mg twice daily for 7 d followed by 5 mg twice daily	—	—
Edoxaban (factor Xa inhibitor)	ENGAGE AF-TIMI 48 (2013)	AF	If CrCl is between 50 and 95 mL/min: 60 mg/d	If CrCl >95: do not use; if CrCl 15–50: 30 mg daily	Avoid use in Child-Pugh B/C
	Hokusai-VTE (2013)	Acute VTE	After initial 5–10 d parenteral anticoagulation, 60 mg once daily if CrCl >50 mL/min or 30 mg once daily if CrCl 30–50 mL/min or body weight ≤ 60 kg	—	—

Abbreviations: CrCl, creatinine clearance; DVT, deep venous thrombosis; PE, pulmonary embolism; TSOACs, target-specific oral anticoagulants; VTE, venous thromboembolism.

Data from Ruff CT, Giugliano RP, Braunwald E, et al. Comparison of the efficacy and safety of new oral anticoagulants with warfarin in patients with atrial fibrillation: a meta-analysis of randomised trials. Lancet 2014;383:955–62; and van der Hulle T, Kooiman J, den Exter PL, et al. Effectiveness and safety of novel oral anticoagulants as compared with vitamin K antagonists in the treatment of acute symptomatic venous thromboembolism: a systematic review and meta-analysis. J Thromb Haemost 2014;12(3):320–28.

Table 3
Comparison of TSOACs and warfarin in AF and VTE

	TSOACs	Warfarin	Relative Risk (95% CI)
Atrial fibrillation			
Ischemic stroke	Same		0.92 (0.83–1.02)
Intracranial hemorrhage	TSOACs better		0.48 (0.39–0.59)
Gastrointestinal bleeding	TSOACs worse		1.25 (1.01–1.55)
Mortality	TSOACs better		0.90 (0.85–0.95)
VTE			
Recurrent VTE	Same		0.88 (0.74–1.05)
Major bleeding	TSOACs better		0.60 (0.41–0.88)
Mortality	Same		0.97 (0.83–1.14)
Special Considerations			
Dosing	Fixed dosing	Adjusted dosing	—
Adherence	Very important	Very important	—
Monitoring	No	Yes	—
Interactions	Fewer	Many	—
Cost	High	Low	—
Reversibility	Preliminary	Yes	—
Special concerns	Renal, liver	Liver	—

Abbreviations: AF, atrial fibrillation; TSOACs, target-specific oral anticoagulants; VTE, venous thromboembolism.
Data from Refs.[26,28,29]

monitor anticoagulation levels, as traditional methods such as activated partial thromboplastin time or INR do not reliably predict anticoagulant effect.[28] Thus, both warfarin and TSOACs have respective pros and cons, and agent selection in multimorbid patients should be informed by a careful evaluation of clinical characteristics, as well as patient goals and values.

Although the focus of this paper is on AF, TSOACs are also used for acute VTE treatment and it is important to note several differences in dosing during the initiation period. Notably, dabigatran and edoxaban are approved for the acute treatment of deep venous thrombosis or pulmonary embolism only if the patient has been treated for 5 to 10 days with a parenteral therapy such as heparin or enoxaparin.[29] The 2 TSOACs that can be started as monotherapy for VTE, rivaroxaban and apixaban, are dosed differently than for AF in the initial VTE treatment period: rivaroxaban is administered at 15 mg twice daily for 3 weeks, after which the dose is reduced to 20 mg daily, and apixaban is administered at 10 mg twice daily for 7 days, followed by 5 mg twice daily thereafter. A metaanalysis of trials studying the acute treatment of VTE showed that TSOACs are comparably effective relative to vitamin K antagonists in reducing VTE recurrence and are associated with a lower risk for major bleeding.[29] However, the mean age of patients in these studies was only about 50 to 60 years, and the efficacy and safety of TSOACs for the extended treatment of VTE, particularly in older adults, are still unknown.

SPECIAL CONSIDERATIONS IN PATIENTS WITH MULTIMORBIDITY

Despite ample clinical trial evidence and consensus guidelines supporting anticoagulation for most older adults with AF, anticoagulation remains greatly underused. Fewer than one-half of AF patients without contraindications to anticoagulation receive treatment.[30] For every advancing decade of life, there is a 14% decrease in warfarin use regardless of other independent risk factors for stroke.[31] Surveys of physicians show that patient age acts as a significant deterrent to the use of anticoagulation in AF.[32]

The complexity of anticoagulation in multimorbid older adults limits the translation of evidence-based recommendations into real-world practice. Clinicians must weigh the benefit of stroke prevention against the significant concerns of bleeding risk, safe administration of the medication, quality of life, and coexisting medical issues. Similar to approaches to cancer screening in older, frail adults, clinicians should account for patient-defined outcomes, competing priorities, and estimated life expectancy.[33]

Net Clinical Benefit of Anticoagulation

Any discussion of the challenges associated with anticoagulation in multimorbid patients is informed by analysis of the net clinical benefit of anticoagulation in AF. The net clinical benefit can be assessed by weighing the absolute benefit (ischemic strokes prevented) against the absolute harm (hemorrhages induced). The Birmingham Atrial Fibrillation Treatment of the Aged (BAFTA) trial quantified this net benefit by randomizing patients over age 75 (mean age, 81.5 years) to either aspirin (75 mg) or warfarin (INR goal, 2.0–3.0).[34] Warfarin considerably reduced the risk of stroke over an average 2.7 years of follow-up, with a relative risk of 0.48 and number needed to treat of 50. There was no difference in bleeding risk between the 2 groups, confirming the effectiveness and safety of warfarin in elderly adults.[35] Although risks associated with anticoagulation increase as patients age, in fact, the net clinical benefit of warfarin accrues over time because patients simultaneously develop additional ischemic stroke risk factors[36] (**Fig. 3**).

Assessment of the net clinical benefit of anticoagulation in patients of advanced age or comorbidity must be informed by competing risks and overall life expectancy. In contrast with patients enrolled in clinical trials, real-world AF patients are frailer and have higher risks of bleeding and more comorbidities, making them subject to additional competing risks.[37] Focusing on stroke as the primary outcome driving treatment may fail to capture other outcomes important to a patient. In multimorbid adults with a

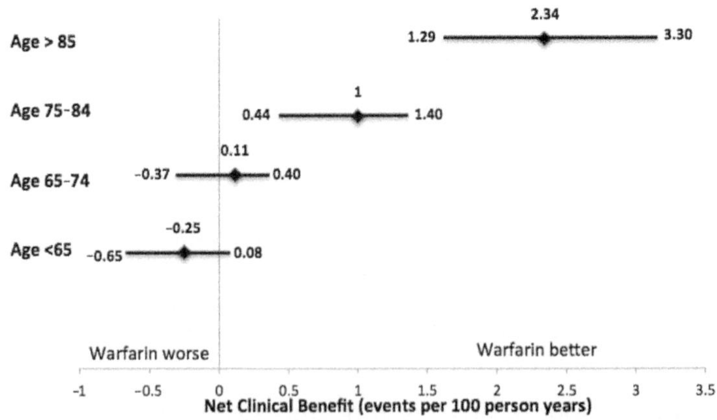

Fig. 3. Net clinical benefit of anticoagulation with warfarin by age. (*Data from* Singer DE, Chang Y, Fang MC, et al. The net clinical benefit of warfarin anticoagulation in atrial fibrillation. Ann Intern Med 2009;151(5):297–305.)

limited life expectancy, calculations of net clinical benefit based on stroke prevention alone may overestimate the benefit of anticoagulation.

Estimating Bleeding Risk of Anticoagulation

Advancing age is an important risk factor for bleeding in AF patients and must be factored into clinical decision making. Elderly patients are at increased risk for both intracranial and extracranial hemorrhage. Among AF patients, each advancing decade in age is associated with a relative increase in hemorrhage rate of 1.3 (95% CI, 1.1–1.6).[38] The most dreaded complication of anticoagulation is intracranial hemorrhage. Intracranial hemorrhages account for 15% to 20% of major warfarin-associated bleeds and are responsible for 90% of fatal bleeds, as well as the majority of disability among survivors.[39] Notably, rates of anticoagulant-associated intracranial hemorrhage increase strikingly above the age of 80.[34]

As in the case of ischemic stroke, the accrual of comorbidities also increases risk of both intracranial and extracranial bleeding in AF patients. Common conditions in the elderly, such as a history of bleeding, anemia, and chronic renal insufficiency, have been linked with major bleeding. Hypertension and history of stroke have also been shown to predict future bleeding.[40] Unfortunately, risk factors for hemorrhage overlap significantly with those for ischemic stroke, underscoring the inherent difficulty that clinicians and patients face in deciding whether to initiate and/or continue anticoagulation (**Fig. 4**).

Akin to stroke risk prediction scores, several bleeding prediction scores incorporating these characteristics have been developed to estimate anticoagulant-associated bleeding risk. Risk models like the HAS-BLED and ATRIA Bleeding Risk scores use clinical risk factors to help clinicians to estimate annual bleeding risk for patients on chronic anticoagulation[41,42] (**Fig. 5**, **Table 4**). Current risk schemes, however, share several drawbacks. A primary limitation is that they were developed using data from patients already taking anticoagulants and thus may not represent the true risk of bleeding in patients who were considered too high risk for anticoagulation. Thus, it is possible that actual bleeding rates in frail elders with a high risk of falls or a history of significant bleeding are greater than what current risk schemes predict.

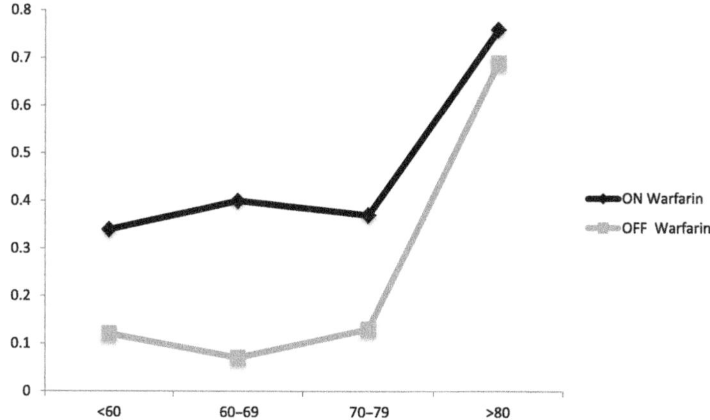

Fig. 4. Unadjusted age-specific rates of intracranial hemorrhage on and off warfarin. (*Data from* Fang MC, Go AS, Hylek EM, et al. Age and the risk of warfarin-associated hemorrhage: the anticoagulation and risk factors in atrial fibrillation study. J Am Geriatr Soc 2006;54:1231.)

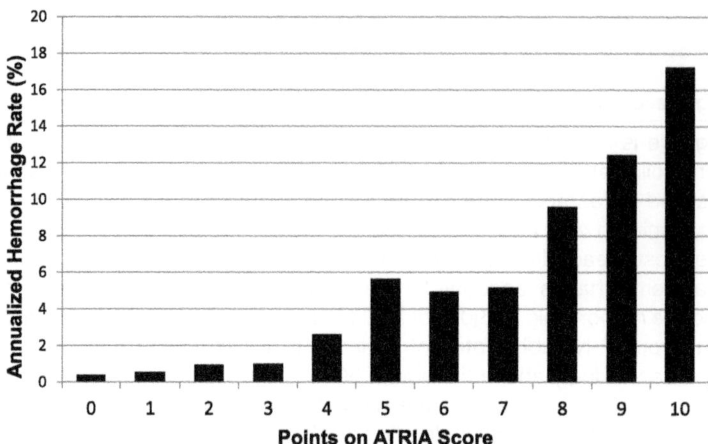

Fig. 5. Annualized rates of major hemorrhage on warfarin by anticoagulation and risk factors in atrial fibrillation (ATRIA) bleeding risk score. (*Adapted from* Fang MC, Go AS, Chang Y, et al. A new risk scheme to predict warfarin-associated hemorrhage the ATRIA (anticoagulation and risk factors in atrial fibrillation) study. J Am Coll Cardiol 2011;58:395–401; and Roalfe A, Bryant T, Davies M, et al. A cross-sectional study of quality of life in an elderly population (75 years and over) with atrial fibrillation: secondary analysis of data from the Birmingham Atrial Fibrillation Treatment of the Aged Study (BAFTA). Europace 2012;14:1420–7.)

Although the most clinically significant risk of anticoagulation is intracranial bleeding, risk scores largely predict extracranial bleeding, and the accuracy of these scores in predicting major bleeding may not be significantly better than physicians' subjective estimates.[43] Furthermore, the available scores are validated mostly in warfarin

Table 4
The HAS-BLED and ATRIA bleeding risk scores

Risk Score	Risk Score Calculation	Risk Categories (Points)	Annualized Bleeding Rates from Validation Cohort (%)
HAS-BLED Score	1 point for each: *h*ypertension, *a*bnormal renal/liver, *s*troke, *b*leeding history or predisposition, *l*abile INR, *e*lderly (>65 years), or *d*rug/alcohol use	Low (0) Intermediate (1–2) High (3+)	1.1 2.9 3.7
ATRIA Bleeding Risk Score	Anemia (3 points) Severe renal disease (3 points) Age > 75 yrs (2 points) Prior bleed (1 point) Hypertension (1 point)	Low (0–3) Intermediate (4) High (5+)	0.8 2.6 5.8

Abbreviations: ATRIA, *an*ticoagulation and *r*isk factors *i*n *a*trial fibrillation study; INR, international normalized ratio.

Data from Fang MC, Go AS, Chang Y, et al. A new risk scheme to predict warfarin-associated hemorrhage the ATRIA (anticoagulation and risk factors in atrial fibrillation) study. J Am Coll Cardiol 2011;58:395–401; and Lip GY, Frison L, Halperin JL, et al. Comparative validation of a novel risk score for predicting bleeding risk in anticoagulated patients with atrial fibrillation: the HAS-BLED (hypertension, abnormal renal/liver function, stroke, bleeding history or predisposition, labile INR, elderly, drugs/alcohol concomitantly) score. J Am Coll Cardiol 2011;57(2):173–80.

patients and there is limited experience applying them to TSOAC patients; this is relevant because TSOACs are associated with lower intracranial hemorrhage risk than warfarin. In light of these limitations, bleeding risk schemes may be most helpful in identifying and minimizing modifiable risk factors, such as controlling hypertension or stopping unnecessary antiplatelet therapy, or when applied to patients at the lower end of stroke risk, where the absolute benefit of anticoagulation is decreased. For multimorbid individuals not represented in the development of bleeding risk scores, clinicians still need to use their best clinical judgment.

Fall Risk

Fear of traumatic intracranial bleeding precipitated by falls significantly influences clinicians in their assessment of the risk–benefit ratio of anticoagulation.[44] Hospitalizations for falls are associated with head injury and increased mortality, particularly among patients taking anticoagulants.[45] The true risk of fall-related intracranial hemorrhage is difficult to determine because those patients at greatest risk of falls are often excluded from clinical studies. One prospective cohort study of adult patients at high risk for falls taking oral anticoagulants did not show a greater risk of major bleeds than patients at low risk of falls.[41] Another study of patients with AF revealed that patients with high fall risk had almost twice the risk of intracranial hemorrhage but still found that the benefits of stroke prevention exceeded the harms when patients were at higher risk for stroke.[46] A commonly cited decision analysis estimated that an average person with AF would need to fall greater than 295 times per year before the risk of traumatic intracranial hemorrhage would outweigh the benefit of ischemic stroke prevention.[47] For patients at the lower end of stroke risk (CHA_2DS_2-VASc scores of 0–3), however, the risks associated with falling may be greater than the benefits. In summary, the available evidence, albeit limited in quality, suggests that the benefits of anticoagulation outweigh the risk of fall-induced intracranial hemorrhage in patients with high stroke risk, but the risks associated with falls are more influential in patients at lower risk of stroke.

Anticoagulants in the Setting of Polypharmacy

Polypharmacy, defined as the prescription of multiple medications, is a common consequence of multimorbidity and another important consideration in prescribing anticoagulation to older adults. Nearly one-half of Medicare beneficiaries report taking 5 or more medications.[34] Increasing numbers of medications compound the risk for drug side-effects and drug–drug interactions. This is especially true of warfarin, for which the range of drug interactions is broad.[48] Polypharmacy also contributes to the cost and complexity of care and can thereby decrease adherence. For example, 1 study describing a hypothetical multimorbid patient found that application of clinical practice guidelines for hypertension, diabetes mellitus, osteoarthritis, chronic obstructive pulmonary disease, and osteoporosis would lead to prescription of 12 medications with complex administration schedules and an out-of-pocket cost of $3797 per year.[49] Given the burden this represents, it is hardly surprising that polypharmacy is associated with an increased likelihood of impaired mobility, morbidity, hospitalizations, nursing home placement, and death.[50]

The negative effects of polypharmacy have led to an increasing emphasis on "deprescribing," a method by which medication lists are culled and simplified to reflect clinical priorities[51] (**Fig. 6**). Because the absolute benefits of anticoagulants increase with older age and additional stroke risk factors, anticoagulants are likely to be among a patient's most beneficial medications. Clinicians should work with patients to determine whether the benefits of anticoagulants are worth the trade-offs of increased

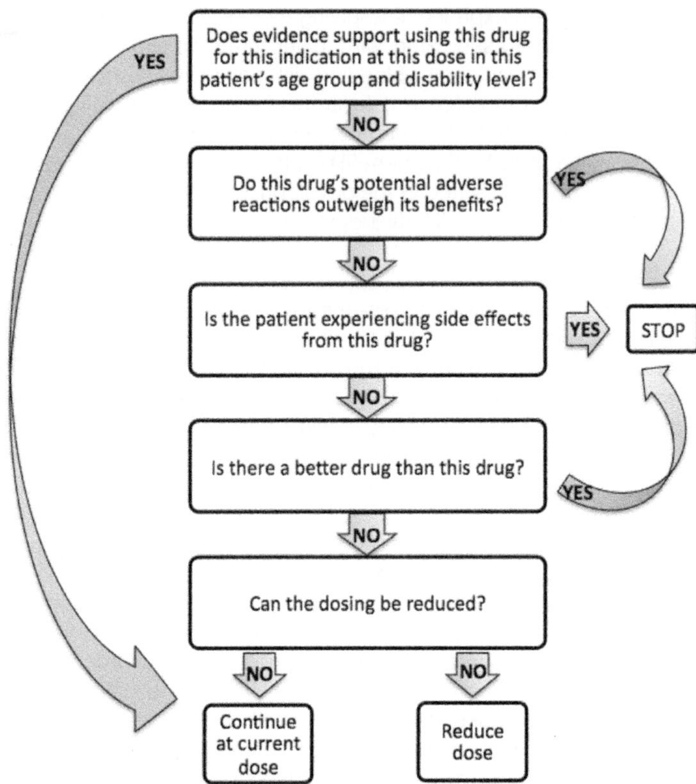

Fig. 6. De-prescribing methodology for improving polypharmacy in the multimorbid elderly. (*Adapted from* Garfinkel D, Mangin D. Feasibility study of a systematic approach for discontinuation of multiple medications in older adults: addressing polypharmacy. Arch Intern Med 2010;170(18):1649.)

bleeding risk, potential drug–drug interactions, and increased complexity of clinical management. Patients should be counseled to wear an alert bracelet, keep an updated and accurate medication list, and ensure familiarity with medications in case of emergencies.

Quality of Life

Anticoagulation holds the promise of both improving and hindering quality of life: it can prevent stroke-related morbidity but also can result in significant adverse effects and affect a patient's lifestyle. Studies that have attempted to quantify the impact of anticoagulants on quality of life have generally found minimal effects.[52] In 1 study, patients who were randomized to long-term warfarin therapy had no differences in daily activities, attitudes, or global quality of life compared with patients not on warfarin.[53] Despite assumptions to the contrary, studies that have compared warfarin with more easily managed medications (such as aspirin or dabigatran) have also not found substantial differences in quality of life.[54,55] In general, taking anticoagulants does not seem to have a significant deleterious impact on measured quality of life; the major impact seems to come from the adverse outcomes of stroke or bleeding.

Selecting the best anticoagulant for a patient with atrial fibrillation

Once a decision is made to recommend anticoagulation, clinicians next have to decide which anticoagulant is best for a given patient. In choosing between warfarin and a TSOAC, key considerations should include the following:

1. The ability to maintain a therapeutic INR range more than 60% of the time, as rates less than this have been associated with lower efficacy and higher risk of bleeding.[56]
2. The willingness of the patient to undergo regular INR monitoring, whether in a clinic, local laboratory, or by using a home INR machine.
3. Coexisting medications, renal function, and factors that may make INR control more difficult, such as interacting medications and variable vitamin K intake.
4. Cost to an individual patient and the health care system.

TSOACs, although associated with fewer drug–drug interactions than warfarin, still may be affected by certain medications such as P-glycoprotein and CYP3A inhibitors and inducers. Prescribers need to thoroughly screen patients' medication lists before prescribing and dosing anticoagulants. Among the TSOACs, there are options for daily or twice daily dosing, which may be important if minimizing pill burden is a concern. The TSOACs each have differences in the degree of renal clearance, with apixaban being the least affected by renal function, and regular assessments of renal function are recommended. Owing to varying degrees of liver clearance, TSOACs should generally be avoided in patients with severe liver dysfunction. When considering TSOACs, prescribers also need to carefully assess a patient's adherence, because discontinuation of these medications has been associated with a higher rate of thromboembolic events. Warfarin's longer half-life makes missed doses less impactful, whereas imperfect adherence to TSOACs make it more likely that patients will have periods of under-anticoagulation. Finally, although reversal agents are beginning to become available (idarucizumab for reversing dabigatran; andexanet alfa as a potential agent for reversing all factor Xa inhibitors), experience with managing bleeding complications from TSOACs is still preliminary. As a consequence, it may be prudent to avoid TSOACs in patients who are likely to have recurrent bleeding events.

SUMMARY

As the number of AF patients with advanced age and multiple coexisting conditions steadily increases, clinicians will increasingly be faced with difficult decisions regarding the appropriateness of anticoagulation and choice of anticoagulant for a given patient. Although multimorbid patients often gain greater absolute benefits from anticoagulation in terms of stroke prevention, they are also at greater risk for complications of therapy and face challenges in safely taking these medications. TSOACs are viable alternatives to warfarin and there is increasing evidence supporting their efficacy and safety. However, clinicians and patients need to be cognizant of unique considerations related to their use, including the risk for bleeding, limited experience with reversibility, the need for attentive adherence, and higher cost. An alliance between patients and clinicians is essential to create an individualized plan for anticoagulation that addresses the myriad issues related to safety and tolerability, all grounded in a patient's own goals for his or her care.

REFERENCES

1. Go AS, Hylek EM, Phillips KA, et al. Prevalence of diagnosed atrial fibrillation in adults: national implications for rhythm management and stroke prevention: the anticoagulation and risk factors in atrial fibrillation (ATRIA) Study. JAMA 2001; 285:2370.

2. Naccarelli GV, Varker H, Lin J, et al. Increasing prevalence of atrial fibrillation and flutter in the United States. Am J Cardiol 2009;104:1534.
3. Office of Information Products and Data Analytics CMMS. CMS administrative claims data, January 2011-December 2011, from the chronic condition warehouse. 2012. Available at: www.ccwdata.org. Accessed July 15, 2014.
4. Risk factors for stroke and efficacy of antithrombotic therapy in atrial fibrillation. Analysis of pooled data from five randomized controlled trials. Arch Intern Med 1994;154(13):1449–57.
5. Sanna T, Diener HC, Passman RS, et al. Cryptogenic stroke and underlying atrial fibrillation. N Engl J Med 2014;370(26):2478–86.
6. Schmidt M, Jacobsen JB, Johnsen SP, et al. Eighteen-year trends in stroke mortality and the prognostic influence of comorbidity. Neurology 2014;82:340–50.
7. Lin HJ, Wolf PA, Kelly-Hayes M, et al. Stroke severity in atrial fibrillation. The Framingham Study. Stroke 1996;27(10):1760–4.
8. Gage BF, Waterman AD, Shannon W, et al. Validation of clinical classification schemes for predicting stroke: results from the national registry of atrial fibrillation. JAMA 2001;285(22):2864–70.
9. Lip GY, Nieuwlaat R, Pisters R, et al. Refining clinical risk stratification for predicting stroke and thromboembolism in atrial fibrillation using a novel risk factor-based approach: the euro heart survey on atrial fibrillation. Chest 2010;137(2): 263–72.
10. You JJ, Singer DE, Howard PA, et al. Antithrombotic therapy for atrial fibrillation: antithrombotic therapy and prevention of thrombosis, 9th ed: American College of Chest Physicians evidence-based clinical practice guidelines. Chest 2012; 141(Suppl 2):e531S–75S.
11. Skanes AC, Healey JS, Cairns JA, et al, Canadian Cardiovascular Society Atrial Fibrillation Guidelines Committee. Focused 2012 update of the Canadian Cardiovascular Society atrial fibrillation guidelines: recommendations for stroke prevention and rate/rhythm control. Can J Cardiol 2012;28:125–36.
12. Camm AJ, Lip GY, DeCaterina R, et al, ESC Committee for Practice Guidelines. 2012 focused update of the ESC guidelines for the management of atrial fibrillation: an update of the 2010 ESC guidelines for the management of atrial fibrillation. Developed with the special contribution of the European Heart Rhythm Association. Eur Heart J 2012;33:2719–47.
13. Fang MC. Implications of the new atrial fibrillation guideline. JAMA Intern Med 2015;175(5):850–1.
14. January CT, Wann LS, Alpert JS, et al. 2014 AHA/ACC/HRS guideline for the management of patients with atrial fibrillation: a report of the American College of Cardiology/American Heart Association Task Force on Practice Guidelines and the Heart Rhythm Society. J Am Coll Cardiol 2014;64(21):e1–76.
15. Friberg L, Rosenqvist M, Lip GY. Evaluation of risk stratification schemes for ischaemic stroke and bleeding in 182 678 patients with atrial fibrillation: the Swedish Atrial Fibrillation Cohort Study. Eur Heart J 2012;33(12):1500–10.
16. Hart RG, Pearce LA, Aguilar MI. Meta-analysis: antithrombotic therapy to prevent stroke in patients who have nonvalvular atrial fibrillation. Ann Intern Med 2007; 146:857–67.
17. Singer DE, Chang Y, Fang MC, et al. Should patient characteristics influence target anticoagulation intensity for stroke prevention in nonvalvular atrial fibrillation? The ATRIA study. Circ Cardiovasc Qual Outcomes 2009;2(4):297–304.
18. Fang MC, Go AS, Chang Y, et al. Predictors of warfarin discontinuation in older patients with atrial fibrillation. J Am Coll Cardiol 2008;51:A238.

19. Kneeland PP, Fang MC. Current issues in patient adherence and persistence: focus on anticoagulants for the treatment and prevention of thromboembolism. Patient Prefer Adherence 2010;4:51–60.
20. Budnitz DS, Lovegrove ML, Shehab N, et al. Emergency hospitalizations for adverse drug events in older Americans. N Engl J Med 2011;365(21):2002–12.
21. Connolly SJ, Ezekowitz MD, Yusuf S, et al. Dabigatran versus warfarin in patients with atrial fibrillation. N Engl J Med 2009;361(12):1139–51.
22. Southworth MR, Reichman ME, Unger EF, et al. Dabigatran and postmarketing reports of bleeding. N Engl J Med 2013;368:1272–4.
23. Patel MR, Mahaffey KW, Garg J, et al. Rivaroxaban versus warfarin in nonvalvular atrial fibrillation. N Engl J Med 2011;365(10):883–91.
24. Granger CB, Alexander JH, McMurray JJ, et al. Apixaban versus warfarin in patients with atrial fibrillation. N Engl J Med 2011;365(11):981–92.
25. Giugliano RP, Ruff CT, Braunwald E, et al. Edoxaban versus warfarin in patients with atrial fibrillation. N Engl J Med 2013;369(22):2093–104.
26. Ruff C, Giugliano RP, Braunwald E, et al. Comparison of the efficacy and safety of new oral anticoagulants with warfarin in patients with atrial fibrillation: a meta-analysis of randomised trials. Lancet 2014;383:955–62.
27. Harrington AR, Armstrong EP, Nolan PE Jr, et al. Cost-effectiveness of apixaban, dabigatran, rivaroxaban, and warfarin for stroke prevention in atrial fibrillation. Stroke 2013;44:1676–81.
28. Weitz JI. Anticoagulation therapy in 2015: where we are and where we are going. J Thromb Thrombolysis 2015;39:264–72.
29. van der Hulle T, Kooiman J, den Exter PL, et al. Effectiveness and safety of novel oral anticoagulants as compared with vitamin K antagonists in the treatment of acute symptomatic venous thromboembolism: a systematic review and meta-analysis. J Thromb Haemost 2014;12(3):320–8.
30. Fang MC, Stafford RS, Ruskin JN, et al. National trends in antiarrhythmic and antithrombotic medication use in atrial fibrillation. Arch Intern Med 2004;164(1): 55–60.
31. Brophy MT, Snyder KE, Gaehde S, et al. Anticoagulant use for atrial fibrillation in the elderly. J Am Geriatr Soc 2004;52(7):1151–6.
32. McCrory DC, Matchar DB, Samsa G, et al. Physician attitudes about anticoagulation for nonvalvular atrial fibrillation in the elderly. Arch Intern Med 1995;155:277.
33. Walter LC, Covinsky KE. Cancer screening in elderly patients: a framework for individualized decision making. JAMA 2001;285(21):2750–6.
34. Fried TR, O'Leary J, Towle V, et al. Health outcomes associated with polypharmacy in community-dwelling older adults: a systematic review. J Am Geriatr Soc 2014;62(12):2261–72.
35. Mant J, Hobbs FD, Fletcher K, et al. Warfarin versus aspirin for stroke prevention in an elderly community population with atrial fibrillation (the Birmingham Atrial Fibrillation Treatment of the Aged Study, BAFTA): a randomised controlled trial. Lancet 2007;370(9586):493–503.
36. Singer DE, Chang Y, Fang MC, et al. The net clinical benefit of warfarin anticoagulation in atrial fibrillation. Ann Intern Med 2009;151(5):297–305.
37. Satagopan JM, Ben-Porat L, Berwick M, et al. A note on competing risks in survival data analysis. Br J Cancer 2004;91(7):1229–35.
38. Fang MC, Go AS, Hylek EM, et al. Age and the risk of warfarin-associated hemorrhage: the anticoagulation and risk factors in atrial fibrillation study. J Am Geriatr Soc 2006;54:1231.

39. Fang MC, Go AS, Chang Y, et al. Death and disability from warfarin-associated intracranial and extracranial hemorrhages. Am J Med 2007;120(8):700–5.
40. Fang MC, Go AS, Chang Y, et al. A new risk scheme to predict warfarin-associated hemorrhage the ATRIA (Anticoagulation and Risk Factors in Atrial Fibrillation) study. J Am Coll Cardiol 2011;58:395–401.
41. Donzé J, Clair C, Hug B, et al. Risk of falls and major bleeds in patients on oral anticoagulation therapy. Am J Med 2012;125(8):773–8.
42. Lip GY, Frison L, Halperin JL, et al. Comparative validation of a novel risk score for predicting bleeding risk in anticoagulated patients with atrial fibrillation: the HAS-BLED (hypertension, abnormal renal/liver function, stroke, bleeding history or predisposition, labile INR, elderly, drugs/alcohol concomitantly) score. J Am Coll Cardiol 2011;57(2):173–80.
43. Donzé J, Rodondi N, Waeber G, et al. Scores to predict major bleeding risk during oral anticoagulation therapy: a prospective validation study. Am J Med 2012; 125(11):1095–102.
44. Pugh D, Pugh J, Mead GE. Attitudes of physicians regarding anticoagulation for atrial fibrillation: a systematic review. Age Ageing 2011;40(6):675–83.
45. Inui TS, Parina R, Chang DC, et al. Mortality after ground-level fall in the elderly patient taking oral anticoagulation for atrial fibrillation/flutter: a long-term analysis of risk versus benefit. J Trauma Acute Care Surg 2014;76:642–50.
46. Gage BF, Birman-Deych E, Kerzner R, et al. Incidence of intracranial hemorrhage in patients with atrial fibrillation who are prone to fall. Am J Med 2005;118(6):612–7.
47. Man-Son-Hing M, Nichol G, Lau A, et al. Choosing antithrombotic therapy for elderly patients with atrial fibrillation who are at risk for falls. Arch Intern Med 1999;159(7):677–85.
48. Holbrook AM, Pereira JA, Labiris R, et al. Systematic overview of warfarin and its drug and food interactions. Arch Intern Med 2005;165(10):1095–106.
49. Boyd CM, Darer J, Boult C, et al. Clinical practice guidelines and quality of care for older patients with multiple comorbid diseases: implications for pay for performance. JAMA 2005;294:716–24.
50. Scott IA, Hilmer SN, Reeve E, et al. Reducing inappropriate polypharmacy: the process of deprescribing. JAMA Intern Med 2015;175(5):827–34.
51. Garfinkel D, Mangin D. Feasibility study of a systematic approach for discontinuation of multiple medications in older adults: addressing polypharmacy. Arch Intern Med 2010;170(18):1648–54.
52. Roalfe A, Bryant T, Davies M, et al. A cross-sectional study of quality of life in an elderly population (75 years and over) with atrial fibrillation: secondary analysis of data from the Birmingham Atrial Fibrillation Treatment of the Aged Study (BAFTA). Europace 2012;14:1420–7.
53. Lancaster TR, Singer DE, Sheehan MA, et al. The impact of long-term warfarin therapy on quality of life. Evidence from a randomized trial. Boston Area Anticoagulation Trial for Atrial Fibrillation Investigators. Arch Intern Med 1991;151(10):1944–9.
54. Gage BF, Cardinalli AB, Owens DK. The effect of stroke and stroke prophylaxis with aspirin or warfarin on quality of life. Arch Intern Med 1996;156(16):1829–36.
55. Monz BU, Connolly SJ, Korhonen M, et al. Assessing the impact of dabigatran and warfarin on health-related quality of life: results from an RE-LY sub-study. Int J Cardiol 2013;168(3):2540–7.
56. Connolly SJ, Pogue J, Eikelboom J, et al. Benefit of oral anticoagulant over antiplatelet therapy in atrial fibrillation depends on the quality of international normalized ratio control achieved by centers and countries as measured by time in therapeutic range. Circulation 2008;118(20):2029–37.

Approach to Evaluating the Multimorbid Patient with Cardiovascular Disease Undergoing Noncardiac Surgery

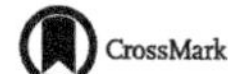

William L. Lyons, MD

KEYWORDS

• Multimorbidity • Preoperative assessment • Geriatric assessment • Frailty

KEY POINTS

- Older, multimorbid patients are at greater risk of negative outcomes after noncardiac surgical procedures.
- Assessment approaches targeting organ-specific diseases (particularly cardiac disease), have been developed for use in the preoperative setting.
- Evaluating patients using a battery of related clinical practice guidelines may lead to overtesting, polypharmacy, and loss of patient-centeredness.
- A better approach is to evaluate patients for cognitive and physical function, mood disorders, mobility, social support, nutritional status, medication use, and frailty, with targeted evaluations for cardiac, pulmonary, and renal disease.
- The best way to perform such a streamlined, practical assessment, and to deliver preoperative optimization based on assessment results, remains to be determined.

Older patients undergo more surgical procedures, in both inpatient and outpatient settings, than do younger individuals.[1] In 2007, those 65 years or older had 2 to 3 times more of such procedures (per capita) than younger persons.[2] The most common major procedures in this population are knee and hip replacement, colectomy, and cardiac surgery,[2] but ambulatory surgeries are becoming more common, with more than 70% of surgical procedures in the United States now performed in the outpatient setting.[3] The older, multimorbid patient is at increased risk of postoperative complications and undesired outcomes,[1,4] including death,[5] and complications are more often medical than surgical.[6] It seems that preoperative comprehensive geriatric assessment, in which risk factors and problems are identified and addressed before surgery,

Disclosure Statement: Author has no conflicts of interest to disclose.
Division of Geriatrics, Department of Internal Medicine, University of Nebraska Medical Center, 986155 Nebraska Medical Center, Omaha, NE 68198-6155, USA
E-mail address: wlyons@unmc.edu

Clin Geriatr Med 32 (2016) 347–358
http://dx.doi.org/10.1016/j.cger.2016.01.007 geriatric.theclinics.com
0749-0690/16/$ – see front matter

may be beneficial in reducing adverse outcomes,[7] but issues of targeting, resource use (particularly time), availability of geriatrically trained clinicians, and general feasibility are unsettled.

In evaluating a multimorbid patient before a contemplated surgery, it may be tempting to catalog various diseases and conditions, and to apply the related clinical practice guidelines cumulatively to preoperative care. Unfortunately, these guidelines are developed for application with individual conditions, not a multimorbid, interacting array of them; they reflect recommendations arising from studies that largely excluded older, frail patients with many diagnoses; they tend to promote polypharmacy; they offer little guidance on how to prioritize recommendations; and they depersonalize medical practice.[8] For multimorbid patients for whom the end of life is in sight, clinicians are advised to focus more on goal-oriented than disease-oriented decision making.[9]

Consulting the literature to provide goal-oriented advice in this population is more easily said than done. Most surgical outcome data, including that in older multimorbid patients, relate to short-term survival, and for older patients there is more to life than this measure.[10] Common top priorities, such as health-related quality of life or maintenance of functional independence, are rarely examined in surgical publications.[4,10,11]

An older, multimorbid patient with particular idiosyncratic health priorities and conditions, and with a problem potentially amenable to surgical treatment, may not necessarily be best served by a trip to the operating room. A prudent approach[4,10] to joint decision making with the patient could be outlined as follows.

- Discuss with the patient global health care goals and priorities: prolonged survival, self-care function and independence, maintenance of cognition, comfort, or something else? Resources are available[12,13] to estimate mortality risk—in the event this is an important consideration—for multimorbid older adults who lack a single dominant life-threatening illness.
- Assess the likelihood that the contemplated surgery can satisfy particular goals and priorities, taking into account both benefits and risks.
- All things considered, if it seems that risk exceeds likely benefit, then recommend nonoperative approaches to care or less invasive procedures.
- Aside from risk, matters of feasibility and burden require consideration. For some patients (and their families or caregivers) the entire course of surgical treatment, including postoperative rehabilitation, medical follow-up visits, and so on, are profoundly complex and burdensome. Patients with scant social support or history of adherence difficulties should be asked about this issue.
- If the benefit seems to exceed the risk, the burden is bearable, and the integrated plan seems feasible, then proceed with a preoperative assessment, with particular focus on physical and cognitive function, nutrition, frailty, medication prescribing and polypharmacy, and selected other issues as described elsewhere in this paper. Preoperative optimization may entail treating multiple comorbidities, medication debridement, "prehabilitation" (involving physical and/or occupational therapy), and nutritional supplementation.

This article concentrates on the type of preoperative assessment with optimization as described. Cardiovascular, pulmonary, and renal conditions are also considered, because diseases in these organs commonly lead to perioperative complications in older adults,[4] but the focus primarily will be on the integrated physiologic, whole person approaches that (probably) produce better results.

COGNITION AND MOOD

In a review[4] of studies involving a variety of surgical procedures, cognitive impairment was shown to be a risk factor for postoperative mortality, with adjusted hazard ratios varying from 1.26 to 5.77. In the preoperative setting early identification of occult cognitive impairment is important, because the trustworthiness of a patient's history and review of symptoms may be questionable,[1] and it may prove necessary to use a surrogate for deliberation and decision making.

In addition to death, preoperative cognitive impairment is also a potent predictor of postoperative delirium, which in turn is associated with longer hospital stay, postoperative functional decline, and delayed recovery.[1,14,15] Estimates of the incidence of postoperative delirium in noncardiac surgeries range from 5% to 52%, with hip fracture repairs and aortic surgeries showing the greatest rates.[11,16] Other risk factors for postoperative delirium, aside from cognitive impairment, include older age, functional impairment, sensory impairment (vision and hearing), depression, preoperative use of psychotropic medications, institutional residence, and greater comorbidity,[16–18] as well as greater severity of postoperative pain.[19]

Postoperative cognitive dysfunction (in which patients demonstrate persistent cognitive deficits after surgery, but do not meet criteria for delirium) affects double the proportion of older than younger patients.[20] Nevertheless, most patients who suffer early postoperative cognitive losses return to their baseline cognitive levels within 3 months of surgery.[21] Postoperative complications and chronic pain may represent modifiable risk factors for persistent cognitive decline.[21]

Experts in geriatric surgery[1,4] recommend performing some form of cognitive screening, such as the Mini-Cog,[22] to gauge patients' preoperative cognitive function. Strategies to reduce the risk of postoperative delirium[4,19] include limiting perioperative use of psychotropic drugs,[23] ensuring patients' glasses and hearing aids are available in the hospital, and meticulous management of postoperative analgesia. **Box 1** summarizes delirium risk factors and preventive measures.

Box 1
Risk factors and preventive measures for postoperative delirium

Risk Factors

- Cognitive impairment
- Older age
- Functional impairment
- Vision, hearing impairment
- Depression
- Preoperative use of psychopharmacologic agents or alcohol
- Residence in an institution (assisted living, nursing home)
- Greater comorbidity

Preventive Measures

- Bring sensory devices (glasses, hearing aids) from home
- Limit use of psychopharmacologic drugs
- Carefully manage postoperative pain

Data from Refs.[1,4,16–19]

Depression predicts not only postoperative delirium, but longer postoperative length of stay, as well as greater pain perception and use of postoperative analgesics.[1] A rapid 2-item screening instrument for depression is the Patient Health Questionnaire-2.[24]

Preoperative alcohol use also predicts the development of postoperative delirium,[18] complications (pneumonia, sepsis, wound infection, increased length of stay), and mortality.[1] A best practices guideline from the American College of Surgeons and the American Geriatrics Society (ACS/AGS)[1] recommend screening patients for alcohol problems preoperatively with a short questionnaire. For those found to have major alcohol-related problems, delay of (elective) surgery with medical detoxification and substance abuse treatment may be in order. Patients with identified alcohol abuse or dependence should be prescribed perioperative multivitamins, folate, and thiamine.

PHYSICAL FUNCTION AND MOBILITY

Functional capacity is a powerful predictor of postoperative outcomes and a vitally important outcome in its own right. Preoperative functional impairment is associated with postoperative complications, morbidity, and mortality.[4,5,25,26] Studies have found that a fellow traveler of functional dependence, residence in an institution, is correlated with postoperative mortality with adjusted odds ratios varying from 1.5 to greater than 3.[4] Not surprisingly, diminished postoperative functional ability is predicted by poor baseline functional status.[27,28] Other predictors of postoperative functional decline include older age, hospital readmission, the occurrence of surgical complications, and postoperative delirium.[1,11,14]

Experts and guidelines[1,4] recommend that clinicians routinely interview patients about their functional abilities as part of a preoperative assessment. In an effort to streamline the preoperative workup, the ACS/AGS guideline[1] suggests that clinicians ask patients 2 basic ADL questions ("Can you get out of bed or chair yourself?" and "Can you dress and bathe yourself?") and 2 instrumental ADL questions ("Can you make your own meals?" and "Can you do your own shopping?"). It also recommends querying patients about falls and difficulty seeing, hearing, or swallowing. An objective (rather than self-reported) measure of mobility is the Timed Up and Go test,[1,4,29] in which the patient is instructed to rise from a chair, walk 10 feet to a fixed point on the floor, turn 180°, walk back to the chair, and sit down. The time required to perform the task is measured. Times in excess of 15 seconds predict increased fall risk.

Preoperative functional or mobility problems should prompt referral to rehabilitation professionals (physical therapy, occupational therapy, or speech therapy, depending on the deficits uncovered) for preoperative care and proactive discharge planning.[1,4] Patients at high risk for functional decline or institutionalization in the wake of surgery deserve a candid discussion of the matter as part of the informed consent process. **Box 2** summarizes key features of function and mobility for preoperative evaluation.

SOCIAL SUPPORT

In studies of the value of geriatric assessment in predicting postoperative outcomes, social support has been shown (as a component of the assessment) to predict 30-day postoperative morbidity.[30] The ACS/AGS guidelines[1] recommend that clinicians evaluating patients in the preoperative setting assess patients' social support systems, because these are critical determinants of discharge disposition. Concerns about insufficient family or other social support may prompt preoperative referral to a social worker. Another key component of the social assessment is the identification of a surrogate decision maker, such as a durable power of attorney for health care.

Box 2
Function-related recommendations for preoperative assessment

- Inquire about preoperative basic and instrumental activities of daily living capabilities
- Inquire about recent falls
- Inquire about difficulties in seeing, hearing, or swallowing
- Perform Timed Up and Go test
- For management of functional problems identified, refer to physical, occupational, speech therapy
- Incorporate risk of functional decline or nursing home admission into informed consent discussion

Surrogates should familiarize themselves with patients' advance directives and health priorities.

NUTRITIONAL STATUS

Preoperative malnutrition has been shown to predict a number of unfortunate postoperative outcomes in older, multimorbid patients: wound dehiscence, anastomotic leaks, infection, delirium, and mortality.[1,4,31] The preoperative assessment should include some form of nutritional screening. The tools with the greatest sensitivity and specificity are the Mini-Nutritional Assessment and the Malnutrition Screening Tool.[32,33] Geriatric surgical experts and guidelines recommend[1,4] asking patients in the preoperative setting about weight loss, calculating body mass index, and measuring serum concentrations of albumin and prealbumin. The following findings suggest severe nutritional risk[34]: unintentional weight loss exceeding 10% to 15% over 6 months; a body mass index of less than 18.5 kg/m^2; and albumin of less than 3.0 g/dL (in the absence of liver or kidney disease). Such high-risk patients should be referred before elective surgery to a dietician, who may design and implement a perioperative nutritional supplementation plan.

The literature supporting benefits of preoperative nutritional supplementation is expanding. A small, controlled study in Japan[35] examined the benefit of liquid dietary supplement provided before operative treatment of esophageal cancer, and patients receiving the supplement suffered fewer postoperative infections, had a shorter hospital duration of stay, and demonstrated better 6-month survival. More generally, in malnourished patients, preoperative nutritional support may reduce the rate of postoperative complications by approximately 10%.[35]

MEDICATION USE

The prescription of inappropriate medications for older, multimorbid patients in the perioperative setting is common,[36] and may be more common on orthopedic than general surgical services. Both polypharmacy and use of psychotropic medications have been associated with development of postoperative delirium.[1,36]

Clinicians evaluating patients before surgery should make a complete review of the as-taken medication list (which may not resemble the formally prescribed regimen), including herbal supplements, over-the-counter drugs, topicals, and ophthalmic drops.[1] The adherence strategies used by the patient or caregivers deserve inquiry as well. The preoperative visit provides an opportunity to perform medication debridement. The Beers List[37] includes potentially inappropriate medications that may be targets for elimination. Meperidine, once a commonly prescribed opiate used in the postoperative setting, should, for all practical purposes, never be used, and there are better antiemetics available (such as ondansetron) than promethazine.[36] More generally, nonessential medications should be stopped, and prescribers should work to ensure a lean, well-justified regimen during the perioperative period. The medication regimens of patients discharged after a surgical hospitalization should similarly be cleansed of unnecessary as-needed agents that may have accumulated during the admission.

PREOPERATIVE ORGAN SYSTEM ASSESSMENT

An evolving evidence base supports organ-specific preoperative evaluations for multimorbid older patients. **Table 1** summarizes risk factors and recommended assessment and preoperative management approaches for the cardiac, pulmonary, and renal systems.

"FRAILTY" AND THE OLDER SURGICAL PATIENT

Frailty is an integrated characteristic, because it encompasses derangements or deficits in multiple physiologic domains. Reflecting a state of increased vulnerability to stressors, it is distinct from comorbidity/multimorbidity (from which it may result) and disability (toward which it leads).[49] The addition of frailty to risk prediction models (such as cardiac risk scores or American Society of Anesthesiologists physical classification category) improves predictive power in evaluating patients before surgery,[50] and using frailty scores in preoperative risk stratification has been described as a "paradigm shift" relative to traditional approaches[51] in the care of multimorbid patients. Older persons may progress along a spectrum from robust to prefrail, to frail, to partially functionally dependent, to completely dependent, and finally to moribund, but progression is not always unidirectional.

Frailty has been shown to predict adverse surgical outcomes, including postoperative complications,[50–52] longer hospital duration of stay,[50] discharge to a facility rather than home,[4,50,53] greater health care costs,[53] readmissions within 30 days,[53] and mortality.[4,52] Unfortunately, frailty remains "an established concept lacking a consensus definition,"[52] and its research application in the perioperative setting has embraced varying measures. **Table 2** illustrates contrasting definitions of the concept. The ACS/AGS guideline[1] recommends determination and documentation of the phenotypic frailty score for patients before surgery. However, some experts[52] have questioned how frailty assessments can best be incorporated into preoperative patient assessments (even if a definition could be agreed on), and have pointed out that clear guidance is still needed on how to intervene on behalf of patients found to be frail.

PREOPERATIVE OPTIMIZATION

Based on the evidence accumulated from application of geriatric assessment approaches to the medical inpatient setting (eg, Acute Care of Elders units, or the Hospital Elder Life Program), preoperative assessment must be linked to preoperative optimization to deliver benefits.[7] Prehabilitation is a term often used to describe such treatments designed to increase patients' functional capacity and reserves in advance of the stress of surgery. The literature is much richer in studies of preoperative assessment (eg, demonstrating the value of risk indices) than prehabilitation programs.

Table 1
Preoperative assessment and management of organ-based medical conditions

Organ System/Issue	Risk Factors/Indications	Assessment/Management
Cardiovascular[1,38–44]		
Risk assessment	• Intrinsic to patient: heart disease, older age, impaired physical function, diabetes mellitus, renal disease • High-risk surgeries: vascular, intrathoracic, intraabdominal, major orthopedic, major urologic	• ACC/AHA Preoperative Algorithm[a,38] • Revised Cardiac Risk Index[40] • American College of Surgery Risk Calculator[b]
Statin use	• If already in use before surgery • Vascular surgery	• Continue at usual dosage if already prescribed • Uncertain drug choice and dosage for new prescription
Beta blockade	• If already in use before surgery • Consider initiating in patients with multiple cardiac risk factors undergoing high-risk surgery	• Continue if already prescribed • Should not be started on day of surgery
Coronary stents	Increased cardiac risk up to 6 mo after placement	Consider scheduling elective surgery after 6-month window
Anemia screening	All older surgical patients	Measure hemoglobin concentration
Electrocardiography	• Other than low-risk surgery • Known ischemic heart disease, arrhythmias, peripheral arterial disease, cerebrovascular disease, heart failure, diabetes mellitus, renal insufficiency, pulmonary disease	Perform preoperative electrocardiography
Pulmonary[1,45–47]		
Risk assessment	COPD, older age, functional dependence, ASA class II or worse, surgical site (near diaphragm, head-and-neck, vascular, neurosurgical), emergency surgery, surgery exceeding 3 h, malnutrition, heart failure, obstructive sleep apnea, pulmonary hypertension, tobacco use, impaired sensorium	• Optimize obstructive lung disease treatment before surgery • Encourage smoking cessation (>4–8 wk preoperatively) • Intensive training of muscles of inspiration • Lung expansion (eg, incentive spirometry) • Selective (not routine) use of nasogastric tubes
Additional testing	• Age >70, acute respiratory process, thoracic abdominal surgery, possible postoperative ICU admission • Unexplained dyspnea, or COPD/asthma not clearly stabilized	• Preoperative CXR • Pulmonary function testing

(*continued on next page*)

Table 1
(continued)

Organ System/Issue	Risk Factors/Indications	Assessment/Management
Renal[1,48]		
Risk assessment	Male sex, older age, preoperative renal insufficiency, diabetes mellitus, active heart failure, hypertension, ascites, intraperitoneal surgery	• Measure preoperative BUN and creatinine for all older patients • Maintain euvolemic fluid status

Abbreviations: ACC, American College of Cardiology; AHA, American Heart Association; ASA, American Society of Anesthesiologists; BUN, blood urea nitrogen; COPD, chronic obstructive pulmonary disease; CXR, chest radiograph; ICU, intensive care unit.

[a] URL is http://content.onlinejacc.org/article.aspx?articleid=1893784.

[b] URL is http://www.riskcalculator.facs.org.

Data from Refs.[1,38–48]

The benefits of prehabilitation have been reported[56,57] in studies of perioperative care of patients with colorectal cancer. Researchers compared prehabilitation with rehabilitation; in each case, patients participated in aerobic and resistance exercise, nutritional counseling with protein supplementation, and relaxation exercises for anxiety reduction. The prehabilitation group received the course of treatment before surgery, whereas the rehabilitation group began immediately afterward. The group receiving prehabilitation showed a greater tendency to return to baseline levels of functional exercise capacity. Postoperative complication rates and hospital duration of stay were similar for the 2 groups.

A more individualized approach is Proactive care of Older People undergoing Surgery (POPS). POPS is described as preoperative comprehensive geriatric assessment coupled with targeted interventions, and a before-and-after study[58] of patients on an orthopedic surgery service demonstrated reduced rates of postoperative delirium and pneumonia, as well as a shorter length of stay.

SUMMARY

Older, multimorbid patients are at increased risk of complications and other undesired outcomes after noncardiac surgery. Improved methods have been developed for

Table 2
Selected components of frailty definitions used in preoperative assessments

Phenotypic (Hopkins/Fried)[54]	Kristjansson et al,[55] 2010	Robinson et al,[51] 2013
• Shrinkage (weight loss) • Weak hand grip • Self-reported exhaustion • Low physical activity • Slow walking speed	• Basic ADL function • Instrumental ADL function • Comorbidity • Polypharmacy • Nutrition (by Mini-Nutritional Assessment) • Cognition (MMSE) • Mood (GDS)	• Mobility (TUG) • Basic ADL function • Comorbidity • Nutrition (by serum albumin) • Cognition (Mini-Cog) • Falls • Anemia

Phenotypic model defines frail as meeting 3 or more components.

Abbreviations: ADL, activities of daily living; GDS, Geriatric Depression Scale; MMSE, Mini Mental State Examination; TUG, Timed Up and Go Test.

Data from Refs.[51,54,55]

assessing this risk, and the best ones take into account holistic, not only disease-specific, factors such as functional capacity, nutritional status, cognitive ability, and frailty. These preoperative assessments are by no means automated and algorithmic, and clinicians must rely heavily on clinical judgment in determining how to collect, weigh, and use their patients' data, as well as how to use clinical practice guidelines.

Many open questions remain for how to manage certain specific physiologic or disease-focused issues in the perioperative context, for example, how best to manage diabetic glucose control, intravenous fluids, or blood transfusions.[8] Less narrowly focused questions requiring further research include the following.

- What is the best overall approach to evaluate a multimorbid patient for noncardiac surgery? The ACS/AGS guideline[1] is an excellent start, but some experts[11,52] have voiced concerns about the feasibility of its broad application given resource constraints of time and expertise.
- Can rapid screening instruments be developed that would allow a significant proportion of comparatively robust, multimorbid older patients to bypass a time-intensive, comprehensive assessment? Such instruments would serve a role analogous to that of the functional screen in the American College of Cardiology/American Heart Association algorithm[38] for preoperative cardiac assessment, in which patients with good physical function bypass the need for additional cardiac testing.
- Which prehabilitation or preoperative intervention strategies improve outcomes, for which patients and for which surgeries? Outcomes of particular interest in such research would be patient-centered (functional capacity, institutional vs community residence, quality of life), not just disease specific.[8,52]
- What are effective methods for communicating with patients (and family) about the critical issues in the preoperative setting? Clarity of language is important, but bluntness (should we tell a patient she is "frail?"; how?) may not help in collaborative decision making.

REFERENCES

1. Chow WB, Rosenthal RA, Merkow RP, et al. Optimal preoperative assessment of the geriatric surgical patient: a best practices guideline from the American College of Surgeons National Surgical Quality Improvement Program and the American Geriatrics Society. J Am Coll Surg 2012;215(4):453–66.
2. Elixhauser A, Andrews RM. Profile of inpatient operating room procedures in US hospitals in 2007. Arch Surg 2010;145(12):1201–8.
3. De Oliveira GS, Holl JL, Lindquist LA, et al. Older adults and unanticipated hospital admission within 30 days of ambulatory surgery: an analysis of 53,667 ambulatory surgical procedures. J Am Geriatr Soc 2015;63:1679–85.
4. Oresanya LB, Lyons WL, Finlayson E. Preoperative assessment of the older patient: a narrative review. JAMA 2014;311(20):2110–20.
5. Hamel MB, Henderson WG, Khuri SF, et al. Surgical outcomes for patients aged 80 and older: morbidity and mortality from major noncardiac surgery. J Am Geriatr Soc 2005;53:424–9.
6. Colorectal Cancer Collaborative Group. Surgery for colorectal cancer in elderly patients: a systematic review. Lancet 2000;356:968–74.
7. Partridge JSL, Harari D, Martin FC, et al. The impact of pre-operative comprehensive geriatric assessment on postoperative outcomes in older patients undergoing scheduled surgery: a systematic review. Anaesthesia 2014;69(Suppl 1):8–16.

8. Akhtar S. Guidelines and perioperative care of the elderly. Int Anesthesiol Clin 2014;52:64–76.
9. Reuben DB. Medical care for the final years of life: "when you're 83, it's not going to be 20 years." JAMA 2009;302(24):2686–94.
10. Van Leeuwen BL, Kristjansson SR, Audisio RA. Should specialized oncogeriatric surgeons operate on older unfit cancer patients? Eur J Surg Oncol 2010;36: S18–22.
11. Schlitzkus LL, Melin AA, Johanning JM, et al. Perioperative management of elderly patients. Surg Clin North Am 2015;95:391–415.
12. Yourman LC, Lee SJ, Schonberg MA, et al. Prognostic indices for older adults: a systematic review. JAMA 2012;307(2):182–92.
13. Department of Geriatrics, University of California, San Francisco. Estimating prognosis for elders. Available at: http://eprognosis.ucsf.edu. Accessed September 26, 2015.
14. Bekker AY, Weeks EJ. Cognitive function after anaesthesia in the elderly. Best Pract Res Clin Anaesthesiol 2003;17:259–72.
15. Wallbridge HR, Benoit AG, Staley D. Risk factors for postoperative cognitive and functional difficulties in abdominal aortic aneurysm patients: a three-month follow-up. Int J Geriatr Psychiatry 2011;26(8):818–24.
16. Dasgupta M, Dumbrell AC. Preoperative risk assessment for delirium after noncardiac surgery: a systematic review. J Am Geriatr Soc 2006;54:1578–89.
17. Kosar CM, Tabloski PA, Travison TG, et al. Effect of preoperative pain and depressive symptoms on the development of postoperative delirium. Lancet Psychiatry 2014;1(6):431–6.
18. Van Meenen LC, Van Meenen DM, De Rooij SE, et al. Risk prediction models for postoperative delirium: a systematic review and meta-analysis. J Am Geriatr Soc 2014;62(12):2383–90.
19. Lynch EP, Lazor MA, Gellis JE, et al. The impact of postoperative pain on the development of postoperative delirium. Anesth Analg 1998;86:781–5.
20. Monk TG, Weldon BC, Garvan CW, et al. Predictors of cognitive dysfunction after major noncardiac surgery. Anesthesiology 2008;1-8:18–30.
21. Nadelson MR, Sanders RD, Avidan MS. Perioperative cognitive trajectory in adults. Br J Anaesth 2014;112:440–51.
22. Borson S, Scanlan J, Brush M, et al. The Mini-Cog: a cognitive 'vital signs' measure for dementia screening in multi-lingual elderly. Int J Geriatr Psychiatry 2000; 15:1021–7.
23. Cleff A, Young JB. Which medications to avoid in people at risk of delirium: a systematic review. Age Ageing 2011;40(1):23–9.
24. Li C, Friedman B, Conwell Y, et al. Validity of the Patient Health Questionnaire 2 (PHQ-2) in identifying major depression in older people. J Am Geriatr Soc 2007;55:596–602.
25. Turrentine FE, Wang H, Simpson VB, et al. Surgical risk factors, morbidity, and mortality in elderly patients. J Am Coll Surg 2006;203(6):865–77.
26. Robinson TN, Eiseman B, Wallace JI, et al. Redefining geriatric preoperative assessment using frailty, disability, and comorbidity. Ann Surg 2009;250:449–55.
27. Lawrence VA, Hazuda HP, Cornell JE, et al. Functional independence after major abdominal surgery in the elderly. J Am Coll Surg 2004;199:762–72.
28. Finlayson E, Zhao S, Boscardin WJ, et al. Functional status after colon cancer surgery in elderly nursing home residents. J Am Geriatr Soc 2012;60(5):967–73.
29. Podsiadlo D, Richardson S. The timed "Up & Go": a test of basic functional mobility for frail elderly persons. J Am Geriatr Soc 1991;39:142–8.

30. Kenig J, Olszewska U, Zychiewicz B, et al. Cumulative deficit model of geriatric assessment to predict the postoperative outcomes of older patients with solid abdominal cancer. J Geriatr Oncol 2015;6(5):370–9.
31. Schiesser M, Kirchhoff P, Muller MK, et al. The correlation of nutrition risk index, nutrition risk score, and bioimpedance analysis with postoperative complications in patients undergoing gastrointestinal surgery. Surgery 2009;145:519–26.
32. Skipper A, Ferguson M, Thompson K, et al. Nutrition screening tools: an analysis of the evidence. JPEN J Parenter Enteral Nutr 2012;36:292–8.
33. Guigoz Y. The Mini-Nutritional Assessment (MNA) review of the literature – what does it tell us? J Nutr Health Aging 2006;10(6):466–85.
34. Weimann A, Braga M, Harsanyi L, et al. ESPEN guidelines on enteral nutrition: surgery including organ transplantation. Clin Nutr 2006;25:224–44.
35. Kubota K, Kuroda J, Yoshida M, et al. Preoperative oral supplementation support in patients with esophageal cancer. J Nutr Health Aging 2014;18(4):437–40.
36. Finlayson E, Maselli J, Steinman MA, et al. Inappropriate medication use in older adults undergoing surgery: a national study. J Am Geriatr Soc 2011;59(11): 2139–44.
37. By the American Geriatrics Society 2015 Beers Criteria Update Expert Panel. American Geriatrics Society 2015 Updated Beers Criteria for potentially inappropriate medication use in older adults. J Am Geriatr Soc 2015;63(11):2227–46.
38. Fleisher LA, Fleischmann KE, Auerbach AD, et al. 2014 ACC/AHA guideline on perioperative cardiovascular evaluation and management of patients undergoing noncardiac surgery: a report of the American College of Cardiology/American Heart Association Task Force on practice guidelines. J Am Coll Cardiol 2014; 64(22):e77–137.
39. Eagle KA, Valshnava P, Froehlich JB. Perioperative cardiovascular care for patients undergoing noncardiac surgical intervention. JAMA Intern Med 2015; 175(5):835–9.
40. Lee TH, Marcantonio ER, Mangione CM, et al. Derivation and prospective validation of a simple index for prediction of cardiac risk of major noncardiac surgery. Circulation 1999;100(10):1043–9.
41. Wijeysundera DN, Duncan D, Nkonde-Price C, et al. Perioperative beta blockade in noncardiac surgery: a systematic review for the 2014 ACC/AHA guideline on perioperative cardiovascular evaluation and management of patients undergoing noncardiac surgery. J Am Coll Cardiol 2014;64:2406–25.
42. Chopra V, Eagle KA. Perioperative mischief: the price of academic misconduct. Am J Med 2012;125:953–5.
43. Holcomb CN, Graham LA, Richman JS, et al. The incremental risk of noncardiac surgery on adverse cardiac events following coronary stenting. J Am Coll Cardiol 2014;64:2730–9.
44. Sinha SS, Eagle KA. Noncardiac surgery <2 years after coronary stent placement was linked to perioperative MI and all-cause mortality. Ann Intern Med 2015; 162(12):JC11.
45. Smetana G. Preoperative pulmonary evaluation. N Engl J Med 1999;340:937–44.
46. Smetana GW. Postoperative pulmonary complications: an update on risk assessment and reduction. Cleve Clin J Med 2009;76:S60–5.
47. Lawrence VA, Cornell JE, Smetana GW. Strategies to reduce postoperative pulmonary complications after noncardiothoracic surgery: systematic review for the American College of Physicians. Ann Intern Med 2006;144(8):596–608.

48. Kheterpal S, Tremper KK, Heung M, et al. Development and validation of an acute kidney injury risk index for patients undergoing general surgery: results from a national data set. Anesthesiology 2009;110(3):505–15.
49. Fried LP, Ferrucci L, Darer J, et al. Untangling the concepts of disability, frailty, and comorbidity: implications for improved targeting and care. J Gerontol A Biol Sci Med Sci 2004;59:255–63.
50. Makary MA, Segev DL, Pronovost PJ, et al. Frailty as a predictor of surgical outcomes in older patients. J Am Coll Surg 2010;210(6):901–8.
51. Robinson TN, Wu DS, Pointer L, et al. Simple frailty score predicts postoperative complications across surgical specialties. Am J Surg 2013;206:544–50.
52. Anaya DA, Johanning J, Spector SA, et al. Summary of the Panel Session at the 38th Annual Surgical Symposium of the Association of VA Surgeons: what is the big deal about frailty? JAMA Surg 2014;149(11):1191–7.
53. Robinson TN, Wu DS, Stiegmann GV, et al. Frailty predicts increased hospital and six-month healthcare cost following colorectal surgery in older adults. Am J Surg 2011;202:511–4.
54. Fried LP, Tangen CM, Walston J, et al. Frailty in older adults: evidence for a phenotype. J Gerontol A Biol Sci Med Sci 2001;56:M146–56.
55. Kristjansson SR, Nesbakken A, Jordhoy MS, et al. Comprehensive geriatric assessment can predict complications in elderly patients after elective surgery for colorectal cancer: a prospective observational cohort study. Crit Rev Oncol Hematol 2010;76:208–17.
56. Li C, Carli F, Lee L, et al. Impact of a trimodal prehabilitation program on functional recovery after colorectal cancer surgery: a pilot study. Surg Endosc 2013;27(4):1072–82.
57. Gillis C, Li C, Lee L, et al. Prehabilitation vs rehabilitation: a randomized control trial in patients undergoing colorectal resection for cancer. Anesthesiology 2014;121(5):937–47.
58. Harari D, Hopper A, Dhesi J, et al. Proactive care of Older People undergoing Surgery (POPS): designing, embedding, evaluating, and funding a comprehensive geriatric assessment service for older elective surgical patients. Age Ageing 2007;36(2):190–6.

Assessing Risks and Benefits of Invasive Cardiac Procedures in Patients with Advanced Multimorbidity

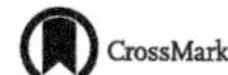

Ariela R. Orkaby, MD[a,b], Daniel E. Forman, MD[c,d,*]

KEYWORDS

• Geriatrics • Cardiology • Multimorbidity • Preoperative assessment

KEY POINTS

- Older adults with multimorbidity face increased challenges in choosing to pursue an invasive cardiovascular procedure because their cardiac disease is only one of many concurrent diseases.
- In older adults, it is often less certain that an invasive cardiac intervention will lead to improvements in symptoms or function because concurrent illnesses or geriatric syndromes may be the principal determinants of the symptoms.
- Concurrent illnesses or geriatric syndromes in old age are more likely to complicate invasive procedures and lead to outcomes that are worse than expected.
- Assessing geriatric syndromes as part of the preoperative assessment provides opportunities to prevent complications, such as delirium and functional decline.
- Understanding what the patient hopes to achieve from the intervention, such as life prolongation versus alleviation of symptoms, is integral to the ideal of shared decision making.

Mr S is an 84-year-old widowed man who lives independently in the community. He presents after being scheduled for an urgent preoperative assessment before a transcatheter aortic replacement (TAVR), scheduled for the coming week. Mr S has had a series of recent falls; his cardiologist attributed the falls to aortic stenosis (AS) and immediately scheduled a TAVR as a way to overcome the falls and also to help Mr S live longer.

Disclosure Statement: Dr D. E. Forman is supported in part by NIA grant P30 AG024827 and VA Office of Rehabilitation Research and Development grant F0834-R.

[a] Division of Cardiology, VA Boston Healthcare System, 400 Veterans of Foreign Wars Pkwy, West Roxbury, MA 02132, USA; [b] Division of Aging, Brigham & Women's Hospital, 1620 Tremont Street, Boston, MA 02120, USA; [c] Section of Geriatric Cardiology, University of Pittsburgh Medical Center, 3471 Fifth Avenue, Suite 500, Pittsburgh, PA 15213, USA; [d] Geriatric Research, Education, and Clinical Center, VA Pittsburgh Healthcare System, University Dr C, Pittsburgh, PA 15240, USA

* Corresponding author. Section of Geriatric Cardiology, University of Pittsburgh Medical Center, 3471 Fifth Avenue, Suite 500, Pittsburgh, PA 15213.

E-mail address: formand@pitt.edu

Clin Geriatr Med 32 (2016) 359–371

http://dx.doi.org/10.1016/j.cger.2016.01.004 geriatric.theclinics.com

0749-0690/16/$ – see front matter

Mr S has been followed by this cardiologist for many years for what initially presented as moderate AS. He also has a past medical history of coronary artery disease (CAD; coronary artery bypass grafting [CABG] in his 70s), myelodysplasia, degenerative joint disease of the right hip, benign prostatic hypertrophy, and chronic kidney disease. Over the past few months he had three falls. In two, there were no significant injuries, but the last one resulted in a rotator cuff strain. Mr S is unable to give many details regarding any of the falls; he states he has "no clear memory." However, he emphasizes that the hip causes lots of pain and as a result he has been stumbling frequently. He wears a life-alert line, which he has never used. He has become increasingly sedentary and anxious, with worsening sleep and appetite. His body mass index is 27, he has lost 3 pounds in 3 months, is relying increasingly on his daughter for shopping, and is having more difficulty with self-care.

After the third fall Mr S was evaluated in the emergency department for his shoulder injury. The emergency room doctor said he probably fell because of hip degenerative joint disease and that he would be better off using a wheelchair. This made Mr S very distressed, especially in the broader context of escalating hip pain, declining mobility, and lack of independence. He confided in his daughter that living like this was "just not worth it anymore," and she became concerned about his well-being and safety. On her advice he returned to the cardiologist.

As part of the cardiologist's assessment, an echocardiogram was performed. Whereas his last echo in 2013 showed aortic valve diameter of 1.2 cm, it was now 1.0 cm. The current echo also showed mean aortic valve gradient of 42 mm Hg and peak gradient of 63 mm Hg. The cardiologist concluded that his falls were caused by syncope from progressing AS, and could be alleviated by a TAVR.

Mr S says he is willing to proceed based mostly on the fact that cardiologist seemed so certain and reassuring. His daughter also urged him to undergo the procedure. Still, he states that he is skeptical TAVR will fix the problem, particularly because he has no symptoms that convince him it is the heart, including no chest pain, shortness of breath, or palpitations. He says that he only really wants his hip to be replaced.

How should the physician approach the decision-making process with regard to Mr S's AS?

THE ALLURE OF SURGERY AND ITS LIMITATIONS IN THE CONTEXT OF MULTIMORBIDITY

With the advent of modern medicine, the ability to "fix" has become a mainstay of clinical practice and an expectation from patients. Nowhere is this clearer than in surgery and surgery-like catheter interventions. From the days of Joseph Lister and the introduction of the sterile technique to modern technological advances, surgery has become progressively safer and is commonly considered the ultimate definitive therapy.

A driving aspect of the professional culture of surgeons and cardiologists is emphasis on and value ascribed to new techniques and innovations as key components of caregiving excellence.[1] Such ethos and investment has contributed to the exponential rise of scope-based, robotic and microscopic interventions that characterize Western medicine. Progressive improvements in cardiopulmonary bypass pumps, minimally invasive options, hemostasis, anesthesia, and procedure time have added to the tolerability, success, and allure of invasive options.[2,3] Increased portability has also been relevant, as surgical options have moved out of tertiary centers, and become progressively more available in local hospitals and even in outpatient offices.

Juxtaposed to technological advances, the burgeoning demographic of older adults has led to the prominent rise of age-related illnesses for which surgery is a therapeutic standard.[4] CAD prevalence, for example, accelerates with advancing age, such that mainstream cardiac procedures, such as CABG, have become strongly linked to broader dynamics of aging. A 2007 estimate noted that 25% of those presenting for CABG were older than age 70 years, with those older than 80 now representing more than 10% of total CABG cases.[5] Moreover, other diseases arise almost exclusively in older adults because they arise from aging physiology. AS, for example, is rare in younger adults, but climbs to 8% among octogenarians.[6] Today's growing interest in aortic valve replacement interventions is propelled primarily by more adults surviving into advanced age when severe AS is able to develop. The average age of those undergoing invasive cardiac procedures for CABG, valve repair, pacemakers and implantable cardioverter-defibrillators, and vascular surgery has risen from 55 to nearly 70 years over the last three decades.[4]

Noncardiac diseases similarly arise with aging.[7] The high prevalence of osteoarthritis with age is linked to the growing application of orthopedic surgeries in those older than age 80.[8] Furthermore, with the aging of the population there has been an overall rise in palliative-oriented procedures for malignancies and other end-stage diseases. An analysis of Medicare data identified that nearly a third of all invasive procedures performed in older adults occur during the last year of life.[9]

Although surgeons and invasive proceduralists focus on technological advances as the rationale for success in older adults, this logic is often flawed. The reliability of surgery and invasive procedures for improving outcomes is often undercut by older adults having multiple medical issues that are active simultaneously or that can become destabilized by one another in the context of surgical stresses. Moreover, even if surgery proceeds as expected, the utility of a procedure to achieve anticipated benefits may do little to overcome the symptoms, morbidity, or mortality that relate to the comorbid diseases. Similarly, entrenched disabilities, frailty, and other limitations rooted in multimorbidity may confound and/or detract from surgical benefits. Therefore, an older adult with multimorbidity faces particular challenges in considering surgical therapeutic options.

MULTIMORBIDITY

In the realm of cardiovascular disease the term comorbidity is often used, identifying the cardiovascular disease as central to the patient's problem list, with all other concurrent diagnoses deemed "comorbid." However, this fails to recognize that other diagnoses and geriatric syndromes may have equal bearing on the patient's sense of health and well-being. "Multimorbidity" implies the interactive effects of two or more "primary" disease processes when they occur together.[10] Moreover, geriatric conditions, such as cognitive changes, deconditioning, falls, sarcopenia, incontinence, and sensory impairments (vision and hearing), are parts of multimorbidity because they further compound vulnerability and complexity.[11] The utility of a surgical intervention must therefore be considered as one concern amid each patient's aggregate clinical status. For example, a patient who has AS is more than just a patient with valvular heart disease. Not only are outcomes of a potential valve replacement fundamentally affected by noncardiac disease processes but from the patient's perspective, noncardiac issues (eg, osteoarthritis and cognitive decline) may constitute much greater concerns and priorities of care.

Reframing the patient's problem list with orientation to multimorbidity rather than one disease is helpful in considering any risk/benefit assessment because it acknowledges that there may be more than one single disease that is determining symptoms, risks, and preferred outcomes. Furthermore, the effects of polypharmacy, limited functional capacities, and decreased physiologic reserves may also affect the older patient with multimorbidity and geriatric syndromes. This leads to additional complexities that transmute clinical decisions because "fixing" one problem may have little benefit for other problems and may lead to additional difficulties (eg, delirium, depression, falls that arise secondary to procedures and medication changes). Incorporating multimorbidity into a decision-making process may not help in identifying who may or may not benefit in respect to the technical aspects of a procedure, but rather in anticipating who will benefit most in the short- and long-term.[12]

Multimorbidity also factors in the assessment of symptoms and the anticipated benefit of surgery to improve symptoms. For example, an 85 year old with severe AS may develop dyspnea on exertion from high cardiac workload associated with even minimal exertion as cardiac pressures quickly mount in response to exercise. For this patient, aortic valve replacement may yield tremendous symptomatic benefit and increased longevity. However, AS in older adults is often associated with concomitant pulmonary hypertension, which can also induce symptoms of dyspnea on exertion. For patients with combined AS and pulmonary hypertension, successful aortic valve repair may do little to improve dyspnea on exertion symptoms. Moreover, chronic obstructive pulmonary disease, sarcopenia, and heart failure are also common in older patients with AS and may additionally compound susceptibility to dyspnea and further complicate management decisions. Differentiating the primary source of symptoms and determining the optimal management strategy is often ambiguous.

Even beyond such relevance of multimorbidity in relation to symptoms and immediate management, awareness of concurrent diseases provides key perspectives regarding the possibility of prolonged recoveries, the utility of rehabilitation, the risk of ventilatory dependency, and the priority of delineating patients' wishes within likely complexity.

MEDICAL COMPLEXITY AND PREOPERATIVE RISK ASSESSMENT

Clinicians have had a long tradition of trying to gauge relative risks to benefits before invasive procedures. Characterization of risks originally centered on the procedure itself (anesthesia, ventilation, bleeding, infection, and techniques), and then evolved to integrate patient-related considerations. More than 70 years ago anesthesiologists developed the American Society of Anesthesiologist Physical Status. Patients were subtyped based on a subjective assessment of their overall health status; six categories were delineated, from healthy to brain dead.[13] Higher American Society of Anesthesiologist scores predicted complications, such as postoperative delirium in patients undergoing colorectal surgery and increased 30-day mortality in those undergoing orthopedic surgery.[14–16]

Over time, surgeons and cardiologists have further refined risk prediction and developed multiple scores. The 2014 updated American College of Cardiology/American Heart Association guidelines for noncardiac surgery stratifies risks inherent in the procedure itself (subdividing into high- and low-risk procedures, and their relative urgency) and risks related to patient characteristics as quantified by the Revised Cardiac Risk Index. This index is a validated tool that was originally developed to predict perioperative cardiac complications in younger patients undergoing major noncardiac surgery.[17,18] Many proponents of the guidelines emphasize the conceptual merits of its integrated procedure-patient perspective. Yet the fact remains that these guidelines still omit consideration of many key risks and parameters pertinent to an older patient, both in regard to the relevance of the risks that are indexed, and especially in respect to the risks that are overlooked. Multimorbidity exemplifies a key danger that is not included. For example, a patient with cognitive impairment and arthritis may have an otherwise favorable preoperative assessment, but this does not include the risks of delirium and inability to participate in intensive rehabilitation, which may significantly impact recovery and survival.

Scoring assessments have also been developed to assess risk in patients anticipating cardiac surgery, and an abundant literature has evolved in which the discriminatory efficacies of these tools are compared. One common tool is the Society of Thoracic Surgeons score, updated in 2008, for predicting mobidity and mortality in patients undergoing coronary artery bypass surgery and valve surgery. This score was developed in a cohort of nearly 800,000 adults, 22% of whom were older than 75 years.[19,20] Assessment takes into account cardiac and noncardiac conditions. Similarly, the EuroSCORE, identifying predictors of postoperative mortality, is another widely used preoperative risk assessment developed in a cohort of 20,000 individuals across Europe undergoing CABG, 10% of whom were older than 75.[21]

Although each tool is distinctive in some respects, they are all similar in that their derivations relied on logistic regression of large surgical databases to determine clinical predictors for surgical and/or mortality outcomes. A critical limitation is that they were developed from existing databases of already collected data, and implicitly limited to parameters that were routinely collected (eg, comorbidities, hemodynamics, morbidity, and mortality). Variables, such as cognition, functional status, quality of life, and social supports, were not and could not be included. Moreover, such outcomes as quality of life, function, and independence were also not considered.

A seminal study of 131 patients by Afilalo and colleagues[22] undergoing aortic valve replacement with an average age of 76 stands out by showing that the addition of gait speed improved the prediction of the STS score on the composite end point of major morbidity and mortality, with the implication that a novel marker of frailty provides key impact on risk prediction in older surgical patients, beyond that afforded by a traditional surgical scoring metric. This study is important because it demonstrates that patient-centered features, such as frailty, may enrich surgical risk assessment (ie, a parameter that is independent of the procedural details). However, it also implicitly raised many questions and challenges. Many surgical candidates cannot walk and/or have walking impediments that confound assessment of gait speed. Perhaps even more important, many surgical candidates may have different therapeutic goals than those that were risk-stratified by gait speed in this study. Moreover, research has not been performed on modifying surgical risk once slow gait speed is identified.

A key value of Afilalo's study[22] was in its quantification of surgical risk with assessments that extended beyond traditional cardiac, pulmonary, and renal parameters, to facilitate perspective of overall condition. In the face of such patient-centered perspective and orientation, it becomes particularly important to assess each patient's goals relative to his or her unique constellation of risks.

Returning to the case of Mr S, the first step is to ascertain his conception of ideal therapeutic goals, followed by consideration of the tradeoffs regarding one therapy versus another to achieve those goals. It is important, for example, to better clarify the differential diagnosis for his falls and the options for his hip pain, in addition to the periprocedure and postprocedure risks associated with TAVR. Time to potential benefit is relevant, but so too is the burden of therapy. Whereas surgeons and interventional proceduralists tend to see technology and procedural refinement as the avenue to improving benefit, for the older adult, it is equally or more important to gauge the patient to see if the goals and holistic substrate can be realistically and reasonably achieved by any particular procedure.

PERTINENT GERIATRIC PERSPECTIVES IN PREOPERATIVE ASSESSMENT

The impact of geriatric domains may often supersede the impact of more traditional parameters of risk, and should be considered as part of preprocedure assessment.

Multimorbidity

Cumulative morbidity in and of itself increases aggregate risk, independent of invasive procedures.[23] One study of Medicare beneficiaries found that for every comorbid condition life expectancy was reduced by 1.8 years compared with those without any chronic illnesses, regardless of race or sex.[24] Similarly, a 75 year old with multiple comorbid conditions is likely to live 3 years less than the average person.[25] Dangers are not merely additive because of the multiplying effects of disease in combination.

An ideal preoperative assessment for older patients with multimorbidity has not been standardized,[26] although likely should include elements of a Comprehensive Geriatric Assessment to fully assess the range of pertinent medical, behavioral, and contextual dynamics. The American College of Surgeons National Surgical Quality Improvement Program (ACS NSQIP) is an evidence-based program aimed at decreasing preventable surgical complications that began as a quality improvement initiative at the Veterans Administration in the 1990s. NSQIP has evolved into a safety program capturing data on surgeries performed at hospitals across the United States.[27] Recognizing that an increasing portion of older adults are being operated on, consensus best practice guidelines for the preoperative assessment of older adults have been developed and published jointly by the American Geriatric Society (AGS) and ACS NSQIP (ACS NSQIP/AGS), including select aspects of a Comprehensive Geriatric Assessment in addition to the usual preoperative studies.[28] Specific components of the Comprehensive Geriatric Assessment that were highlighted include cognitive and functional assessment.

A prospective study identified 100 patients aged 70 and older who were undergoing TAVR.[29] In addition to calculating preoperative risk using the STS and Euroscore score, each patient underwent a geriatric assessment, including measures of cognition, function, and nutrition. These components were used to create a frailty index to identify frail individuals preoperatively. Fifty percent of the cohort was identified as frail. The study found that the preoperative geriatric assessment identified those at risk of mortality similarly well as traditional risk scores.

Other studies have also demonstrated that identifying frailty preoperatively can distinguish those at increased risk of prolonged hospitalization and institutionalization. Importantly, these preoperative assessments were not performed by a single surgeon but by a multidisciplinary team that included a surgeon, cardiologist, geriatrician, and often also involved social workers and nurses.[30] This team-based approach helps to balance the workload and can better support the patient and their family as they go through the decision process. For those being assessed for valve repair current recommendations include evaluation by a multidisciplinary "heart team" that should include at least a cardiologist, cardiac surgeon, and imaging specialists.[31] This team sometimes includes a geriatrician, neurologist, or other specialist, although the inclusion of a geriatrician is not mentioned in the US team-care guidelines[28] nor required in the European guidelines.[32] For elders undergoing orthopedic surgery studies demonstrate that a comanagement team involving a geriatrician improves outcomes.[33] Whether this model is beneficial for the older cardiac surgery patient remains to be proven.

Frailty

Frailty is a critical marker of poor surgical outcomes, including increased complications, prolonged hospitalization, dependency, postoperative institutionalization, and mortality.[34–36] This is particularly relevant for the older adult with multimorbidity because frailty delineates risk more specifically than risk assessments based exclusively on cumulative medical conditions.

In 2001 Fried and colleagues[37] developed one of the first constructs of frailty using a physical phenotype defined by having at least three of five components: weight loss, slow gait speed, weakness, low physical activity, and exhaustion. One of the criticisms of the Fried frailty phenotype is that it does not include assessment of mood or cognition, both of which are likely contributors to the syndrome of frailty and certainly contribute to poor outcomes.

Another operationalized definition of frailty is the cumulative deficit model developed by Rockwood and Mitnitski.[38] This theory postulates that over time the accumulation of deficits across multiple health domains, such as comorbidities, functional measurements, and mood assessment, leads to the clinically recognized frailty syndrome. There is significant controversy on the relationship between disability, comorbidity, and frailty with some suggesting that each domain is separate from the other and others who believe that the three are closely interrelated.[39,40]

To date there is no consensus on the definition of frailty, although there is consensus that it is an important syndrome that predisposes to poor outcomes.[41] The test of gait speed, measured over 4 to 6 m, is often applied as a simple, convenient marker of frailty that can be used in the office or home to discern and even track frailty, and its bearing on poor outcomes.[42] In patients who are unable to walk, measurement of grip strength using a dynamometer has been suggested.[43] Other proxies of frailty, such as dependence in activities of daily living, dementia, and general difficulty with mobility, have been correlated with poor outcomes after cardiac surgery, including institutionalization and 2-year mortality.[44]

Returning to the case of Mr S, it is unclear how much of his functional limitation is caused by his AS, degenerative joint disease, or general frailty and deconditioning. For many patients being assessed for cardiac surgery it may not be possible in the preoperative setting to tease out the culprit of their physical limitation, which may well be their cardiovascular disease. A total of 45% of those who participated in the PARTNER trial were nonambulatory, although many of these individuals did benefit from the TAVR.[45,46]

Cognition

Cognitive impairment is associated with increased risk of morbidity and mortality in surgical patients and increased risk of frailty and postoperative delirium.[47–49] Nonetheless, cognitive impairment is often underdiagnosed.[50] Although there are many cognitive screening tools available, the Mini-Cog (consisting of three word recall and clock draw) is a quick and easy test that can be performed in multiple languages, takes less than 2 minutes, is easy to interpret, and has been validated in the preoperative setting,[47] providing a convenient and sensitive measure of cognition.

The ACS NSQIP/AGS guidelines recommend that cognitive testing be the first step in a preoperative assessment.[28] First, this helps clarify the patients' capacity to understand and can help clinicians to tailor information to optimize and best ensure shared decision-making. Insights regarding cognition also enable clinicians to consider reversible causes, including depression, sleep apnea, and medication effects, and to take steps to modify these circumstances. Similarly, clinicians can select procedural strategies (eg, anesthesia, surgical approaches), perioperative management (eg, pain, sleep, hydration and bowel regimens, transfers, clinician consistency), and postoperative management (eg, rehabilitation, home supports, medication monitoring) to optimize the procedural components in which cognitive limits can be most detrimental.[51,52]

Although there has been considerable concern around the risks of cognitive decline associated with cardiac surgery, this remains controversial. A systematic review of older adults (mean age, 68; majority men) who had undergone cardiac procedures, such as CABG or carotid endarterectomy, did not find conclusive evidence that changes to either intermediate- or long-term cognition were common.[53] The overall quality of available evidence was low, particularly because few studies have assessed cognition as an outcome. Still, even without clear evidence, the authors recommend that patients should be counseled on the possible risk of cognitive changes after invasive procedures.

Over time, procedural and anesthesia techniques have advanced to moderate some aspects of cognitive risks in relation to surgery and other procedures. Shorter procedures, reduced vascular trauma, reduced anesthesia burden, and improved oxygenation have all helped. However, it is also clear that elements of care external to the procedure (transfers, pain, polypharmacy, baseline cognition, sensory limitations) have considerable bearing on cognitive ramifications of surgery.

BEYOND THE PROCEDURE

Beyond the immediate procedural risks, broader risks of management are also critical. Early mobility, aspiration pneumonia precautions, and delirium prevention are complementary priorities of care.

Mobilization

Short- and long-term recovery are directly related to the ability of the patient to mobilize as early as possible postoperatively and to thereby minimize risks of thromboembolism, depression, sarcopenia, respiratory failure, delirium, and infections. Choosing a minimally invasive cardiac procedure, such as TAVR, over an open repair, if appropriate, can improve chances that a patient will mobilize sooner in the postoperative period. Similarly, a radial approach may be preferred over a femoral approach for those undergoing catheterization. Ironically, an older patient is often considered "safe" when lying in bed after a procedure (often with the well-meaning intentions to provide rest or minimize falling risks); however, immobilization increases the risk of overall complications and morbidity. However, to achieve early mobilization benefits, appropriately trained nursing staff and therapists are also fundamental. A patient's personal support system, including family members, can also be a resource for the hospital and the patient.

Cardiac Rehabilitation

Cardiac rehabilitation and rehabilitation in general are underused in older adults undergoing cardiac surgery, even though studies have shown clear benefit, especially in those with multimorbidity.[54,55] Structured rehabilitation programs provide exactly the supervision, supports, and opportunities for encouragement that are crucial for older adults struggling with the complexity of multimorbid processes and debilitating symptoms. Even simpler exercise programs lacking all the enriching behavioral and lifestyle components of cardiac rehabilitation have particular benefits for older surgical patients (cardiac and noncardiac).

Therefore, just as risk assessment of older complex patients must start with determination of each patient's goals of care, the anticipation of fitting rehabilitation and effective convalescence is equally fundamental. Rehabilitation is an interconnected part of aggregate therapy, especially for older adults with baseline multimorbidy compounded by frailty, deconditioning, and/or functional limitations.

DECIDING IF A CARDIAC PROCEDURE IS WORTH THE RISK

Predicting who will benefit from a cardiac procedure is notoriously difficult. Life expectancy models have been suggested to help guide clinical decision making.[56] Methods such as these are often used to differentiate between chronologic and biologic age.[57] A robust 85 year old may be physiologically closer to a 75 year old and conversely a frail 75 year old may physiologically be more similar to an 85 year old, and such perspective may help guide decisions whether or not to pursue surgery and/or how to best facilitate it.

A systematic review identified six factors that predict mortality in 6 months in those with advanced illnesses not caused by cancer.[58] These include a decline in performance status, advanced age, malnutrition, multimorbidity, organ dysfunction, and hospitalization caused by acute decompensation. However, such focus on life expectancy alone does not necessarily address the patient's goals for choosing to pursue a procedure. If the goal is to alleviate symptoms and/or generally improve quality of life, life expectancy may be less useful as the basis of the decision making process.

Lag time to benefit, or when the patient can expect to experience any benefits of an intervention, is also an important consideration.[59] Patients with severe AS that is a source of chest pain and physical incapacity may have immediate relief postoperatively. However, an older adult with an asymptomatic slowly expanding abdominal aortic aneurysm, multimorbidity, and frailty may not benefit from a surgical repair in a practical timeframe. Making the issues more complex, for the later patient, options for newer techniques (eg, endovascular aneurysm repair) may change the risk/benefit calculation.

For many patients with advanced disease, it is often appropriate to involve a specialist palliative care team to help manage symptoms and guide goals of care discussions. Advanced disease does not necessarily preclude surgery, because many patients may still desire interventions that can moderate symptoms or improve function. However, palliative care experts can help highlight the limits and complexities of surgery, and the benefits of alternative approaches to management.

In all patients, and particularly in the older patient with multimorbidity, the ideal approach to medical decision-making involves a shared process that includes considering the patients goals and wishes, short- and long-term.[10,60] Patients may be faced with decisions that can improve one disease process at the possible risk of worsening another. For example, undergoing catheterization to treat angina may improve the patient's pain, but the necessary contrast may worsen renal function. Patients may also fundamentally differ in their worldviews and support systems. Individualized care planning by clinicians and patients is essential.

In some cases patients may request a cardiac procedure where the risks may seem excessive to their providers, and even irrational. It becomes reasonable for treating clinicians (who are bound by the ethical principle of *primum non nocere*, first do no harm) to discuss such differences frankly with their patients. Such discussion often helps elucidate more fundamental reasons for patients' requests (eg, fear of dying, fear of pain), and opportunities (by clinicians) to provide clear explanations, teaching, and reassurance. Such dialogue often serves as the crux of shared decision-making.

SUMMARY

In the older adult with multimorbidity, the decision to pursue an invasive cardiac procedure is not only limited to the inherent risks of the intervention. Classically operative success has focused on technical, major associated morbidity, and mortality rates; however, in this population, success or failure is often extended beyond these metrics. With advances in technical ability, a patient may survive a procedure, but whether they will derive benefit, and how that benefit is assessed can only be done by giving attention to the individual patient's narrative. Refocusing the assessment from disease-centric to a holistic patient-centric approach can help in the decision-making process. A patient may consider a procedure successful if they are able to maintain their prior level of function and cognitive abilities. For one patient this may imply added years of vitality, but for another, this might primarily mean increased comfort and self-worth for a few months within the course of a known terminal disease. For patients who choose to pursue invasive cardiac procedures, specific management choices can help to reduce risks of the procedure and recovery, and improve the probability that patients will meet their personal therapeutic goals.

REFERENCES

1. Aho JM, Schaff MS, Thiels CA, et al. A history of innovation: cardiac surgery in Minnesota. Minn Med 2015;98(1):32–5.
2. Cooley DA, Frazier OH. The past 50 years of cardiovascular surgery. Circulation 2000;102(20 Suppl 4):IV87–93.
3. Schmitto JD, Mokashi SA, Cohn LH. Minimally-invasive valve surgery. J Am Coll Cardiol 2010;56(6):455–62.
4. Nicolini F, Agostinelli A, Vezzani A, et al. The evolution of cardiovascular surgery in elderly patient: a review of current options and outcomes. Biomed Res Int 2014;2014:736298.
5. Natarajan A, Samadian S, Clark S. Coronary artery bypass surgery in elderly people. Postgrad Med J 2007;83(977):154–8.
6. Likosky DS, Sorensen MJ, Dacey LJ, et al. Long-term survival of the very elderly undergoing aortic valve surgery. Circulation 2009;120(11 Suppl):S127–33.
7. Anderson GF. Medicare and chronic conditions. N Engl J Med 2005;353(3): 305–9.
8. Yoshihara H, Yoneoka D. Trends in the incidence and in-hospital outcomes of elective major orthopaedic surgery in patients eighty years of age and older in the united states from 2000 to 2009. J Bone Joint Surg Am 2014;96(14):1185–91.
9. Kwok AC, Semel ME, Lipsitz SR, et al. The intensity and variation of surgical care at the end of life: a retrospective cohort study. Lancet 2011;378(9800):1408–13.
10. American Geriatrics Society Expert Panel on the Care of Older Adults with Multimorbidity. Patient-centered care for older adults with multiple chronic conditions: a stepwise approach from the American Geriatrics Society: American Geriatrics Society Expert Panel on the Care of Older Adults with Multimorbidity. J Am Geriatr Soc 2012;60(10):1957–68.
11. Boyd C, Fortin M. Future of multimorbidity research: how should understanding of multimorbidity inform health system design? Public Health Rev 2010;32:451–74.

12. Guiding principles for the care of older adults with multimorbidity: an approach for clinicians. Guiding principles for the care of older adults with multimorbidity: an approach for clinicians: American Geriatrics Society Expert Panel on the Care of Older Adults with Multimorbidity. J Am Geriatr Soc 2012;60(10):E1–25.
13. Daabiss M. American Society of Anaesthesiologists physical status classification. Indian J Anaesth 2011;55(2):111–5.
14. Rix TE, Bates T. Pre-operative risk scores for the prediction of outcome in elderly people who require emergency surgery. World J Emerg Surg 2007;2:16.
15. Tei M, Wakasugi M, Kishi K, et al. Incidence and risk factors of postoperative delirium in elderly patients who underwent laparoscopic surgery for colorectal cancer. Int J Colorectal Dis 2016;31(1):67–73.
16. Yeoh CJ, Fazal MA. ASA grade and elderly patients with femoral neck fracture. Geriatr Orthop Surg Rehabil 2014;5(4):195–9.
17. Fleisher LA, Fleischmann KE, Auerbach AD, et al. 2014 ACC/AHA guideline on perioperative cardiovascular evaluation and management of patients undergoing noncardiac surgery: executive summary: a report of the American College of Cardiology/American Heart Association Task Force on Practice Guidelines. Circulation 2014;130(24):2215–45.
18. Lee TH, Marcantonio ER, Mangione CM, et al. Derivation and prospective validation of a simple index for prediction of cardiac risk of major noncardiac surgery. Circulation 1999;100(10):1043–9.
19. Shahian DM, O'Brien SM, Filardo G, et al. The Society of Thoracic Surgeons 2008 cardiac surgery risk models: part 1–coronary artery bypass grafting surgery. Ann Thorac Surg 2009;88(1 Suppl):S2–22.
20. O'Brien SM, Shahian DM, Filardo G, et al. The Society of Thoracic Surgeons 2008 cardiac surgery risk models: part 2–isolated valve surgery. Ann Thorac Surg 2009;88(1 Suppl):S23–42.
21. Leontyev S, Walther T, Borger MA, et al. Aortic valve replacement in octogenarians: utility of risk stratification with EuroSCORE. Ann Thorac Surg 2009;87(5):1440–5.
22. Afilalo J, Eisenberg MJ, Morin JF, et al. Gait speed as an incremental predictor of mortality and major morbidity in elderly patients undergoing cardiac surgery. J Am Coll Cardiol 2010;56(20):1668–76.
23. Salive ME. Multimorbidity in older adults. Epidemiol Rev 2013;35:75–83.
24. DuGoff EH, Canudas-Romo V, Buttorff C, et al. Multiple chronic conditions and life expectancy: a life table analysis. Med Care 2014;52(8):688–94.
25. Cho H, Klabunde CN, Yabroff KR, et al. Comorbidity-adjusted life expectancy: a new tool to inform recommendations for optimal screening strategies. Ann Intern Med 2013;159(10):667–76.
26. Wozniak SE, Coleman J, Katlic MR. Optimal preoperative evaluation and perioperative care of the geriatric patient: a surgeon's perspective. Anesthesiol Clin 2015;33(3):481–9.
27. Ingraham AM, Richards KE, Hall BL, et al. Quality improvement in surgery: the American College of Surgeons National Surgical Quality Improvement Program approach. Adv Surg 2010;44:251–67.
28. Chow WB, Rosenthal RA, Merkow RP, et al. Optimal preoperative assessment of the geriatric surgical patient: a best practices guideline from the American College of Surgeons National Surgical Quality Improvement Program and the American Geriatrics Society. J Am Coll Surg 2012;215(4):453–66.
29. Stortecky S, Schoenenberger AW, Moser A, et al. Evaluation of multidimensional geriatric assessment as a predictor of mortality and cardiovascular events

after transcatheter aortic valve implantation. JACC Cardiovasc Interv 2012;5(5): 489–96.
30. Lindman BR, Alexander KP, O'Gara PT, et al. Futility, benefit, and transcatheter aortic valve replacement. JACC Cardiovasc Interv 2014;7(7):707–16.
31. Kappetein AP, Head SJ, Généreux P, et al. Updated standardized endpoint definitions for transcatheter aortic valve implantation: the Valve Academic Research Consortium-2 consensus document. J Thorac Cardiovasc Surg 2013; 145(1):6–23.
32. Kristensen SD, Knuuti J, Saraste A, et al. 2014 ESC/ESA Guidelines on non-cardiac surgery: cardiovascular assessment and management: the joint task force on non-cardiac surgery: cardiovascular assessment and management of the European Society of Cardiology (ESC) and the European Society of Anaesthesiology (ESA). Eur J Anaesthesiol 2014;31(10):517–73.
33. Fisher AA, Davis MW, Rubenach SE, et al. Outcomes for older patients with hip fractures: the impact of orthopedic and geriatric medicine cocare. J Orthop Trauma 2006;20(3):172–8 [discussion: 179–80].
34. Klein BE, Klein R, Knudtson MD, et al. Frailty, morbidity and survival. Arch Gerontol Geriatr 2005;41(2):141–9.
35. Xue QL. The frailty syndrome: definition and natural history. Clin Geriatr Med 2011;27(1):1–15.
36. Makary MA, Segev DL, Pronovost PJ, et al. Frailty as a predictor of surgical outcomes in older patients. J Am Coll Surg 2010;210(6):901–8.
37. Fried LP, Tangen CM, Walston J, et al. Frailty in older adults: evidence for a phenotype. J Gerontol A Biol Sci Med Sci 2001;56(3):M146–56.
38. Rockwood K, Mitnitski A. Frailty in relation to the accumulation of deficits. J Gerontol A Biol Sci Med Sci 2007;62(7):722–7.
39. Fried LP, Ferrucci L, Darer J, et al. Untangling the concepts of disability, frailty, and comorbidity: implications for improved targeting and care. J Gerontol A Biol Sci Med Sci 2004;59(3):255–63.
40. Abellan van Kan G, Rolland Y, Bergman H, et al. The I.A.N.A Task Force on frailty assessment of older people in clinical practice. J Nutr Health Aging 2008;12(1): 29–37.
41. Abellan van Kan G, Rolland Y, Houles M, et al. The assessment of frailty in older adults. Clin Geriatr Med 2010;26(2):275–86.
42. Abellan van Kan G, Rolland Y, Andrieu S, et al. Gait speed at usual pace as a predictor of adverse outcomes in community-dwelling older people an International Academy on Nutrition and Aging (IANA) Task Force. J Nutr Health Aging 2009;13(10):881–9.
43. Leong DP, Teo KK, Rangarajan S, et al. Prognostic value of grip strength: findings from the Prospective Urban Rural Epidemiology (PURE) study. Lancet 2015; 386(9990):266–73.
44. Kwon S, Symons R, Yukawa M, et al. Evaluating the association of preoperative functional status and postoperative functional decline in older patients undergoing major surgery. Am Surg 2012;78(12):1336–44.
45. Green P, Arnold SV, Cohen DJ, et al. Relation of frailty to outcomes after transcatheter aortic valve replacement (from the PARTNER trial). Am J Cardiol 2015; 116(2):264–9.
46. Green P, Cohen DJ, Genereux P, et al. Relation between six-minute walk test performance and outcomes after transcatheter aortic valve implantation (from the PARTNER trial). Am J Cardiol 2013;112(5):700–6.

47. Robinson TN, Wu DS, Pointer LF, et al. Preoperative cognitive dysfunction is related to adverse postoperative outcomes in the elderly. J Am Coll Surg 2012; 215(1):12–7 [discussion: 17–8].
48. Hu CJ, Liao CC, Chang CC, et al. Postoperative adverse outcomes in surgical patients with dementia: a retrospective cohort study. World J Surg 2012;36(9): 2051–8.
49. Millar K, Asbury AJ, Murray GD. Pre-existing cognitive impairment as a factor influencing outcome after cardiac surgery. Br J Anaesth 2001;86(1):63–7.
50. Connolly A, Gaehl E, Martin H, et al. Underdiagnosis of dementia in primary care: variations in the observed prevalence and comparisons to the expected prevalence. Aging Ment Health 2011;15(8):978–84.
51. Yue J, Tabloski P, Dowal SL, et al. NICE to HELP: operationalizing National Institute for Health and Clinical Excellence guidelines to improve clinical practice. J Am Geriatr Soc 2014;62(4):754–61.
52. American Geriatrics Society Expert Panel on Postoperative Delirium in Older Adults. American Geriatrics Society abstracted clinical practice guideline for postoperative delirium in older adults. J Am Geriatr Soc 2015;63(1):142–50.
53. Fink HA, Hemmy LS, MacDonald R, et al. Intermediate- and long-term cognitive outcomes after cardiovascular procedures in older adults: a systematic review. Ann Intern Med 2015;163(2):107–17.
54. Suaya JA, Shepard DS, Normand SL, et al. Use of cardiac rehabilitation by Medicare beneficiaries after myocardial infarction or coronary bypass surgery. Circulation 2007;116(15):1653–62.
55. Menezes AR, Lavie CJ, Forman DE, et al. Cardiac rehabilitation in the elderly. Prog Cardiovasc Dis 2014;57(2):152–9.
56. Available at: http://eprognosis.ucsf.edu/%C2%A0. Accessed January 21, 2015.
57. Seco M, Edelman JJ, Forrest P, et al. Geriatric cardiac surgery: chronology vs. biology. Heart Lung Circ 2014;23(9):794–801.
58. Salpeter SR, Luo EJ, Malter DS, et al. Systematic review of noncancer presentations with a median survival of 6 months or less. Am J Med 2012;125(5):512.e1–6.
59. Lee SJ, Leipzig RM, Walter LC. Incorporating lag time to benefit into prevention decisions for older adults. JAMA 2013;310(24):2609–10.
60. Epstein RM, Peters E. Beyond information: exploring patients' preferences. JAMA 2009;302:195–7.

Integrating Care Across Disciplines

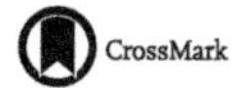

Nina L. Blachman, MD*, Caroline S. Blaum, MD, MS

KEYWORDS

- Interdisciplinary care • Geriatrics • Heart failure • Team

KEY POINTS

- The goal of the interdisciplinary team is to work in a patient-centered manner to manage patient symptoms and prevent complications and readmissions.
- Members of the interdisciplinary care team include physicians, nurses, social workers, pharmacists, dietitians, and physical and occupational therapists.
- Interdisciplinary care can take place in the hospital, outpatient clinic, at home, or remotely via telemonitoring.
- In patients with heart failure, interdisciplinary teams are effective at preventing exacerbations and readmissions, and can improve the quality of care.

INTRODUCTION

Interdisciplinary teams (IDTs) are found throughout modern complex health care systems.[1] They function in acute care hospitals, ambulatory care clinics, home care settings, nursing homes, and hospices. They are often found in disease-specific areas, such as diabetes or cardiovascular clinics, or in cancer centers, and in site-based care programs, such as home care or postacute transitional care programs. IDTs are key components of patient-centered medical homes in primary care[2] and in some specialty care settings, and multiple types of IDTs are part of the infrastructure of organized systems of care such as managed and accountable care organizations.[3] This article focuses on those IDTs in care settings that deal with older adults with cardiovascular disease (CVD) and multiple chronic conditions (MCCs). It reviews the history and structure of such IDTs, and the components of effective IDT care and its barriers. This article provide an overview of team care in CVD, and discusses heart failure (HF) IDTs in some detail because IDT care in HF has been extensively studied and widely implemented, and evidence for efficacy and effectiveness is available.[4]

Division of Geriatric Medicine and Palliative Care, Department of Medicine, New York University School of Medicine, 550 First Avenue, BCD 615, New York, NY 10016, USA
* Corresponding author.
E-mail address: nina.blachman@nyumc.org

Clin Geriatr Med 32 (2016) 373–383
http://dx.doi.org/10.1016/j.cger.2016.01.010 geriatric.theclinics.com

The health care professionals comprising IDTs work together to implement a coordinated plan for each patient.[5] Historically, a distinction was made between IDTs and multidisciplinary teams, which were considered to involve members working separately and without collaborating on a treatment plan. However, given the rapidly increasing complexity of the health care system, the aging of the population, and the increase in the number of older adults with MCCs, it is now clear that IDT–based health care in which team members work together to meet the complex needs of patients is essential to safe and effective patient care. IDTs bring together practitioners with a diverse set of skills and specialties (such as physicians, nurse practitioners, social workers, and physical therapists), and can provide measurable value to patients.[6] Multiple providers are needed on the care team because no single profession provides practitioners with the resources or educational background to handle all aspects of care for a patient.[7] In a 2006 position paper, the American Geriatrics Society noted that interdisciplinary care is important for older adults with complex comorbidities.[8] More recently, principles and models of effective team-based care were described by an Institute of Medicine discussion paper (2012),[1] and IDT care is fostered and promoted by national organizations such as the Patient-Centered Primary Care Collaborative and the Interprofessional Education Collaborative.[9–11]

HISTORY OF INTERDISCIPLINARY CARE FOR OLDER ADULTS

Geriatrics has been on the leading edge of the development of IDT care. Since the 1940s, IDTs have been instrumental in managing geriatric patients at home.[11] Team training in health care was adopted early by geriatric medicine and gerontology, and the Health Resources and Services Administration was issuing grants related to teaching collaboration and teamwork in geriatrics as far back as the 1980s.[12] On the inpatient side, IDTs in geriatrics began in the 1970s, even before Medicare reforms, because hospitals experienced bed shortages when patients had extended lengths of stay waiting for nursing home placement. The geriatric IDTs of that era helped to facilitate discharge planning and ease this problem.[13]

Geriatrics also developed comprehensive geriatric assessment (CGA) in the inpatient, ambulatory and home care settings[14–16] in the 1990s. Many types of comprehensive assessments with variable methods of assessing and managing problems were tested. This early geriatrics model advanced the approach to care of complex patients by pioneering patient evaluation in multiple domains, including medical, pharmacologic, and psychosocial. Importantly, CGA pointed out the importance of functional and cognitive evaluation of older adults, and is foundational to many care models that are now in widespread use. IDTs were and are a fundamental component of CGA because the complementary skills of different team members improve the quality of assessments.

Cardiologists dealing with older patients with HF and complex health care status also realized the importance of IDTs for these patients. HF clinics began to appear in 1983, but became more respected and widespread after a seminal study by Rich and colleagues[17] in 1993 found that patients who were part of a HF IDT clinic intervention had both fewer readmissions and decreased length of stay. In 2004, Naylor and colleagues[19] showed that nurse care coordination can improve the transition from hospital to home and reduce complications.[18,19] This nurse care coordination can also address lapses in communication among providers and between providers and patients and caregivers. For example, physicians may not properly educate patients and caregivers on medication regimens, and/or may not recognize enhanced vulnerabilities of older patients with HF because of their comorbidities, cognitive impairment, and deficits in their ability to perform activities of daily living.[18] Comprehensive discharge planning and nurse care coordination can help ensure that patients' medical information is communicated not only to the patients and caregivers but also to the outpatient physician to allow close follow-up.[20]

Over the past 20 years, the complexity of health care has increased dramatically and shows no signs of slowing down. Team-based care has become essential in many areas of the health care system and is recognized as particularly important for older adults with MCCs and CVD.

GENERAL CHARACTERISTICS OF INTERDISCIPLINARY TEAMS

Table 1 shows potential members of an IDT that would be organized to provide comprehensive interdisciplinary care to older patients. The table lists the roles different team members may play, and the multiple varied issues that must be addressed in older adults with MCCs. Although articulated nearly 20 years ago, information in this table remains a useful guide to the complex needs of multimorbid patients.[5] Advanced practice nurses (APNs), social workers, and pharmacists are becoming more common in primary care clinics, particularly with the advent of the patient-centered medical home in primary care (discussed later), and are often found in geriatrics ambulatory clinics. Different teams in different clinical settings can be composed of different disciplines, depending on the site and goal of the IDT-based care.

In 2012, the Institute of Medicine developed a discussion paper on the *Core Principles & Values of Team-Based Care*.[1] That paper, whose investigators included providers of multiple disciplines and also patients, articulated several principles of team-based health care, including shared goals, clear roles, mutual trust, effective communication, and measureable outcomes. It cited examples of several well-functioning teams around the country, and many of these teams focused on the care of older patients and/or patients with MCCs.

IDT care of older adults, although becoming increasingly available, still faces many of the same barriers it has faced for the past 30 years.[21] It is not reimbursed under usual fee-for-service payment systems. In the setting of managed care and in newer forms of health care delivery associated with shared savings, such as accountable care organizations, creative ways to reimburse team-based care are being developed. Another common barrier concerns the challenges team members can face as they strive to work together.

Effective team-based care requires many kinds of personal interactions, trust in the competence of other team members, and clear articulation of the roles and responsibilities of each team member. In general, most types of health care professional training do not teach much, if anything, about working in teams, so training in effective teamwork to help address these challenges is important. Over the years, core competencies of interdisciplinary training have been described and tools and curricula are available, but there is often insufficient opportunity for IDT training to help members work together effectively.

INTERDISCIPLINARY TEAM CARE IN CARDIOVASCULAR DISEASE

Older patients with CVD and MCCs experience IDT care in multiple settings and care models. Many of these care settings use IDT care to focus specifically on cardiovascular problems.[22] IDTs are now so common in CVD care that the American College of Cardiology issued a position paper in 2015 that explored the types of IDT care currently used, advantages and evidence for team-based care, and barriers to effective team-based care.[23] Examples of IDT care in cardiology include teams that work

Table 1
IDT roles

Role	Consult For
Physician Assessment Pathologic diagnosis and treatment Medications Prognosis Medical management	Changes in cognition Impairments in ADLs Depression Delirium vs dementia Severe malnutrition Stage IV pressure sores Polypharmacy Follow-up care
Clinical nurse specialist Facilitates communication Provides assessment and interventions for frail elderly Counseling Teaching Coordinates discharge planning Provides case management	Assessment of functional status Assessment of interventions for common geriatric syndromes (falls, incontinence, poor nutrition, high-risk medications, delirium vs dementia, depression) Assistance with end-of-life decision making Case management Complex family issues Palliative care Compliance issues Patients with frequent readmissions Assistance with ethical decision making Need for patient/family conference Assistance with discharge planning and follow-up needed Education of patients/families
Nurse Assesses patient function and develops plan of care Monitors response to nursing and medical plan of care Coordinates patient care Supports health maintenance and health promotion Provides support to patients and families Provides education to patients, caregivers and IDT members	Functional concerns (baseline vs current function) Falls Risk/presence of pressure ulcers Continence Behavior problems (delirium vs dementia) Palliative care issues Resource to family/caregiver Education treatments, prevention/health maintenance information, medications, and so forth Compliance issues Plan of care
Social worker Assesses and makes referrals for discharge needs Acts as liaison with home care agencies, rehabilitation, skilled facilities, and community agencies Provides counseling and support Provides coordination of care Financial planning/reimbursement Case management	Assessment of high-risk older adults (cognitive impairment, depression, lives alone, lack of supports, frequent readmission, impairment) Lack of finances for care Patient and caregiver relationship issues Care coordination Need for hospice care Patients from skilled facilities Suspected abuse or neglect of older patient Education (eg, on available resources, services, payment options)

(*continued on next page*)

Table 1
(*continued*)

Role	Consult For
Physical therapist Provides assessment of mobility including bed/chair transfers and gait Interventions focus on lower extremities ROM, strength, and coordination Provide exercises for specific areas of weakness Assesses need for assistive devices and prostheses Provides education to patients, caregivers, and IDT members Provides relief from pain caused by postural and muscular imbalance	Unsteady gait Weakness Balance problems Falls history Orthostasis Mobility safety concerns Changes in weight-bearing status Patients at risk for functional decline caused by acute or chronic problems Need for assistive device Education (eg, transfer techniques, how to get up from a fall) Need for exercises/ROM because of immobility Recommendations for discharge disposition
Occupational therapist Assessment of self-care activities (ADLs and IADLs) Targets upper extremities for ROM, strength, and endurance Fine motor coordination Assesses for adaptive equipment (eg, reachers, splints, orthotics) Provides education to patients, caregivers, and IDT members	Impairments/suspected impairments in self-care Safety concerns in performing self-care activities Patients with cognitive impairments Limitations in ADLs and IADLs with lack of supports Patients at risk of functional decline caused by acute or chronic problem Need for adaptive equipment Education
Dietitian Nutritional assessment Evaluates adequacy of diet in light of acute illness and patient's ability to consume nutrients and fluids Provides education to patients, caregivers, and IDT members	Lack of appetite Recent weight loss (10% or greater) Albumin level less than 3.6 mg/dL Enteral nutrition Supplement recommendations Diet recommendations Education (diet changes, changes in diet routines–small frequent meals)

Abbreviations: ADL, activities of daily living; IADL, instrumental activities of daily living; ROM, range of motion.

From Kresevic D, Holder C. Interdisciplinary care. Clin Geriatr Med 1998;14(4):790–1; with permission.

with patients with devices and arrhythmias, such as in settings involving pacemakers, implantable cardiac defibrillators (ICDs), and cardioversion.

Widespread team-based programs, often with major nursing and APN staffing, include coagulation clinics that manage patients taking anticoagulant drugs. Other conditions besides CVD require anticoagulation, but such clinics are usually within cardiology departments, and cardiologists generally provide physician input. Preventive cardiology team-based care is also increasingly being implemented, in which the IDT provides self-management support to patients working to control risk factors for CVD. Cardiovascular rehabilitation after acute coronary syndrome, before or after valve surgery or in the setting of HF, also requires a strong IDT. Most common are IDTs that focus on patients with HF and that function in several care settings.

HF IDTs have been well studied and evidence about their composition and function is available, so the special case of HF is discussed in detail later.

Many patients with CVD and MCCs are cared for in primary care as well as ambulatory cardiology, and because they have a substantial and varied disease burden they also receive care in multiple other settings. Therefore, patients with CVD and MCCs experience the types of IDT care that are in widespread use to care for complex patients. Complex patients with MCCs may be cared for in care coordination programs, advanced primary care models such as the patient-centered medical home, transitional care programs provided after hospitalizations, home care, nursing home care, and palliative care. Clearly, discussion of these common care delivery methods, all of which use IDT care, is beyond the scope of this article. Palliative care is discussed in more detail elsewhere in this issue (See Pak E, Wald J, Kirkpatrick JN: Multimorbidity and End of Life Care in Patients with Cardiovascular Disease).

THE CASE OF HEART FAILURE

It is instructive to specifically consider HF to see how critical a role interdisciplinary care can play in the care of older adults with multimorbidity. Based on the diagnosis-related group codes, HF is the most common discharge diagnosis among hospitalized patients in the United States.[24] The prevalence of HF increases with age, and approximately 12% of men and women aged 80 years and older are living with the condition.[25] As the population gets older, the number of patients over 80 years old with HF is projected to increase 66% by 2030, which means that more than 8 million people will be living with the condition.[25] After age 65, the incidence of HF is approximately 10 per 1000.[26]

In the United States and the Western world, most cases of HF are caused by coronary artery disease, dilated cardiomyopathy, valvular disease, and hypertension.[25] Symptoms of HF range from decreased exercise tolerance to exertional dyspnea and orthopnea. In 2010, there were 676,000 emergency room visits for HF.[26] The total cost of HF to the United States each year is estimated to be $32 billion.[26] HF is a major cause of death in this country, and patients' 5-year mortality is 50%.[26]

Although many patients die of sudden death, others require repeated hospital admissions in their last year of life.[27] In a review of Medicare claims from 2007 to 2009, 35% of readmissions were for HF.[4] For patients with HF, the 6-month readmission rate to the hospital is cited to be in the range of 25%-50%.[28] Most readmissions occur within a month of discharge from the hospital.[29] This finding indicates that the transition process from hospital to home needs to be improved.

Complex older adults with HF and multimorbidity, in particular, have more complications with transitions from hospital to home than younger patients, and a care team can help improve that passage.[7] In one study, 53% of readmissions were related to medication nonadherence or diet.[17] These issues are potentially preventable through vigilant monitoring by nonphysician team members such as nurses and pharmacists. Addressing social barriers like poor health literacy and lack of help at home can also fix these problems.[30] Interdisciplinary care for HF requires multiple specialists and providers who bring diverse skill sets to these complex patients.

The IDT can share the goals of managing symptoms, reducing costs, and improving patient satisfaction.[4] Patients with HF often shuttle between settings, mandating coordinated care among multiple providers. Care for patients with HF can take place in hospitals and rehabilitation facilities, as inpatients, outpatients, at home, and by telephone.[31,32] In the case of HF, adherence to specific regimens of care (diet, fluid balance, and exercise) can make a critical difference between a patient remaining stable at home and requiring readmission to a hospital.[33] Multiple providers, working as a team, can counsel patients on these issues to prevent readmissions. **Box 1** enumerates the complexities involved in successfully caring for patients with HF.

In recent years, payers such as Medicaid and Medicare have prioritized containing the costs involved in HF admissions.[4] The Centers for Medicare & Medicaid Services (CMS) focused specifically on 30-day readmission for HF as a measure of quality of care.[34] In October 2012, CMS instituted a program under which hospitals with an excessive number of readmissions began to see a decrease in reimbursement.[4] Thus, the need for better management of patients with HF is not just about quality of care for the patients, but also about the fiscal sustainability of hospitals.

As a result of the complexities of these patients, care transition teams have become a focal point to reduce 30-day readmissions. The programs start the discharge planning process early, coordinate with patients and family members to educate them about the plan, and review medication management issues.[25] In the inpatient setting, IDTs for multimorbid older adults help reduce nursing home admissions, decrease hospital length of stay, reduce the use of health care services, and improve quality of life.[8] The transition from hospital to home is often fraught with preventable complications.[18] There are systems issues with hospital discharges and lapses in communication among providers. For example, physicians may not properly educate patients and caregivers on medication regimens. The elderly are most vulnerable to poor outcomes because of comorbidities, including cognitive impairment and deficits in their ability to perform activities of daily living.[18] Comprehensive discharge planning can help ensure that patients' medical information is communicated to the outpatient physician to allow close follow-up.[20]

Box 1
Barriers to effective HF management

Multiple comorbid conditions
- Coronary heart disease
- Hypertension
- Diabetes
- Renal insufficiency
- Chronic lung disease
- Arthritis

Polypharmacy
- Medication compliance
- Adverse drug reactions

Dietary compliance issues

Psychosocial concerns
- Social isolation
- Depression

Financial constraints

Physical limitations
- Reduced visual and auditory acuity
- Neuromuscular deficits (eg, stroke, Parkinsonism)
- Arthritis

Cognitive dysfunction

From Rich MW. Heart failure disease management: a critical review. J Card Fail 1999;5(1):65; with permission.

Once home, as outpatients, it is particularly beneficial to provide a team approach to care.[4] The reason behind this may be at least in part that compliance rates among patients receiving home visits have been found to be highest immediately after hospital discharge.[27] IDTs in the outpatient setting help patients maintain function, improve adherence with medications, prevent adverse drug events, and reduce the use of home services.[8] As patients require more medications and increasing doses of existing medications, compliance can worsen, and physicians often do not suspect that a patient is not adhering to a medication regimen.[18] Cardiac nurses can spend more time with patients reviewing medications and gauging responses to therapy, information that can be invaluable to physicians.[6] In a multisite randomized controlled trial, APNs who collaborated with physicians were able to prolong the time until readmission in older adults with MCCs.[18,25]

Patients who are too frail or who are unable to travel to outpatient clinics can benefit from home visits.[19] The correct timing for a home visit is difficult, because patients are often readmitted to the hospital in the short time frame between the hospitalization and the scheduled visit, but that should not limit the team's efforts.[35] When providers visit patients' homes, they can more readily identify potential barriers to compliance and are better able to optimize care.[4] A team viewing the patient's home circumstances can also offer more focused patient education.[36] In a study by Rich and colleagues,[37] not living alone was a predictor of adherence. Although home visits do not replace another person living in the patient's residence, they can help. A meta-analysis found that home visits had a positive effect on 30-day and 3-month to 6-month readmission rates for patients with HF.[29] Because patients with HF experience acute episodes in which they require changes in medication and treatment, having this support is valuable.

The typical agenda for a home visit is a team review of medications, diet, and fluid management in order to help patients adhere to the recommended treatment plan. Ensuring that cognitively impaired patients who need help with medications have adequate home support is key. The team members involved in the home visit might be a physician or a resident in training, nurse, pharmacist, physical therapist, and social worker.

Studies have shown the benefits of a HF nurse specifically in preventing readmissions, shortening length of stay, and reducing costs.[4] HF nurses help educate patients and family members about many issues, including diet and fluid balance, and are thus able to help prevent HF exacerbations.[19] For instance, some patients benefit from devices such as ICDs, biventricular pacing, and ventricular assist devices.[19] Those interventions are managed most directly by the cardiologists on the team.

Clinical pharmacists are critical for patient education and medication adherence, and have been shown to reduce patient mortality.[4] In prior studies, 44% of elderly patients had been inappropriately prescribed medications after a hospitalization.[31] The presence of a clinical pharmacist can help to combat these potentially life-threatening errors. Up to 50% of patients with HF also have cognitive impairment, further highlighting the importance of minimizing adverse drug events for this population.[31] Because of altered pharmacokinetics and pharmacodynamics in older individuals, especially in those with renal impairment, drugs for patients with HF must be titrated to a safe dose, and a clinical pharmacist's involvement in care from the start can improve prescribing practices.[19]

Physical therapists are also critical for enabling patients to improve functional status and thus prevent readmission to hospitals for deconditioning.[4] When patients lose mobility, physical therapists can help restore function in a rehabilitation setting.[19] Patients may simply need an at-home evaluation to remove potential fall risks or install assistive devices such as grab bars in the shower. For those, the physical or occupational therapists take the lead.

In addition, depression is present in approximately 20% of patients with HF.[31] Depression can negatively affect a patient's health and functional status, and thus the inclusion of a psychologist on a HF team can help prevent depression from being overlooked and untreated by other providers.[4]

Social workers are also pivotal members of the team, particularly to set up services at home and help with transitions of care.[4] In addition, registered dietitians are essential for managing patients with HF, especially those at risk of malnutrition.[19] Many patients with HF require counseling on the sodium and fluid changes that are needed to comply with a HF diet, and the more multimorbid patients, with conditions such as diabetes, need even more support.

In addition, a newer development in managing patients with HF has been telemonitoring, which allows patients to be followed remotely and prevents HF exacerbations from occurring.[35] It is an important tool in HF team management, and has been shown to reduce readmissions.[38] In a Cochrane Review, telemonitoring reduced the rate of both hospital admission and death.[39] Information on patients' weights, blood pressures, respiratory rates, and oxygen saturations can all be obtained remotely, helping to guide treatment decisions.[19] Based on the weight changes, the nurses can inform patients of diuretic dosage adjustments.[37] Although telephone support was shown in a systematic review not to have an impact on 30-day readmission, it did affect 3-month to 6-month readmission rates.[29]

SUMMARY

Most patients with CVD and coexisting MCCs are treated in primary care settings, and IDTs are critical to treating these patients effectively. Cardiologists and geriatricians have a long history of using IDTs, and they have proliferated throughout the health care system around the country. Patients with HF are more complex as they age, and a collaborative team approach is most beneficial to provide patient-centered care. Evidence suggests that interdisciplinary care prevents readmissions. In a large study by the Agency for Healthcare Research Quality, the 3 interventions that proved to reduce readmissions over 3 to 6 months were outpatient HF clinics, home visits, and telemonitoring.[40] These interventions should be implemented in the management of elderly patients with HF.

REFERENCES

1. Mitchell P, Wynia M, Golden R, et al. Core principles & values of effective team-based health care. Discussion paper. Washington, DC: Institute of Medicine; 2012. Available at: www.iom.edu/tbc.
2. American Academy of Family Physicians (AAFP) AAoPA, American College of Physicians (ACP), and American Osteopathic Association (AOA). Joint principles of the patient-centered medical home. Available at: http://www.aafp.org/dam/AAFP/documents/practice_management/pcmh/initiatives/PCMHJoint.pdf. Accessed December 16, 2015.
3. Meyers D, Peikes D, Genevro J, et al. The roles of patient-centered medical homes and accountable care organizations in coordinating patient care. AHRQ Publication No. 11-M005-EF. Rockville (MD): Agency for Healthcare Research and Quality; 2010.
4. Feltner C, Jones CD, Cene CW, et al. Transitional care interventions to prevent readmissions for persons with heart failure: a systematic review and meta-analysis. Ann Intern Med 2014;160(11):774–84.
5. Kresevic D, Holder C. Interdisciplinary care. Clin Geriatr Med 1998;14(4):787–98.

6. Schmitt MH, Farrell MP, Heinemann GD. Conceptual and methodological problems in studying the effects of interdisciplinary geriatric teams. Gerontologist 1988;28(6):753–64.
7. Flaherty E, Hyer K, Fulmer T. Team care. Chapter 26. In: Halter JB, Ouslander JG, Tinetti ME, et al, editors. Hazzard's geriatric medicine and gerontology. 6th edition. New York: McGraw-Hill; 2009.
8. Mion L, Odegard PS, Resnick B, et al. Interdisciplinary care for older adults with complex needs: American Geriatrics Society Position Statement. J Am Geriatr Soc 2006;54(5):849–52.
9. Interprofessional Education Collaborative Expert Panel. Core competencies for interprofessional collaborative practice: report of an expert panel. Washington, DC: Interprofessional Education Collaborative; 2011.
10. Principles of successful teamwork and team competencies. In: Program GITT, editor. Chicago (IL): Rush University Medical Center; 2008.
11. Baldwin DC Jr. Some historical notes on interdisciplinary and interprofessional education and practice in health care in the USA. J Interprof Care 2007; 21(Suppl 1):23–7.
12. Institute of Medicine. Retooling for an aging America: building the health care workforce. Washington, DC: National Academy Press; 2008.
13. Wieland D, Kramer BJ, Waite MS, et al. The interdisciplinary team in geriatric care. Am Behav Sci 1996;39(6):655.
14. Stuck AE, Siu AL, Wieland GD, et al. Comprehensive geriatric assessment: a meta-analysis of controlled trials. Lancet 1993;342(8878):1032–6.
15. Rubenstein LZ, Josephson KR, Wieland GD, et al. Effectiveness of a geriatric evaluation unit. N Engl J Med 1984;311(26):1664–70.
16. Rubin CD, Sizemore MT, Loftis PA, et al. The effect of geriatric evaluation and management on Medicare reimbursement in a large public hospital: a randomized clinical trial. J Am Geriatr Soc 1992;40(10):989–95.
17. Rich MW, Vinson JM, Sperry JC, et al. Prevention of readmission in elderly patients with congestive heart failure: results of a prospective, randomized pilot study. J Gen Intern Med 1993;8:585–90.
18. Stewart S, Marley JE, Horowitz JD. Effects of a multidisciplinary, home-based intervention on unplanned readmissions and survival among patients with chronic congestive heart failure: a randomised controlled study. Lancet 1999;354(9184): 1077–83.
19. Naylor MD, Brooten DA, Campbell RL, et al. Transitional care of older adults hospitalized with heart failure: a randomized, controlled trial. J Am Geriatr Soc 2004; 52(5):675–84.
20. Phillips CO, Wright SM, Kern DE, et al. Comprehensive discharge planning with postdischarge support for older patients with congestive heart failure: a meta-analysis. JAMA 2004;291(11):1358–67.
21. Wynia MK, Von Kohorn I, Mitchell PH. Challenges at the intersection of team-based and patient-centered health care: insights from an IOM working group. JAMA 2012;308(13):1327–8.
22. Bellam N, Kelkar AA, Whellan DJ. Team-based care for managing cardiac comorbidities in heart failure. Heart Fail Clin 2015;11(3):407–17.
23. Brush JE Jr, Handberg EM, Biga C, et al. 2015 ACC health policy statement on cardiovascular team-based care and the role of advanced practice providers. J Am Coll Cardiol 2015;65(19):2118–36.

24. Costantini O, Huck K, Carlson MD, et al. Impact of a guideline-based disease management team on outcomes of hospitalized patients with congestive heart failure. Arch Intern Med 2001;161(2):177–82.
25. Heidenreich PA, Albert NM, Allen LA, et al. Forecasting the impact of heart failure in the United States: a policy statement from the American Heart Association. Circ Heart Fail 2013;6(3):606–19.
26. Mozaffarian D, Benjamin EJ, Go AS, et al, American Heart Association Statistics Committee and Stroke Statistics Subcommittee. Heart disease and stroke statistics–2015 update: a report from the American Heart Association. Circulation 2015;131(4):e29–322.
27. Inglis SC, Pearson S, Treen S, et al. Extending the horizon in chronic heart failure: effects of multidisciplinary, home-based intervention relative to usual care. Circulation 2006;114(23):2466–73.
28. Coons JC, Fera T. Multidisciplinary team for enhancing care for patients with acute myocardial infarction or heart failure. Am J Health Syst Pharm 2007;64(12):1274–8.
29. McDonald K, Ledwidge M, Cahill J, et al. Heart failure management: multidisciplinary care has intrinsic benefit above the optimization of medical care. J Card Fail 2002;8(3):142–8.
30. Rich MW, Beckham V, Wittenberg C, et al. A multidisciplinary intervention to prevent the readmission of elderly patients with congestive heart failure. N Engl J Med 1995;333(18):1190–5.
31. Cooper LB, Hernandez AF. Assessing the quality and comparative effectiveness of team-based care for heart failure: who, what, where, when, and how. Heart Fail Clin 2015;11(3):499–506.
32. Creaser JW, DePasquale EC, Vandenbogaart E, et al. Team-based care for outpatients with heart failure. Heart Fail Clin 2015;11(3):379–405.
33. Jaarsma T. Inter-professional team approach to patients with heart failure. Heart 2005;91(6):832–8.
34. Department of Health and Human Services. Federal register, Part II. US Government Publishing Office Web site. 2011. Available at: http://www.gpo.gov/fdsys/pkg/FR-2011-08-18/pdf/2011-19719.pdf. Accessed March 2, 2016.
35. Chaudhry SI, Mattera JA, Curtis JP, et al. Telemonitoring in patients with heart failure. N Engl J Med 2010;363(24):2301–9.
36. Holland R, Battersby J, Harvey I, et al. Systematic review of multidisciplinary interventions in heart failure. Heart 2005;91(7):899–906.
37. Rich MW, Gray DB, Beckham V, et al. Effect of a multidisciplinary intervention on medication compliance in elderly patients with congestive heart failure. Am J Med 1996;101(3):270–6.
38. Konstam MA, Greenberg B. Transforming health care through the medical home: the example of heart failure. J Card Fail 2009;15(9):736–8.
39. Takeda A, Taylor SJ, Taylor RS, et al. Clinical service organisation for heart failure. Cochrane Database Syst Rev 2012;(9):CD002752.
40. Feltner C, Jones CD, Cené CW, et al. Transitional care interventions to prevent readmissions for people with heart failure. Rockville (MD): Agency for Healthcare Research and Quality (US); 2014.

Multimorbidity and End of Life Care in Patients with Cardiovascular Disease

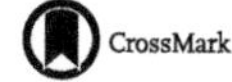

Esther Pak, MD[a], Joyce Wald, DO[b], James N. Kirkpatrick, MD[c,*]

KEYWORDS

• End of life • Withdrawal of cardiac devices • Decision-making

KEY POINTS

- Care of patients with cardiovascular disease (CVD) and multimorbidity is complicated.
- There are significant challenges in prognostication in end-stage CVD that further complicate the difficulties of care at the end of life.
- Nuances in end of life decision-making are inherent in multimorbidity, but they are compounded by particular issues raised by cardiac device therapy.
- Early palliative care involvement as part of a multidisciplinary approach (before end stage) can improve end of life care.
- The end of life care of patients with cardiovascular disease who have multiple other morbid conditions is complex and best served with early palliative care involvement as part of a multidisciplinary team.

INTRODUCTION

Best practices in end of life care for patients with cardiovascular disease (CVD) and multiple comorbidities have not been comprehensively studied.[1–3] The number of patients with CVD and multimorbidity continues to grow with the aging of the population, as discussed elsewhere in this issue (See Bell SP, Saraf AA: Epidemiology of Multimorbidity in Older Adults with Cardiovascular Disease, in this issue). Patients with CVD suffer from a high burden of symptoms, even before diagnosis of severe cardiac disease, and especially at end of life.[4] The prevalence of multimorbidity in patients with CVD may complicate efforts to diagnose and treat symptoms. Prevalence of cognitive impairment in patients with CVD is particularly underappreciated as a complicating factor in decision making and self-care.[5–7]

[a] Palliative Care, Hospital of the University of Pennsylvania, Ravdin 2, 3400 Spruce Street, Philadelphia, PA 19104, USA; [b] Cardiology, Perelman Center for Advanced Medicine, Hospital of the University of Pennsylvania, East Pavilion, 2nd Floor, 3400 Civic Center Boulevard, Philadelphia, PA 19104, USA; [c] Cardiology, Bioethics and Humanities, Regional Heart Center, University of Washington Medical Center, 1959 Pacific Avenue Northeast, Seattle, WA 98125, USA
* Corresponding author.
E-mail address: kirkpatj@cardiology.washington.edu

Clin Geriatr Med 32 (2016) 385–397
http://dx.doi.org/10.1016/j.cger.2016.01.005 geriatric.theclinics.com
0749-0690/16/$ – see front matter

Despite a high mortality among patients with end-stage heart failure (HF),[8,9] difficulty in prognostication complicates advance care planning and may serve as a significant barrier to receiving palliative care and transitioning to hospice. As a result, patients with CVD tend to receive aggressive care[10] and to use large amounts of health care resources[11] in the terminal stages. Hospice agencies traditionally have had limited experience with patients with end-stage CVD, and costly palliative end-stage cardiac therapies, such as inotropes, may complicate hospice admissions.[12]

CHALLENGES IN PROGNOSTICATION

Validated instruments are available to help determine prognosis in patients with severe CVD. Data, such as the 6-minute-walk test, maximal oxygen consumption, and laboratory parameters, such as creatinine and brain natriuretic protein, can help predict mortality in a variety of risk scoring systems (**Table 1**). Some of these tools may help determine if and when patients with CVD may benefit from hospice. The simple "surprise" question ("Would I be surprised if this patient was to die in the next 6 to

Table 1
Summary of prognostic tools in CVD

Prognostic Tool	Variables	End Point
Seattle Heart Failure Model[13]	Age Sex New York Heart Association class Weight Ejection fraction Systolic blood pressure Cause of heart failure Medication use Diuretic dose Anemia % Lymphocytes	Death at 1 y, 2 y, 3 y
Heart failure survival score[14]	Ischemic cardiomyopathy Resting heart rate Ejection fraction Mean resting blood pressure Intraventricular conduction delay Maximal oxygen consumption Serum sodium Pulmonary capillary wedge pressure	Death at 1 y
Heart failure risk scoring system[15]	Age Respiratory rate Systolic blood pressure Blood urea nitrogen Serum sodium Comorbid conditions: dementia, cerebrovascular disease, chronic obstructive pulmonary disease, cirrhosis, cancer, anemia	Death at 30 d, 1 y
Acute decompensated heart failure national registry[16]	Systolic blood pressure Blood urea nitrogen Creatinine	Death in hospital

Adapted from Adler ED, Goldfinger JZ, Kalman J, et al. Palliative care in the treatment of advanced heart failure. Circulation 2009;120:2600.

12 months?") seems to accurately identify many patients at end of life.[17,18] Nonetheless, the variable trajectory with decompensation and improvement[19–22] makes prognostication difficult. Determination of end of life and time to death from clinical parameters is not always clear for individuals.

Furthermore, patients with CVD often have comorbidities that increase functional impairment[20] and total mortality.[23] Diabetes, chronic kidney disease, cerebrovascular disease, depression, functional impairment, and cognitive impairment were found to be associated with greater total mortality risk in patients with severe CVD.[24] Accounting for other comorbidities, as in the multimorbidity index,[25] may provide more accurate prognoses.

Technologies, such as cardiac implantable electronic devices, interventions for structural disease, such as transcatheter aortic valve replacement (TAVR), and mechanical circulatory support (MCS) devices can radically alter disease course and further complicate prognostication. Implanted defibrillators increase survival in patients with HF.[26,27] Cardiac resynchronization therapy not only increases survival, but can also help improve symptoms.[28,29] TAVR can improve symptoms and quality of life in select patients.[30] MCS, such as ventricular assist devices (VADs), improve quality of life and increase survival in select patients.[31]

The presence of multimorbidity influences treatment options for patients with CVD. For example, frailty, reflective of aging and presence of multimorbidity, is associated with increased mortality and higher rates of poor outcomes after TAVR.[32] In MCS, advanced age is a risk factor for death, even after VAD implantation.[33] Although advanced age itself is not a contraindication to MCS, it is associated with comorbidities that increase risk. Although technologies may improve quality of life, patients with CVD and multimorbidity experience increased risk of mortality before and after interventions, including from noncardiovascular causes.

Accurate prognostication is paramount not only for timely consideration of interventions, but also for determining hospice eligibility. Inaccurate prognosis can result in late referrals to hospice, worse caregiver satisfaction with hospice services, lack of awareness of when death will occur, and unmet needs.[34] Because of formidable challenges in prognostication, variable illness trajectory, and the increased risk of mortality in patients with CVD and multimorbidity, elucidation of patient goals and advance care planning should take place early in the disease course.

PALLIATIVE CARE AND HOSPICE AT END OF LIFE

Challenges in prognostication and complex symptoms warrant early incorporation of palliative care expertise in patient management. The likelihood of meaningful impact on patients' quality of life is increased by earlier palliative care involvement.[35] Consideration of palliative care consultation is appropriate when in accordance with patient wishes and when risks of therapies outweigh benefits. The Centers for Medicare and Medicaid Services[36] have instituted a requirement that a palliative care expert play a role in the multidisciplinary team caring for patients considered for VAD implantation as destination therapy. Although the elements of that role remain undefined, this requirement implies recognition of the value of palliative care in the management of this patient group.

Palliative care consultation may be particularly helpful in implementation of advance care plans and appropriate referrals to hospice.[37] **Box 1** shows criteria for hospice admission in patients with CVD. Other factors associated with decreased survival include decline in functional status, need for intermittent or continuous intravenous therapy, unclear benefit from advanced therapies, frequent admissions, and worsening renal function.[38]

Box 1
Hospice criteria

Criteria for hospice

Optimally treated for heart disease or not a candidate for surgery

AND

New York Heart Association class IV and symptomatic at rest despite optimal treatment with diuretics and vasodilators, preferably angiotensin-converting enzyme inhibitors and angiotensin receptor blockers

Other supporting, but not required factors

Symptomatic supraventricular tachycardias

Ventricular arrhythmias refractory to antiarrhythmic medications and appropriate interventions

History of cardiac arrest

History of resuscitation

History of unexplained syncope

History of brain embolism of cardiac origin

Concomitant human immunodeficiency virus

Palliative care involvement and appropriate referrals to hospice may result in increased survival through special attention and better medication adherence. Patients with HF who were enrolled in hospice were found to have increased survival compared with those not in hospice.[39] In fact, discharge from hospice may be possible for patients who undergo initiation or successful uptitration of cardiac medications. Hospice referral may be premature for patients not optimally treated. Early palliative care involvement may also encourage collaboration between multiple specialties in the complex care of patients with CVD, resulting in noncardiovascular specialists implementing optimal medical therapy.[4]

MULTIMORBIDITY AND NUANCES IN END OF LIFE CARE

Symptom Management

Unlike management in other diseases, such as cancer, life-prolonging cardiovascular therapies often have a beneficial effect on symptoms and quality of life.[4] It may be argued that the distinction between disease-modifying therapy and palliative therapy has less relevance in end-stage CVD than in other disease states. The neurohormonal derangements associated with end-stage CVD contribute to classic HF symptoms, such as dyspnea and fatigue, but these patients often experience noncardiac symptoms. Although optimal medical therapy may improve symptoms, quality of life, and longevity, adjustment of medication regimens should take into consideration benefits, burdens of medications, and potential consequences of abrupt withdrawal.[4] Additionally, the presence of certain comorbidities may preclude safe use of individual cardiac medications.[40] **Table 2** summarizes treatment options for prevalent symptoms and examples of comorbidities that may complicate treatments. Although cardiovascular specialist involvement in end of life care results in increased use of cardiac medications, lack of palliative care involvement is associated with limited use of palliative mediations, such as opioids and benzodiazepines.[53]

Table 2
Treatment options for common symptoms

Symptom	Therapy	Caution in Comorbidities
Dyspnea	Diuretics Low-dose opioids[41–43] Oxygen[44] Palliative milrinone or dobutamine[45]	Chronic kidney disease[46–48]
Pain	Opioids Angina pain Nitrates[49] β-Blockers[50] Ranolazine[51] Coronary revascularization	Chronic obstructive pulmonary disease[40] Chronic kidney disease
Depression	Selective serotonin reuptake inhibitors Serotonin-norepinephrine reuptake inhibitors Tricyclic antidepressants	Arrhythmias
Fatigue	Evaluate for secondary causes Treat sleep apnea Methylphenidate may increase risk of arrhythmia and ischemia[52] Palliative milrinone or dobutamine[45]	—

Inotropes

Inotropic infusions with milrinone and dobutamine can help ameliorate refractory HF symptoms, improve quality of life, and reduce hospitalizations.[45] Inotropes bridge patients to transplant and/or MCS, but they also provide relief from symptoms for patients who are at the end of life and who are not candidates for advanced therapies. Risks of arrhythmia and sudden cardiac death are increased with use of inotropes[45] and longevity may be reduced, particularly in patients with multiple comorbidities. These risks are further compounded by renal failure, which results in accumulation of inotrope levels.[54] Other complications are associated with intravenous access, including infection. The choice to begin inotropes for end-stage palliation of HF symptoms can therefore involve complicated advance care planning, particularly in the tradeoff between longevity and symptom relief. In a sense, inotropes as terminal palliation are much more like opioid drips in using the principle of double effect: they are used with the intent to address symptoms, but they may have the unintended consequence of shortening lifespan. Many hospice agencies are limited in their ability to provide inotropes because of lack of experience and cost considerations.[12] Palliative care providers can play an important role in providing care for patients with inotropic dependence.[55]

Withdrawal of Cardiac Medications and Device Therapies

The benefits (symptom relief, longevity) and risks (side effects, undesired outcomes, hassle) of optimal medical therapy and cardiac device interventions must be carefully considered.[56] As diseases progress, palliation of symptoms plays a more prominent role than preventive and life-prolonging therapy, and there are multiple points at which discontinuation of therapies may be appropriate (**Fig. 1**). Yet decision-making about which therapies to continue and which to stop can be complicated.

Withdrawal of cardiac medications is appropriate in circulatory and/or renal dysfunction.[57] Withdrawal of β-blockers may be appropriate in symptomatic bradycardia, hypotension, and severe fatigue, or the development of severe reactive airway

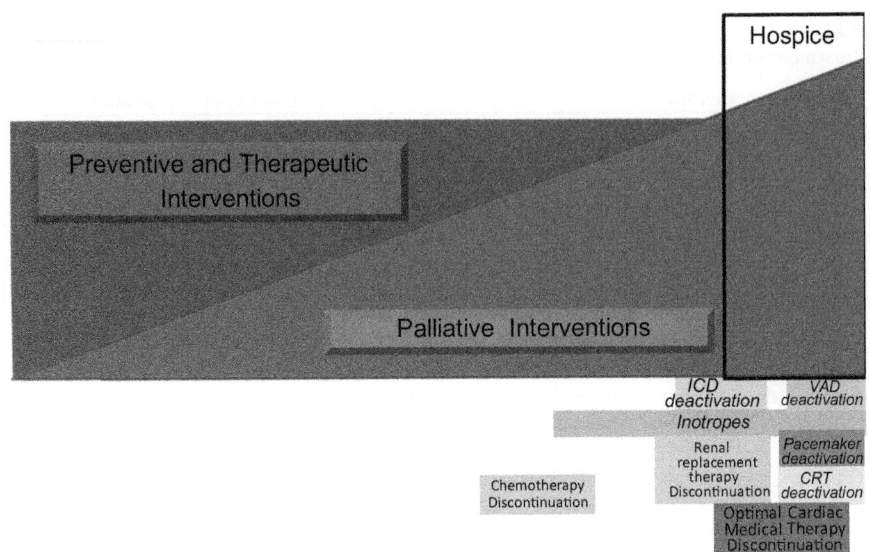

Fig. 1. Care of patients with cardiovascular disease and multimorbidity at the end life. CRT, Cardiac Resynchronization Therapy; ICD, Implantable Cardiac Defibrillator; VAD, Ventricular Assist Device. (*Adapted from* National Consensus Project for Quality Palliative Care. Clinical practice guidelines of quality palliative care, 3rd edition. Available at: http://www.nationalconsensusproject.org/NCP_Clinical_Practice_Guidelines_3rd_Edition.pdf. Accessed March 8, 2016.)

disease. The use of angiotensin-converting enzyme inhibitors and angiotensin receptor blockers may be complicated in hypotension, hyperkalemia, and renal failure. In patients on anticoagulation therapy for atrial fibrillation, the risks of bleeding should be weighed carefully against risk of thromboembolic events.[58]

As patients approach end of life, it is important to assess their goals to make decisions about discontinuation of defibrillation, pacing, and resynchronization therapies. Because patients with CVD and multimorbidity tend to die of noncardiovascular etiologies in progressive metabolic decline, the original intent of cardiac device therapies may no longer apply. Device reprogramming and/or deactivation are important considerations at the time of inotrope initiation because inotropes increase arrhythmogenicity. **Table 3** summarizes considerations in cardiac device therapy at end of life. Unfortunately, most patients have not discussed the possibility of modifying or deactivating their devices with their providers.[64–67] Although palliative care and hospice providers are usually well-versed in guiding patients in advance care planning, they may require the expertise of an electrophysiologist in determining the best course of action concerning an individual patient's cardiac implantable electronic devices. Furthermore, traditionally, few hospices have had protocols to address deactivation.[68] Recent data suggest that educational interventions can reduce the number of patients who are shocked in hospice.[69]

Care of patients with VADs at the end of life raises complex medical, technical, psychosocial, and ethical issues. Published reports on the experience with end of life care for patients with VADs are limited. Older data suggest hospice agencies admit few patients with VADs[19]; and many hospice agencies likely remain unfamiliar with the complexities of care for patients with VADs, including dressing changes, and death in the setting of a device that supports cardiac function. Adding to the potential ethical and

Table 3
Cardiac implantable electronic devices in end of life: considerations

	Issues in Continuing Device Therapy		Issues in Withdrawing Device Therapy	
Device	**Benefits**	**Risks**	**Benefits**	**Risks**
ICD	Prevention of sudden cardiac death	No prevention of death caused by progressive HF or noncardiac disease Pain Anxiety Increased mortality[59,60] Unnecessary shocks in terminal stages	Avoidance of shocks Accordance with patient preferences	Death from arrhythmias
ATP	Prevention of sudden cardiac death Control of arrhythmias	Likelihood of dysfunction on inotropy	Accordance with patient preferences	—
CRT	Improvement in symptoms[61] Does not necessarily prolong dying process[62,63]	—	—	Worsening of symptoms, quality of life

Abbreviations: ATP, antitachycardia pacing; CRT, cardiac resynchronization therapy; ICD, intracardiac defibrillation therapy.

medical complexities, some patients develop complicated relationships with their implanted devices, viewing their VADs with gratitude and even giving them names.[25] This device anthropomorphization may complicate decisions about deactivation. In addition, caregivers of patients with VADs experience significant stress, leading to reduced quality of life, and they may feel conflicted as surrogate decision-makers in end of life situations.[25]

Complications associated with VADs that can occur at any point after implantation include infection, bleeding, thrombotic events, and mechanical pump failure. Multimorbidity interacts with these complications in complex ways. Immunosuppression, bleeding and clotting diatheses, renal failure, and severe peripheral atherosclerotic disease can raise the risks for complications. Cognitive decline impairs a patient's ability to manage the technical components of VAD care. Patients may also experience irritation, infection, and significant discomfort where the pump is placed or where the driveline exits the skin to attach to the device controller.

Causes of death in patients with VAD include infection, bleeding, right HF, embolic stroke, intracranial hemorrhage, device malfunction, and multisystem failure.[70] Mechanical dysfunction of VADs can lead to rapid decompensation and death.[56] Multimorbidity increases the likelihood of death from noncardiovascular causes in patients with VAD as in other populations with CVD. Patients, families, and clinicians have complex views of VAD deactivation and death.[71] After a VAD is turned off, patients may die right away or after a period of time, depending on residual cardiac function.

Given these complexities, coupled with the high risk of neurologic events with potential adverse effects on decision-making capacity, it is important to engage in advance care planning before the terminal phase, and ideally preimplantation.[72]

Advance care plans or "preparedness plans" can even specify under what circumstances or in which conditions a VAD should be deactivated, potentially alleviating some of the stress experienced by surrogate decision-makers at the end of life. These plans may need to acknowledge what a VAD means to an individual patient. In light of all the complexities of VADs and patients with VADs, a strong relationship among the patient, caregivers, VAD team, and multidisciplinary team are crucial in the intricate decision-making processes and implementation of decisions and goals. Frequently, difficult decisions, such as discontinuing MCS, are made jointly by patients, caregivers, and providers, easing the burden on designated surrogate decision-makers.

EARLY AND ITERATIVE MULTIDISCIPLINARY CARE

Optimal end of life care of patients with CVD and other comorbidities requires dexterous use of cardiac medications and therapies, and discernment in the appropriate withdrawal of life-sustaining interventions and the application of palliative measures. The complexities inherent in this population necessitate a nuanced understanding of the benefits and burdens of cardiovascular therapies, coupled with an appreciation that many life-prolonging measures also alleviate symptoms. Individualized plans must incorporate these nuances with the goals, values, and preferences of individual patients. Team-based care with primary care, cardiology, palliative care, and other subspecialties should promote effective and comprehensive care of these complex patients. The context of a multidisciplinary team may facilitate improved communication among team members and patients, prioritization of competing treatments, and coordination of services.[73] An emphasis on this collaboration early in the disease process facilitates effective treatment plans that look ahead to the tough choices and the dynamic changes that happen when patients are dying.[4] Disease management teams are already familiar in cardiology, particularly in the management of candidates for VAD and TAVR. Involvement of palliative care clinicians before end of life, not simply as a pro forma inclusion on teams evaluating candidacy, may improve the quality of life and reduce the suffering of patients who do poorly despite aggressive therapies. For patients who are deemed poor candidates for advanced therapies, such as VAD, heart transplant, TAVR, and high-risk surgery, palliative care consultation can ensure that patients receive aggressive interventions to address symptoms and facilitate timely and appropriate referrals to hospice.[56]

Fig. 1 depicts care over the course of illness for a patient with CVD and multimorbidity based on the current model of palliative care.[74] As the disease burden progresses, changes in focus occur, but palliative care should play a role alongside preventive and life-prolonging interventions. Decisions about withdrawal of certain therapies may face different patients at different times but may optimally serve as signposts in a transition from life-prolongation to palliation. Initially, cardiovascular clinicians and other specialists take a central role in directing care with the appropriate application of medications and devices that prolong life and lessening symptom burden. Nonetheless, primary care and palliative care clinicians play an important role in symptom control, management of comorbidities, and advance care planning. Each discipline can provide specific and invaluable input, with each service taking a more or less prominent role at different times, depending on the clinical circumstances, in what amounts to a continuously iterative process. As patients approach end of life, cardiovascular clinicians and other subspecialists may serve more supportive roles in the provision of palliative interventions but are still essential for determining appropriate continuation and/or withdrawal of medications and device therapies.

SUMMARY

The care of patients with severe CVD and multimorbidity entails complex medical decision making, especially at the end of life. Because of the vicissitudes in the course of CVD and the success of therapies to forestall mortality, prognosis is difficult. The transition to end of life is similarly not always easy to identify. Continuation and dynamic modification of life-sustaining cardiac medications and therapies confers benefits in symptom control and quality of life, even at the end of life, but these interventions may have unintended consequences in the presence of other comorbidities. Proven therapies must be incorporated into the context of patient preferences, values, and goals to achieve effective titration of medications and appropriate initiation and withdrawal of cardiac device therapies. As patients decline in the terminal stages, it is especially important to modify medical and device therapies in accordance with goals and values, and with hemodynamic changes, increasing multimorbidity, and accumulating symptom burden. The increasing prevalence of multimorbidity among patients with severe CVD also argues for a comprehensive approach to coordinating multidisciplinary care, and early involvement of palliative care. All patients will die, and the provision of effective end of life care for those with CVD and multimorbidity increasingly requires cooperation between palliative care, specialty care, and primary care.

REFERENCES

1. Derfler MC, Jacob M, Wolf RE, et al. Mode of death from congestive heart failure: implications for clinical management. Am J Geriatr Cardiol 2004;13(6):299–304.
2. Emerging Risk Factors Collaboration, Di Angelantonio E, Kaptoge S, Wormser D, et al. Association of cardiometabolic multimorbidity with mortality. JAMA 2015; 314(1):52–60.
3. Ekundayo OJ, Muchimba M, Aban IB, et al. Multimorbidity due to diabetes mellitus and chronic kidney disease and outcomes in chronic heart failure. Am J Cardiol 2009;103(1):88–92.
4. Goodlin SJ. Palliative care in congestive heart failure. J Am Coll Cardiol 2009; 54(5):386–96.
5. Gaviria M, Pliskin N, Kney A. Cognitive impairment in patients with advanced heart failure and its implication on decision-making capacity. Congest Heart Fail 2011;17:175–9.
6. Leto L, Feola M. Cognitive impairment in heart failure patients. J Geriatr Cardiol 2014;11(4):316–28.
7. Nordlund A, Berggren J, Holmström A, et al. Frequent mild cognitive deficits in several functional domains in elderly patients with heart failure without known cognitive disorders. J Card Fail 2015;21(9):702–7.
8. Slaughter MS, Rogers JG, Milano CA. Advanced heart failure treated with continuous flow left ventricular assist device. N Engl J Med 2009;361:2241–51.
9. Smith GL, Vaccarino V, Kosiborod M, et al. Worsening renal function: what is a clinically meaningful change in creatinine during hospitalization with heart failure. J Card Fail 2003;9:13–25.
10. Tanvetyanon T, Leighton JC. Life-sustaining treatments in patients who died of chronic congestive heart failure compared with metastatic cancer. Crit Care Med 2003;31(1):60–4.
11. Setoguchi S, Glynn RJ, Stedman M, et al. Hospice, opiates, and acute care service use among the elderly before death from heart failure or cancer. Am Heart J 2010;160(1):139–44.

12. Sindone AP, Keogh AM, Macdonald PS, et al. Continuous home ambulatory intravenous inotropic drug therapy in severe heart failure: safety and cost efficacy. Am Heart J 1997;134:889–900.
13. Levy WC, Mozaffarian D, Linker DT, et al. The seattle heart failure model: prediction of survival in heart failure. Circulation 2006;113:1424–33.
14. Aaronson KD, Schwartz JS, Chen TM, et al. Development and prospective validation of a clinical index to predict survival in ambulatory patients referred for cardiac transplant evaluation. Circulation 1997;95:2660–7.
15. Lee DS, Austin PC, Rouleau JL, et al. Predicting mortality among patients hospitalized for heart failure: derivation and validation of a clinical model. JAMA 2003; 290:2581–7.
16. Fonarow GC, Abraham WT, Yancy CW, et al, ADHERE Scientific Advisory Committee, Study Group, and Investigators. Risk stratification for in-hospital mortality in acutely decompensated heart failure: classification and regression tree analysis. JAMA 2005;293:572–80.
17. Schneider N, Oster P, Hager K, et al. Identifying elderly patients with advanced heart failure at the end of life. Int J Cardiol 2011;153(1):98–9.
18. Schwarz ER, Baraghoush A, Morrissey RP, et al. Pilot study of palliative care consultation in patients with advanced heart failure for cardiac transplantation. J Palliat Med 2012;15(1):12–5.
19. Goodlin SJ, Kutner J, Connor S, et al. Hospice care for heart failure patients. J Pain Symptom Manage 2005;29:525–8.
20. Teno JM, Weitzen S, Fennell ML, et al. Dying trajectory in the last year of life: does cancer trajectory fit other diseases? J Palliat Med 2001;4(4):457–64.
21. Vader JM, Rich MW. Team-based care for managing noncardiac conditions in patients with heart failure. Heart Fail Clin 2015;11(3):419–29.
22. Wiegand DL, Kalowes PG. Withdrawal of cardiac medications and devices. AACN Adv Crit Care 2007;18(4):415–25.
23. Glynn LG, Buckley B, Reddan D, et al. Multimorbidity and risk among patients with established cardiovascular disease: a cohort study. Br J Gen Pract 2008; 58(552):488–94.
24. Murad K, Goff DC Jr, Morgan TM, et al. Burden of comorbidities and functional and cognitive impairments in elderly patients at the initial diagnosis of heart failure and their impact on total mortality: the cardiovascular health study. JACC Heart Fail 2015;3(7):542–50.
25. Kheirbek RE, Alemi F, Fletcher R. Heart failure prognosis: comorbidities matter. J Palliat Med 2015;18(5):447–52.
26. Moss AJ, Hall WJ, Cannom DS, et al. Improved survival with an implanted defibrillator in patients with coronary disease at high risk for ventricular arrhythmia. Multicenter automatic defibrillator implantation trial investigators. N Engl J Med 1996; 335(26):1933–40.
27. Moss AJ, Zareba W, Hall WJ, et al. Prophylactic implantation of a defibrillator in patients with myocardial infarction and reduced ejection fraction. N Engl J Med 2002;346(12):877–83.
28. Bristow MR, Saxon LA, Boehmer J, et al. Cardiac-resynchronization therapy with or without an implantable defibrillator in advanced chronic heart failure. N Engl J Med 2004;350(21):2140–50.
29. Chao CT, Tsai HB, Wu CY, et al. Cumulative cardiovascular polypharmacy is associated with the risk of acute kidney injury in elderly patients. Medicine (Baltimore) 2015;94(31):e1251.

30. Reynolds MR, Magnuson EA, Wang K, et al. Health-related quality of life after transcatheter or surgical aortic valve replacement in high-risk patients with severe aortic stenosis: results from the PARTNER trial. J Am Coll Cardiol 2012;60: 548–58.
31. Rogers JG, Aaronson KD, Boyle AJ. Continuous flow left ventricular assist device improves functional capacity and quality of life of advanced heart failure patients. J Am Coll Cardiol 2010;55:1826–34.
32. Green P, Arnold SV, Cohen DJ, et al. Relation of frailty to outcomes after transcatheter aortic valve replacement (from the PARTNER trial). Am J Cardiol 2015; 116(2):264–9.
33. Holman WL, Kormos RL, Naftel DC, et al. Predictors of death and transplant in patients with a mechanical circulatory support device: a multi-institutional study. J Heart Lung Transplant 2009;28:44–50.
34. Teno JM, Shu JE, Casarett D, et al. Timing of referral to hospice and quality of care: length of stay and bereaved family members' perceptions of the timing of hospice referral. J Pain Symptom Manage 2007;34(2):120–5.
35. Temel JS, Greer JA, Muzikansky A, et al. Early palliative care for patients with metastatic non-small-cell lung cancer. N Engl J Med 2010;363:733–42.
36. Centers for Medicare and Medicaid Service Eligibility. Available at: https://www.cms.gov/Medicare/Eligibility-andEnrollment/OrigMedicarePartABEligEnrol/index.html. Accessed September 20, 2015.
37. Campbell ML, Frank RR. Experience with an end-of-life practice at a university hospital. Crit Care Med 1997;25(1):197–202.
38. Setoguchi S, Stevenson LW, Schneeweiss S. Repeated hospitalizations predict mortality in the community population with heart failure. Am Heart J 2007; 154(2):260–6.
39. Connor SR, Pyenson B, Fitch K, et al. Comparing hospice and nonhospice patient survival among patients who die within a three-year window. J Pain Symptom Manage 2007;33(3):238–46.
40. Hawkins NM, Virani S, Ceconi C. Heart failure and chronic obstructive pulmonary disease: the challenges facing physicians and health services. Eur Heart J 2013; 34(36):2795–803.
41. Currow DC, Abernethy AP. Pharmacological management of dyspnoea. Curr Opin Support Palliat Care 2007;1:96–101.
42. Doust JA, Pietrzak E, Dobson A, et al. How well does B-type natriuretic peptide predict death and cardiac events in patients with heart failure: a systematic review. BMJ 2005;330:625.
43. Booth S, Wade R, Johnson M, et al. The use of oxygen in the palliation of breathlessness. A report of the expert working group of the Scientific Committee of the Association of Palliative Medicine. Respir Med 2004(98):476.
44. Booth S, Wade R, Johnson M, et al. The use of oxygen in the palliation of breathlessness. A report of the expert working group of the scientific committee of the Association of Palliative Medicine. Respir Med 2004;98:476.
45. Hauptman PJ, Mikolajczak P, George A, et al. Chronic inotropic therapy in end-stage heart failure. Am Heart J 2006;152:1096–8.
46. Ahmed A, Rich MW, Sanders PW, et al. Chronic kidney disease associated mortality in diastolic versus systolic heart failure: matched study. Am J Cardiol 2007; 99:393–8.
47. Go AS, Chertow GM, Fan D, et al. Chronic kidney disease and the risks of death, cardiovascular events, and hospitalization. N Engl J Med 2004;351:1296–305.

48. Hillege HL, Girbes AR, de Kam PJ, et al. Renal function, neurohormonal activation, and survival in patients with chronic heart failure. Circulation 2000;102(2): 203–10.
49. Cotter G, Metzkor E, Kaluski E, et al. Randomized trial of high-dose isosorbide dinitrate plus low-dose furosemide versus high-dose furosemide plus low-dose isosorbide dinitrate in severe pulmonary oedema. Lancet 1998;351:389–93.
50. Hjalmarson A, Goldstein S, Fagerberg B, et al. Effects of controlled-release metoprolol on total mortality, hospitalizations, and well-being in patients with heart failure: the Metoprolol CR/XL Randomized Intervention Trial in congestive heart failure (MERIT-HF). JAMA 2000(283):1295–302.
51. Banon D, Filion KB, Budlovsky T, et al. The usefulness of ranolazine for the treatment of refractory chronic stable angina pectoris as determined from a systematic review of randomized controlled trials. Am J Cardiol 2014;113(6):1075–82.
52. Prommer E. Methylphenidate: established and expanding roles in symptom management. Am J Hosp Palliat Care 2012;29(6):483–90.
53. Rutten FH, Heddema WS, Daggelders GJ, et al. Primary care patients with heart failure in the last year of their life. Fam Pract 2012;29(1):36–42.
54. Cox ZL, Calcutt MW, Morrison TB, et al. Elevation of plasma milrinone concentrations in stage D heart failure associated with renal dysfunction. J Cardiovasc Pharmacol Ther 2013;18(5):433–8.
55. López-Candales AL, Carron C, Schwartz J. Need for hospice and palliative care services in patients with end stage heart failure treated with intermittent infusion of inotropes. Clin Cardiol 2004;27(1):23–8.
56. Goldfinger JZ, Adler ED. End-of-life options for patients with advanced heart failure. Curr Heart Fail Rep 2012;7:140–7.
57. Adler ED, Goldfinger JZ, Kalman J, et al. Palliative care in the treatment of advanced heart failure. Circulation 2009;120:2597–606.
58. Poli D, Antonucci E, Grifoni E, et al. Bleeding risk during oral anticoagulation in atrial fibrillation patients older than 80 years. J Am Coll Cardiol 2009;54: 999–1002.
59. Sears SF Jr, Conti JB. Quality of life and psychological functioning of ICD patients. Heart 2002;87:488–93.
60. Seder DB, Patel N, McPherson J, et al. Geriatric experience following cardiac arrest at six interventional cardiology centers in the United States 2006-2011: interplay of age, do-not-resuscitate order, and outcodmes. Crit Care Med 2014;42(2): 289–95.
61. Cleland JG, Daubert JC, Erdmann E, et al. The effect of cardiac resynchronization on morbidity and mortality in heart failure. N Engl J Med 2005;352:1539–49.
62. Sobanski P, Jaarsma T, Krajnik M. End-of-life matters in chronic heart failure patients. Curr Opin Support Palliat Care 2014;8(4):364–70.
63. Stortecky S, Schoenenberger AW, Moser A, et al. Evaluation of multidimensional geriatric assessment as a predictor of mortality and cardiovascular events after transcatheter aortic valve implantation. JACC Cardiovasc Interv 2012;5:489–96.
64. Goldstein NE, Lampert R, Bradley E, et al. Management of implantable cardioverter defibrillators in end-of-life care. Ann Intern Med 2004;141(11):835–8.
65. Kirkpatrick JN, Gottlieb M, Sehgal P, et al. Deactivation of implantable cardioverter defibrillators in terminal illness and end of life care. Am J Cardiol 2012; 109:91–4.
66. Kramer DB, Kesselheim AS, Brock DW, et al. Ethical and legal views of physicians regarding deactivation of cardiac implantable electrical devices: a quantitative assessment. Heart Rhythm 2010;7(11):1537–42.

67. Lampert R, Hayes DL, Annas GJ, et al. HRS expert consensus statement on the management of cardiovascular implantable electronic devices (CIEDs) in patients nearing end of life or requesting withdrawal of therapy. Heart Rhythm 2010;7(7):1008–26.
68. Goldstein N, Carlson M, Livote E, et al. Brief communication: management of implantable cardioverter-defibrillators in hospice: a nationwide survey. Ann Intern Med 2010;152(5):296–9.
69. Kraynik SE, Casarett DJ, Corcoran AM. Implantable cardioverter defibrillator deactivation: a hospice quality improvement initiative. J Pain Symptom Manage 2014;48(3):471–7.
70. Kirklin JK, Naftel DC, Pagani FD, et al. Sixth INTERMACS annual report: a 10,000-patient database. J Heart Lung Transplant 2014;33:555–64.
71. Swetz KM, Cook KE, Ottenberg AL, et al. Clinicians' attitudes regarding withdrawal of left ventricular assist devices in patients approaching the end of life. Eur J Heart Fail 2013;15(11):1262–6.
72. Swetz KM, Kamal AH, Matlock DD, et al. Preparedness planning before mechanical circulatory support: a 'How-To' guide for palliative medicine clinicians. J Pain Symptom Manage 2014;47(5):926–35.
73. Fendler TJ, Swetz KM, Allen LA. Team-based palliative and end-of-life care for heart failure. Heart Fail Clin 2015;11:479–98.
74. Bonow RO, Ganiats TG, Beam CT, et al. ACCF/AHA/AMA-PCPI 2011 performance measures for adults with heart failure: a report of the American College of Cardiology Foundation/American Heart Association task force on performance measures and the American Medical Association-physician consortium for performance improvement. J Am Coll Cardiol 2012;59(20):1812–32.

Future Research Directions for Multimorbidity Involving Cardiovascular Diseases

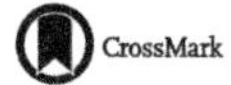

Marcel E. Salive, MD, MPH

KEYWORDS

• Multimorbidity • Aging • Chronic disease • Multiple morbidities

KEY POINTS

- A research agenda focused on cardiovascular disease (CVD) in the context of multimorbidity (2 or more chronic conditions) can address broad scientific issues that are important to the populace.
- Systematic understanding of the molecular mechanisms underlying complex and potentially interacting chronic diseases can be developed to improve strategies for treatment and prevention.
- Clinical trials should ascertain comorbid disease, enroll multimorbid persons to study applicable interventions, and examine patient-centered outcomes relevant to health benefits and harms.
- By eliciting and addressing patient goals of care, the treatment of complex patients with cardiovascular and other chronic illnesses can optimize person-centered outcomes.
- Guideline development must systematically approach the most common and salient disease combinations and, in the case of an absence of evidence, outline high-priority research questions.

INTRODUCTION

Multimorbidity, or multiple chronic conditions (MCCs), is defined as the coexistence of 2 or more chronic conditions and has been observed in approximately two-thirds of older adults in many population studies, making it the "most common chronic condition."[1] Although MCCs lacks a standardized definition in some respects, considerable research has been published demonstrating its substantial human burden in terms of symptoms, medications, treatment costs, and quality of life.[2] Multimorbidity is increasing faster than any single disease and is increasing across all age groups.[3]

Disclosure Statement: The author has nothing to disclose. The views expressed in this article do not necessarily reflect the view of the National Institutes of Health, Department of Health and Human Services, or the United States government.
Division of Geriatrics and Clinical Gerontology, National Institute on Aging, National Institutes of Health, 7201 Wisconsin Avenue, Suite 3c307, MSC 9205, Bethesda, MD 20892-9205, USA
E-mail addresses: msalive@msn.com; Marcel.salive@nih.gov

Clin Geriatr Med 32 (2016) 399–407
http://dx.doi.org/10.1016/j.cger.2016.01.008
0749-0690/16/$ – see front matter Published by Elsevier Inc.

No core list of chronic conditions has been widely accepted to define MCCs; however, most population-based studies of the topic are dominated by persons with hypertension, hyperlipidemia, coronary artery disease, and other CVDs. This article advances a set of future research directions for multimorbidity involving CVDs, using an interdisciplinary patient-centered (not disease-centered) approach, with the intent of moving the field forward by translating evidence into policy and practice.

Geriatricians and general internists have previously developed research agendas related to multimorbidity in an effort to broaden the focus from single diseases or organ systems.[4–6] Subsequently, the Department of Health and Human Services released *Multiple Chronic Conditions: A Strategic Framework* in 2010. Although a major focus has been on the strategic framework's Goal 4, "Facilitate research to fill knowledge gaps about, and interventions and systems to benefit, individuals with MCC," substantial work has addressed the other goals: (1) foster health system change, (2) empower individuals, and (3) equip clinicians.[6] In the spirit of a cycle approach to health from staying healthy to treating conditions to reducing pain and suffering, this article approaches the research on CVDs but from a patient-centered multimorbidity perspective. With this broad scope, it must be recognized that any set of research directions is subjective and not definitive. Available sources that were examined include prior published research agendas, recent meetings, and grant portfolio analyses. A research agenda focused on CVDs in the context of multimorbidity can address broad scientific issues that are important to the populace.

FRAMEWORK FOR MULTIMORBIDITY AND CARDIOVASCULAR DISEASES

This article uses the prominent frameworks for multimorbidity. Although some studies of multimorbidity have analyzed several diseases and conditions at once, other studies have evaluated interactions between just 2 or 3 conditions (dyads and triads), for example, hypertension and diabetes. Another approach is the comorbidity paradigm, where research focuses on an index condition and its coexisting conditions (eg, comorbidities of coronary artery disease).[7] Among comorbid conditions, concordant conditions have similar underlying pathophysiology and may be more the focus of the same disease management plans; for example, diabetes is considered concordant with hypertension, coronary artery disease, and peripheral vascular disease.[8] Atherosclerotic vascular disease is another salient example, which manifests in the body systems as cerebrovascular, cardiovascular, and peripheral artery diseases, although they commonly co-occur. Conversely, discordant conditions are not directly related in either pathology or management, such as discordance of coronary artery disease with low back pain, prostate cancer, and arthritis. Another important concept among the multimorbid conditions is that one condition may be clinically dominant, such as an end-stage disease, or one severely symptomatic, such as class IV congestive heart failure. Finally, some research uses the true multimorbidity approach, where the diseases are considered equally without ranking, and the focus is the impact on the patient.

The frameworks themselves raise several researchable questions. Although a widely accepted definition of multimorbidity is 2 or more chronic conditions, this could achieve wider consensus, and alternatives, such as 3 or more conditions, could be examined and rejected. Which conditions should be included on a universal list of chronic conditions? Should obesity, hyperlipidemia, urinary incontinence, and other geriatric syndromes (cognitive impairment, and delirium) be on that list?[2] How should atherosclerosis be included? Should CVDs be grouped with stroke? How should the framework for research on combinations of CVDs and MCCs be optimized? Which dyads and triads including CVDs are most in need of new research?

Much of the focus of basic science is on identifying underlying causes of multimorbid diseases and understanding the role of aging (**Fig. 1**). Aging, as well as certain etiologic factors, may lead to loss of reserve and organ dysfunction. Some of the causes interact with aging and the diseases as they progress may feed back onto the causal factors. A substantial research agenda includes methods and analytic development to distinguish the effects of aging from factors that cause disease or make it progress or increase in severity.[9]

Within a multimorbid patient, there may be disease-disease interactions, such as the hypertrophic remodeling of the right ventricle (cor pulmonale) that may accompany a variety of chronic respiratory diseases. Other disease-disease interactions may be identified by systematically examining the molecular mechanisms underlying complex diseases. This search includes whether the pathways of one disease may perturb those of another disease, resulting in shared clinical and pathobiological characteristics.

Most chronic diseases have available drug interventions, which give rise to concerns about the potential for interactions. Serious drug adverse events might be viewed as a type of drug-disease interaction, and overall such events cause considerable mortality and health care utilization. Persons with multimorbidity may be at risk of another drug-disease interaction, sometimes referred to as "therapeutic competition," arising when the treatment of one disease adversely affects (competes with) another coexisting condition.[10] Drugs recommended for one condition can be contraindicated or recommended to be avoided in the presence of the other condition. Two well-publicized examples of therapeutic competition are the effects of a cyclooxygenase 2 inhibitor for arthritis on heart disease and rosiglitazone for diabetes increasing heart failure symptoms. Disease-treatment interaction may also arise for therapeutic procedures or subsequent to device implantations. Within the multimorbid person, diseases may progress, become more severe, and lead to both disease-specific and universal (patient-centered) outcomes. Universal outcomes are those that occur across multiple conditions and are less disease specific, such as self-rated health, symptom burden, functional status, and quality of life.

A proposed research agenda is discussed and is listed in the Key Points and in **Table 1**.

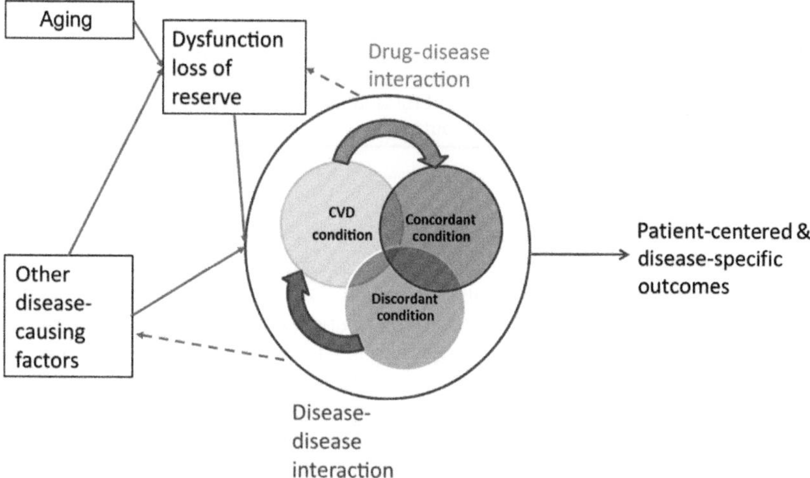

Fig. 1. Model of interaction of aging, underlying causes, modifiers, and chronic conditions in multimorbidity.

Table 1
Research directions for multimorbidity that includes cardiovascular disease

Overarching topics	Develop research programs on high priority dyads and triads of conditions. Obtain consensus on multimorbidity definition and which CVD conditions to routinely include.
Basic science	Examine biological pathways and systems for underlying causes of specific combinations of chronic conditions. Develop and evaluate therapeutic approaches for dyads based on mechanistic studies. Develop methods to distinguish effects of aging from factors causing disease and increasing its severity. Elucidate basic science of behavior to improve self-management of chronic disease.
Clinical trials	Reduce exclusions based on comorbid chronic disease for most trials. Evaluate tailored interventions for older persons with multimorbidity and CVD. Increase use of universal outcomes in CVD clinical trials. Develop and test multimorbidity outcome that could be applied to prevention trials.
Practice/implementation	Develop a minimal phenotyping approach to chronic conditions that can be used in longitudinal studies and linkable electronic health records. Develop methods to identify patient goals and incorporate them into care of persons with multimorbidity and CVD, including use in shared decision-making tools. Develop and validate risk prediction instruments that include outcomes of importance to patients, including comorbid conditions as predictors. Develop and evaluate self-management approaches to multimorbidity for dyads and triads.
Guidelines and quality measures	Translate research on high-priority dyads and triads into CVD guidelines. Evaluate guideline dissemination approaches on CVD guidelines that have incorporated the dyad and triad information in primary care. Develop approach for guidelines to deal with conditions that are discordant to CVD, such as depression and chronic pain. Develop and refine quality measures for persons with MCCs and CVD that can be used for quality improvement programs in primary and specialty outpatient care.

BASIC SCIENCE AND DISCOVERY

Among the most frequent co-occurring chronic conditions, the elucidation of common underlying pathways is a high priority that might lead to broad clinical applications. The interdisciplinary field of geroscience aims to understand the relationship between aging biology and age-related diseases. Aging is a universally experienced risk factor underlying the development of most chronic diseases and can also accelerate disease occurrence at the levels of the cell, tissue, organ, and entire human. Is it possible to characterize the chronic diseases more fully and enable personalization of treatments? For most diseases, an intermediate or preclinical phenotype is either not identified or well defined. Can subtypes of a chronic disease be identified, and does subtyping enable identification of additional concordant chronic conditions? What are the common or underlying mechanisms or metabolic pathways that are involved? What interventions can be developed and tested to alter the pathogenesis?

Mechanistic studies need to be systematically focused on multimorbid phenotypes, so that disease mechanisms are better understood and to help identify the molecular basis of the pathobiological relationships between diseases.[11] Interventions can be developed for these underlying mechanisms and studied for broader impact on multiple disease outcomes. Animal models that pertain to combinations of chronic conditions have been targeted but with limited success. Better animal models are needed for multimorbidity; otherwise, many of these complex studies will need to be conducted on humans.

CLINICAL TRIALS

Many chronic disease interventions have been evaluated in randomized clinical trials (RCTs) for safety, efficacy, and sometimes effectiveness. At present, the paradigm for therapeutics development focuses on one disease at a time. Important aspects of interventional clinical trials related to multimorbidity and CVDs include increasing the enrollment of multimorbid persons in such trials, expanding the use of universal outcome measures, and developing trials that target multmorbidity itself. Selected head-to-head comparative effectiveness and safety trials in persons with prevalent dyad or triad disease combinations that include CVDs are a high priority.

Applying the multimorbidity framework to clinical research, in particular RCTs, can be challenging. Few studies, in particular clinical trials of cardiovascular interventions, explicitly enroll multimorbid persons; rather, they may exclude many specific chronic conditions, most of which increase with age. Clinical trials should ascertain comorbid disease, enroll multimorbid persons to study applicable interventions, and examine patient-centered outcomes relevant to health benefits and harms.

Meaningful outcomes are required for clinical trials in persons with multimorbidity. The persistence and progression of diseases and courses of treatments affect health status in multiple dimensions, such as physical and mental health, pain, and other symptoms; therefore, well-validated universal outcome measures across diseases are needed for research and practice. A minimum senior data set might include such outcomes as general health; pain; fatigue; physical health, mental health, and social role function; and measured gait speed.[12]

Multimorbidity itself can be a focus for intervention trials, in selected instances. The choice of which conditions to include, however, in a composite endpoint MCCs, must be made strategically. This approach is fraught with risks, not least of which is that it differs from the single condition treatment approach traditionally adopted by regulatory agencies. In particular, a strong rationale for the likelihood that a specific intervention could prevent or treat several major chronic conditions would be required. Furthermore, parsimony in choosing conditions and similarity of the perceived importance of the conditions may be considered in developing a composite. Nevertheless, some candidates may emerge, and a large successful trial using a multimorbidity outcome of, for example, CVDs, cancer, and dementia could develop strong evidence that would potentially have a major public health impact.

PRACTICE-BASED RESEARCH

There is a great need for research based in clinical practice involving the care of persons with multimorbidity and CVDs. Common dyads and triads are particularly well suited for this type of research. By eliciting and addressing patient goals of care, the treatment of complex patients with cardiovascular and other chronic illnesses can optimize the person-centered outcomes. Coordinating the care of the MCCs can be done in various ways, and optimizing those approaches in practice would achieve significant health benefits. It is well-known that persons with MCCs are among the highest users of medical resources, yet the treatment of multimorbid patients is fraught with complexity with issues, such as polypharmacy and the limitations of practice guidelines that have not adequately considered potential disease-drug interactions. Clinical decision support tools that address the complex issues of combinations could be developed and tested in a variety of care settings. Interventions that encourage deprescribing of certain dangerous, ineffective, or nonrecommended drugs could be developed and tested.

Self-management can be transformed into a holistic multimorbidity management tool that avoids a disease-specific approach and instead addresses prevention and patient goals.

Much of this work will also involve development of and testing new models of health care, because these patients are the most difficult to manage. An overarching and important issue is how to deal with complexity and optimize care coordination. Ultimately this approach involves the transformation of specialty and primary care.

POPULATION-BASED RESEARCH

Although RCTs remain the gold standard for comparative studies, exclusions as well as resource limitations compel continued use of observational studies for many comparative-effectiveness research questions. Well-known susceptibility to bias, as well as confounding by indication, gives impetus to consideration of several key factors in interpreting the results of observational drug studies, including biologic plausibility, magnitude of differences, new-user design, validity of endpoints, and replication of findings.[13] New outcome measures may be developed for big-data surveillance of drug-drug and drug-disease interactions and adverse effects.

One novel incremental approach to addressing gaps in the observational data on multimorbidity involves increasing data linkage along with selective new data collection (**Fig. 2**). Building blocks for this approach include existing CVD registries,

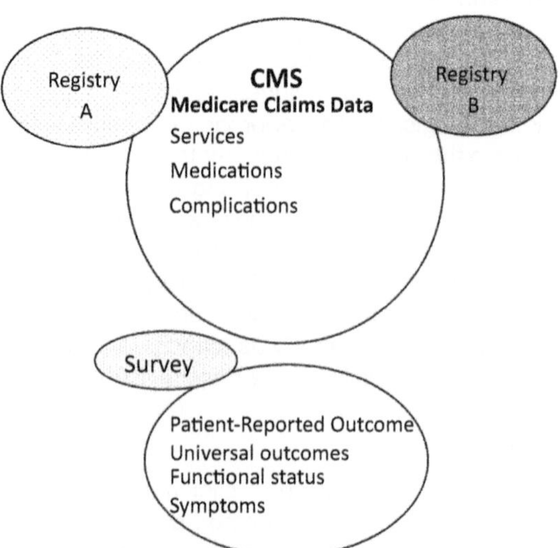

Fig. 2. Proposed approach to improve multimorbidity study linking multiple data sources.

which may be populated with persons who have a specific CVD, procedure, implant, or surgical procedure. They should be enhanced by adopting a standardized approach to phenotyping the chronic conditions. Using 2 or more such registries might enable inclusions of multiple treatment options for a specific condition (eg, surgical and medical management of a common underlying condition). The linkage to Medicare administrative claims data may enable ascertainment of a variety of pharmacologic, rehabilitation, and other services potentially involved in the treatment. Direct data collection will be required for ascertainment of patient reported outcomes, such as symptoms and quality of life. This infrastructure is beginning to be applied to studies of multimorbid persons, but its extension and generalization as part of the big data era may produce substantial advances in knowledge. In particular, the ascertainment of multimorbidity can be cross-validated to reduce the persistent misclassification and biases that may exist in previous research.

Methods development is also needed in the pursuit of multimorbidity research. Alternative statistical methods could be developed for evaluating these programs and interventions that involve greater complexity. Better methods are needed to study decision making under uncertainty and also to incorporate variation in patient preferences.

GUIDELINES

Few clinical guidelines offer an approach to managing the problems of multimorbidity; rather, they focus on a single disease. This problem cannot be addressed, however, in isolation because it reflects a paucity of applicable research/evidence. Therefore, acknowledging multimorbidity is just a first step before it can be included more fully in the guideline development process.[14] Specific combinations, such as common dyads or triads, may require tailored guidance. Common discordant conditions may, however, raise a serious challenge, particularly when the relationship between the 2 conditions is not fully established or understood, such as with coexisting depression and CVD. Ultimately, guideline change will be driven by the entire body of relevant clinical research evidence enabled by linkage of high-quality data, incorporating at least relevant drug-disease interactions and the evaluation of risks and benefits for persons with complex combinations of conditions.[15]

QUALITY MEASUREMENT

With the stated intention of some payers to transition to a payment system that pays for value and outcomes rather than service delivery comes a need for measures of value and outcomes that are applicable to multimorbidity. Universal outcome measures for multimorbidity might be suitable as quality measures if they are shown to be valid, responsive, and feasible and can be applied with few exclusions in clinical practice.[12] Most quality measures at present are disease specific and process oriented. Quality measure development of tools suitable for multimorbidity that are not disease specific will need to rest on a foundation of evidence. Eventually, the improvement of meaningful health outcome measures will drive health care and innovation.

SUMMARY

Future research on multimorbidity would be facilitated through development of a consensus definition of MCCs that can be used in linked medical records. In addition, etiologic studies of multimorbidity should expand to include co-occurrence of cardiovascular and other physical and mental health conditions. Methodologic development should be extended for observational studies of comparative treatment effectiveness among multimorbid older adults with CVD and complex treatment regimens. Clinical trial evidence guiding treatment of complex, older adults can be improved by eliminating upper age limits for study inclusion, by reducing the use of eligibility criteria that disproportionately affect multimorbid older patients, and by evaluating outcomes that are highly relevant to older individuals. Pragmatic trials of treatment strategies for multimorbidity that use universal health outcomes as primary or secondary endpoints may be particularly fruitful.

Research infrastructure grants can be an effective platform for observational studies of multimorbidity, polypharmacy, and comparative effectiveness, and for pragmatic interventional trials. Many funding agencies support this research, including foundations, the Agency for Healthcare Research and Quality, several institutes of the National Institutes of Health, and the Patient-Centered Outcomes Research Institute. The potential for public health impacts of a program of research on multimorbidity cannot be overstated.

REFERENCES

1. Tinetti ME, Fried TR, Boyd CM. Designing health care for the most common chronic condition–multimorbidity. JAMA 2012;307(23):2493–4.
2. Salive M. Multimorbidity in older adults. Epidemiol Rev 2013;35:75–83.
3. Pefoyo A, Bronskill S, Gruneir A, et al. The increasing burden and complexity of multimorbidity. BMC Public Health 2015;15:415.
4. Norris S, High K, Gill T, et al. Health care for older Americans with multiple chronic conditions: a research agenda. J Am Geriatr Soc 2008;56(1):149–59.
5. Boyd C, Ritchie C, Tipton EF, et al. From bedside to bench: summary from the American geriatrics Society/National Institute on aging research Conference on Comorbidity and multiple morbidity in older adults. Aging Clin Exp Res 2008; 20(3):181–8.
6. Parekh A, Goodman R, Gordon C, et al, HHS Interagency Workgroup on Multiple Chronic Cond. Managing multiple chronic conditions: a strategic framework for improving health outcomes and quality of life. Public Health Rep 2011;126(4): 460–71.
7. Feinstein A. The pre-therapeutic classification of co-morbidity in chronic disease. J Chronic Dis 1970;23:455–68.
8. Piette J, Kerr E. The impact of comorbid chronic conditions on diabetes care. Diabetes Care 2006;29(3):725–31.
9. Fabbri E, Zoli M, Gonzalez-Fieire M, et al. Aging and multimorbidity: new tasks, priorities, and frontiers for integrated gerontological and clinical research. J Am Med Dir Assoc 2015;16(8):640–7.
10. Lorgunpai S, Grammas M, Lee D, et al. Potential therapeutic competition in community-living older adults in the U.S.: use of medications that may adversely affect a coexisting condition. PLoS One 2014;9(2):e89447.
11. Menche J, Sharma A, Kitsak M, et al. Disease networks. Uncovering disease-disease relationships through the incomplete interactome. Science 2015; 347(6224):1257601.
12. Working Group on Health Outcomes for Older Persons with Multiple Chronic Conditions. Universal health outcome measures for older persons with multiple chronic conditions. J Am Geriatr Soc 2012;60(12):2333–41.

13. Hennessy S. When should we believe nonrandomized studies of comparative effectiveness? Clin Pharmacol Ther 2011;90(6):764–6.
14. Boyd C, Kent D. Evidence-based medicine and the hard problem of multimorbidity. J Gen Intern Med 2014;29(4):552–3.
15. Uhlig K, Leff B, Kent D, et al. A framework for crafting clinical practice guidelines that are relevant to the care and management of people with multimorbidity. J Gen Intern Med 2014;29(4):670–9.

Index

Note: Page numbers of article titles are in **boldface** type.

Clin Geriatr Med 32 (2016) 409–414
http://dx.doi.org/10.1016/S0749-0690(16)30022-2 geriatric.theclinics.com
0749-0690/16/$ – see front matter

D

E

F

G

H

I

K

L

M

Moving?

Make sure your subscription moves with you!

To notify us of your new address, find your **Clinics Account Number** (located on your mailing label above your name), and contact customer service at:

Email: journalscustomerservice-usa@elsevier.com

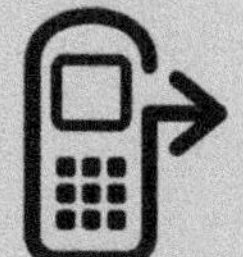

800-654-2452 (subscribers in the U.S. & Canada)
314-447-8871 (subscribers outside of the U.S. & Canada)

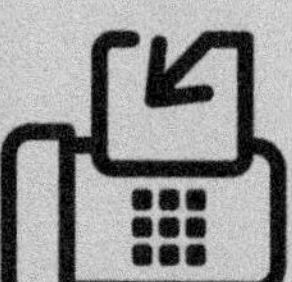

Fax number: 314-447-8029

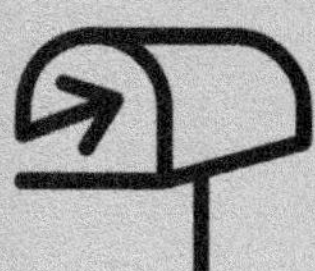

Elsevier Health Sciences Division
Subscription Customer Service
3251 Riverport Lane
Maryland Heights, MO 63043

*To ensure uninterrupted delivery of your subscription, please notify us at least 4 weeks in advance of move.

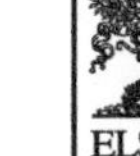

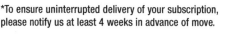

Printed and bound by CPI Group (UK) Ltd, Croydon, CR0 4YY
07/10/2024
01040504-0001